Lead in the
Human

A Report Prepared by the

COMMITTEE ON LEAD IN THE
HUMAN ENVIRONMENT
Environmental Studies Board
Commission on Natural Resources
National Research Council

NATIONAL ACADEMY OF SCIENCES

Washington, D.C.   1980

Library of Congress Cataloging in Publication Data

National Research Council. Committee on Lead in the
  Human Environment.
  Lead in the human environment.

  Includes bibliographies.
    1. Lead-poisoning. 2. Lead—Environmental
aspects. 3. Lead in the body. 4. Lead—Environmental
aspects—United States. I. Title. [DNLM: 1. Environmental pollutants. 2. Lead poisoning]
RA1231.L4N39 1980   615.9'25688   80–14734
ISBN 0-309-03021-8

Available from:

National Academy Press
National Academy of Sciences
2101 Constitution Avenue, N.W.
Washington, D.C.   20418

Printed in the United States of America

Preface

In response to the Lead-Based Paint Poisoning Prevention Act of 1971, the U.S. Department of Housing and Urban Development (HUD) organized the Lead-Based Paint Poisoning Prevention Research Program. In 1977 to 1978, HUD reviewed the effectiveness of its research program, in order to determine what future directions the research should take (Billick and Gray 1978). At the same time, HUD asked the National Research Council to assist in this review and evaluation. The Committee on Lead in the Human Environment was established by the Environmental Studies Board of the Commission on Natural Resources in the summer of 1978 to respond to HUD's request.

The Environmental Studies Board and HUD asked the Committee to conduct a comprehensive review of the state of knowledge about environmental issues related to the hazards and prevention of lead poisoning, to evaluate information gaps and identify research needs, and to examine the lead-related research programs of HUD and other federal agencies and evaluate their appropriateness to the indicated needs. Among other topics, the Committee was asked specifically to evaluate the state of knowledge about the relative contributions of lead from different sources of exposure to the total body burden, and to compare alternative strategies for reducing exposures. Although it was recognized that effects of lead on plants, animals, and ecosystems also are important, this study was to emphasize hazards of lead to humans.

The study was conducted in two phases: an initial information-gathering phase, followed by an assessment phase. In September 1978, the Committee sponsored a workshop that brought together more than 100 research scientists and government officials with expert knowledge on some aspect of lead in the environment. The purposes of the workshop were to bring the Committee into contact with the most recent developments in lead research and the management of lead hazards, and to help the Committee identify and rank critical issues for its own assessment. Major topics of discussion at the workshop included identification of populations at risk, contributions of specific sources and routes of exposure to total exposure to lead, relationships between exposure to lead and human health, methods of reducing exposure, and costs and benefits of potential control measures.

A month later, the Committee met with representatives from federal agencies with substantial lead research programs to discuss the topics being studied and the levels of effort in the various agencies. Additional information on these and other federal research programs on lead in the environment was gathered subsequently by the Committee's staff, and is summarized in Appendix B.

The contract with HUD anticipated that the study would rely substantially on available review documents. In its early deliberations, the Committee recognized that the scientific literature on lead in the environment is extensive, and that several relatively comprehensive recent reviews and assessments of knowledge on the subject are available. The Committee determined that, in light of the objectives of the study, efforts should not be directed toward preparing another review of what is known about lead in the environment and its possible effects on human health. Instead, we identified a need to assess *what is not known*, but needs to be known to support decisions about exposures to lead. This orientation has tended to create a rather negative tone in parts of the report, where statements that emphasize gaps in knowledge often predominate. This is simply a matter of emphasis; the Committee is not so pessimistic about the state of knowledge as the tenor of the report may at times seem to imply.

The Committee agreed with the suggestion of one of its members, Emil Pfitzer, that the assessment of the state of knowledge should be organized around a set of critical issues that are most pertinent for decision making on lead in the environment. That approach culminated eventually in the nine-step model of the decision process, described in Chapter 1, that provides the organizing framework for much of the report. We believe that the systematic approach used here is one valuable way to conduct assessments in support of decisions about exposure to lead, and we recognize that other approaches are also feasible and useful. The method used here emphasizes the need to define specific populations with exposures to lead (the target groups for control measures). Since it was not possible to consider all interesting populations in detail, the Committee selected three cases that illustrate a range of exposure conditions. The report assesses each case, following the steps of our systematic approach, and within that framework examines what is known and what still needs to be known for making decisions. We apologize to readers for the redundancy introduced by the presentation of three parallel case studies, but we believe that the value of this systematic approach more than offsets the sometimes tedious reading.

The report consists of five major chapters and five appendixes. Chapter 1 describes a systematic approach to making decisions on lead-related environmental problems. Chapter 2 examines the state of knowledge of lead in the environment and its effects on health for both the high exposures experienced by urban children and exposures that are typical for most Americans today, and compares these exposure levels to what is known of the natural occurrence of lead in the environment and in humans. Chapter 3 reviews some recent regulatory activities of the federal government, in order to see how unknowns and uncertainties have affected the scientific basis used to support policy decisions. Chapters 4 and 5 present the Committee's findings and recommendations, respectively.

Throughout its study, the Committee was concerned with both the state of knowledge and the nature and quality of evidence, but elected to emphasize the former. This choice was in keeping with the central charge to the Committee, which is to identify research needs and recommend topics and approaches for studies to pursue needed information. In order to identify gaps in knowledge, it was necessary to summarize what is known, and to specify the nature of controversial issues. On controversial topics, however, our objective was generally to suggest research that could help resolve the questions, and not to attempt to produce more definitive resolutions than those already available. Consequently, this report contains relatively few references to specific results of recent research. Instead, most citations are to major summary documents. Synopses of more than a dozen major recent reviews and assessments of the literature on lead are presented in Appendix A, as an initial guide to the literature on most topics. The principal exceptions are in cases where no satisfactory review documents are available, or where important recent results have been published since the major reviews were compiled.

The Committee recognizes that the review documents that we have relied upon heavily were prepared for a number of different purposes. We have used the documents primarily to demonstrate the extent of available assessments of problems, and to guide readers to sources of more detailed discussion and references to primary literature. The Committee does not necessarily agree, or disagree, with all of the conclusions reached by the authors of the various review documents. We encourage readers who are not already familiar with those major reference documents and the primary literature on which they are based to consult those sources, if they wish to critically weigh the findings and recommendations of this report.

An alternative statement by one member of the Committee, Clair Patterson, follows Chapter 5. In his statement, Dr. Patterson addresses several topics that he felt were inadequately considered in the charge to the Committee and in the approach taken by the majority. Those issues include the large excess of typical modern levels of exposure to lead compared to the natural occurrence of the element; the implications of the current lack of knowledge of the biological effects of lead at typical modern levels of exposure; the historical and technological roots of the current global lead pollution problem; and the failure of present approaches to environmental management either to define the problem properly or to deal with it effectively.

The Committee met approximately monthly from November 1978 to June 1979 to develop its approach and to discuss and evaluate current knowledge of critical issues. Drafts of sections of the report were prepared by Committee members, consultants, and staff and discussed at the meetings. A first draft compiled by the chair and staff was reviewed by the Committee at its April meeting, and a completed, revised draft was discussed at the June meeting.

ACKNOWLEDGMENTS

The Committee appreciates the time, thoughtful suggestions, and information provided by a wide range of individuals from universities, government, industry, and public interest organizations to this effort. In particular, we wish to express our gratitude to the individuals who participated as panel members at the workshop meeting, and to all who attended the workshop and participated in the general discussion sessions. Many of those individuals, and others, also submitted written comments or reprints of scientific papers (see Appendix E). We also thank the representatives of federal agencies who presented information on their lead-related research programs to the Committee, and the many others who subsequently were contacted for additional information (also listed in Appendix E). The draft report was reviewed by 25 individuals at the request of the Committee, the Environmental Studies Board, the Commission on Natural Resources, and the NRC's Report Review Committee. The many critical evaluations and constructive suggestions we received from these reviews have significantly improved the quality of our product. We wish to thank the consultants to the Committee, George Provenzano, Ruth Kelly, and Nolen Provenzano, for work devoted to preparing Appendix C; and further gratitude is due George Provenzano for his advice to the Committee on cost–benefit aspects of lead issues, rendered throughout the study. Finally, we reserve our deepest thanks for the staff of the National Research Council, including Robert Rooney, Raphael Kasper, Christina Olson, Estelle Miller, David Savage, Barbara Brown, Marsha Elliott, Judith Cummings, Shirley Bebee, James Charleton and especially the staff to this Committee, Sally Campbell, Adele King, and Ned Groth. Dr. Groth devoted his skill and very much of his time and effort to the incorporation of the Committee's discussion, concepts, and ideas into parts of the draft and into revisions, as well as to the vast correspondence associated with the work of the Committee. Without his dedication, completion of the report would certainly have been much further delayed.

BEN B. EWING, *Chairman*
Committee on Lead in the Human Environment

REFERENCE

Billick, I.H. and V.E. Gray (1978) Lead Based Paint Poisoning Research: Review and Evaluation, 1971–1977. Office of Policy Development and Research. Washington, D.C.: U.S. Department of Housing and Urban Development.

Contents

Lead in the
Human
Environment

Summary

INTRODUCTION

Lead, a useful but toxic metal, is an integral part of the economy of the United States; American industry consumes about 1.3 million tons of lead annually. Various end uses ultimately release about 600,000 tons of lead into the environment each year in this country, and additional discharges occur in mining, smelting, manufacturing, and recycling processes. As a result, the environment of the United States is pervasively contaminated with lead. This effect is most evident in urban areas, where sources of lead are densely concentrated, but rural and remote areas also are contaminated with lead well above natural background levels.

Every member of the general population of the United States is exposed to elevated levels of lead in air, drinking water, and foods, that are present because of human activities. Some groups of people are exposed to additional and occasionally very large doses of lead from other, more specific sources. For instance, young children may ingest soil and dust that contain lead deposited from the air or from paint on walls; and some children eat paint chips directly. Some adults are exposed to lead in workplace environments. Populations with relatively intense exposures require special attention and protection beyond that given to the commonplace exposures of the general population to lead.

It is well established that lead is toxic to humans at high doses, and that levels of exposure encountered by at least some members of the population are high enough to constitute a hazard to health. Because of

3

demonstrable or likely hazards, six federal agencies, acting under authority of at least eight separate laws, have developed regulations or administer programs intended to protect the public health from lead hazards. Four major regulatory decisions were rendered in 1978, and others are pending. Despite this level of government activity, substantial questions exist about the adequacy of scientific knowledge upon which such decisions are based. What level of lead in the environment constitutes a hazard? Will recent actions provide adequate protection for all sectors of the public? Are additional control measures needed? If so, what sources or routes of exposure to lead are most important in causing excessive body burdens, and what are the most cost-effective ways to reduce total exposure? If clear answers to these questions are unavailable, what research could provide information of significant value? How does the needed research compare with present federal research programs on lead in the environment and its effects on health?

Questions such as these prompted the U.S. Department of Housing and Urban Development (HUD) to ask the National Research Council to conduct this study. In response, the Committee on Lead in the Human Environment first defined the array of information that would ideally be used to make decisions about lead in the environment (Chapter 1). We used a systematic approach to assess the need for scientific evidence pertaining to amounts of lead in the environment and in people, relationships between specific environmental sources and body burdens and between body burdens and biological effects, and costs and effectiveness of various measures that can reduce exposures or lower body burdens. It is recognized as well that government decision makers also need to make subjective judgments, such as what degree of biological change is detrimental to health, whether and to what extent the population may tolerably be exposed to a risk of detrimental effects, and what amount of resources society can afford to commit to preventive measures.

Having defined what one would like to know, the Committee next assessed what is presently known and not known about lead in the environment (Chapter 2). Because of the recent regulatory activities noted above, several extensive summaries and assessments of the available literature have been prepared in the last few years (Appendix A). Rather than attempt to refine further what is already known, the Committee focused its assessment on the limitations and uncertainties of current understanding of critical processes and effects, and of the values associated with them. The state of knowledge was examined, using a systematic approach, for three separate cases: urban children, representing a population at elevated risk; the general population of the United States; and the natural background occurrence of lead, which provides a baseline against which the effects of human activities can be measured.

THE STATE OF KNOWLEDGE

Case I: URBAN CHILDREN

The hazards of lead to the health of children in the urban environment are well understood in qualitative terms. Sources that result in exposures to lead are largely known, and the inherent sensitivity of young children is well established. Most urban children are exposed to lead in the air, in their diets, in urban soil and dust, and in drinking water, and many are exposed to lead paints on building surfaces. Characteristics of the family environment and the individual child's age, health, nutrition, and behavior all can affect the degree to which a child exposed to environmental sources of lead will develop an elevated body burden of the element. A few percent of young children, especially those who ingest substantial amounts of soil, dust, or paint, are in danger of severe overexposure to lead.

Recent data suggest that mean blood lead levels in children 1 to 3 years old are 15 to 20 μg/100 ml and that about 6 to 7 percent of the children tested in cities with childhood blood lead screening programs meet the criteria for undue lead absorption (blood lead concentration greater than 30 μg/100 ml, combined with the elevated concentration of erythrocyte protoporphyrin in the blood).

Convincing evidence exists that the biosynthesis of heme is inhibited significantly at blood lead levels above 25 to 30 μg/100 ml, and a few data suggest that these effects may occur at levels as low as 15 μg/100 ml. Prudent medical judgment regards such biochemical changes as the early stages of a continuous process that could culminate in a disease condition. Less persuasive, but growing, evidence suggests that commonplace exposures to lead in urban environments may be associated with detrimental effects on the intellectual development and behavior of children; unusually high exposures are convincingly linked to such effects. To guard against risks to children's health, several federal agencies—HUD, HEW, CPSC, EPA, and FDA—currently administer programs or are developing regulations designed to reduce the amount of lead to which children are exposed.

The central issues HUD asked the Committee to examine were the quantitative contributions of different sources of lead in urban environments to levels of lead in children's bodies, and the implications of that information for control strategies. The Committee's conclusion is that these questions cannot be answered precisely or convincingly, chiefly because of gaps in present knowledge. Additional research can strengthen the assumptions and data base now available for use in exposure/absorption models, and we feel such information should be pursued. However, it is clear that the relative contributions of different sources of lead to total exposure vary substantially among different specific groups of children. In our judgment, it would be unsound to base policies on any single, general estimate of relative source contributions, since such an estimate would apply imprecisely if at all to many specific human populations.

Different sources of lead are dominant causes of exposure for different children; in order to afford reasonable protection to all children, control strategies must recognize that fact, and pursue coordinated control of all important sources. The Committee concluded that a relatively small fraction of all urban children, who have seriously elevated body burdens of lead, can be effectively protected only by identification and removal of lead hazards, especially lead-based paints, in their environments. A much larger number of children, at less severe but still significant risk, can be protected by more general controls that reduce the amounts of lead from paints, gasoline, and other sources that contaminate soils, dust, air, water, and foods to which children are exposed.

Recent federal regulatory activities have focused attention on the need for quantitative information on dose–effect relationships, in order to define the minimal amount of lead in children's bodies that is detrimental to health, and for more exact estimates of the degree of health protection that can be attained by implementing specific control measures. The Committee concluded that these questions cannot be answered precisely now, and in our judgment, the methodological limitations inherent in research on such questions will always preclude the elimination of uncertainties. We recommend several research approaches that can increase the precision of information on these topics (see Chapter 5). Nevertheless, in our judgment, recent and future policy actions have been made and should continue to be made on the basis of numerous sound, properly qualified conclusions that can be supported with available knowledge.

Current laws assign regulatory authority for different sources of children's exposure to lead to different agencies; no single policy-making body is empowered to deal with total exposure in an integrated fashion. As a result, policies to protect children from excessive exposure to lead have been fragmented and sometimes inconsistent. There is a clear need for continuing, coherent, and well-coordinated efforts to reduce hazards to the health of urban chidren posed by lead in their environment.

Case II: GENERAL ADULT POPULATION

In qualitative terms, the greatest source of general exposure to lead is the diet. Air and drinking water can be significant additional sources at some locations, and tobacco smoke may contribute to the total exposure of heavy smokers. In general, dust, soil, and paint are rarely ingested in any significant amounts by adults.

Recent surveys of adult populations indicate that the range of typical blood lead levels is about 10 to 40 μg/100 ml; the mean for most groups is between 10 and 20 μg/100 ml, and in about 3.5 percent of the population, levels may exceed 30 μg/100 ml.

Typical levels of lead in adults are not associated with obvious illness; however, as in children, heme synthesis may be inhibited in some individuals by lead at concentrations above about 20 to 30 μg/100 ml. In addition, recent evidence from studies of populations with occupational exposure to lead has associated a number of effects with blood lead levels in the range of 30 to 40 μg/100 ml. Effects include chromosomal abnormalities, toxicity to the fetus, increased risk of miscarriage or stillbirth, and interference with male and female reproductive functions. Current understanding of dose–effect and dose–response relationships involving blood lead levels of less than 50 μg/100 ml is too inconclusive to estimate the risk of toxic effects in asymptomatic members of the general population. Nevertheless, it seems prudent to conclude that, at best, there is a narrow margin between typical and toxic levels; and pregnant women may be considered a group at special risk.

Some measures already in effect have reduced general exposures to lead. Further reductions should be pursued and can be achieved, particularly if the lead content of foods can be significantly lowered. As in the case of urban children, definitive dose–response data and precise information about the range of human variation in exposure to lead are not available, and regulatory decisions will require substantial judgments in the face of irreducible uncertainties.

Case III: NATURAL OCCURRENCE OF LEAD

Humans have been mining and smelting lead for more than 40 centuries, and the element has been extensively redistributed in the environment by human activities. Estimates of natural (pretechnological) levels of lead in the environment and in people are useful for judging the magnitude of perturbations that have occurred in the natural biogeochemical cycle of the element, and can offer additional insight into the possible risk of biological effects of typical present-day exposures.

Natural levels of lead in the atmosphere can be estimated by several geochemical techniques to be 1 to 2 orders of magnitude lower than current "background" levels, and 3 to 4 orders of magnitude lower than levels in the air at urban sites. Deposition of lead from the atmosphere has increased the amounts of the element in soils, sediments, and surface waters; however, too little is known of rates of movement and chemical behavior of lead in these media to permit precise quantitative estimates of changes that have occurred. Lead appears to enter aquatic and terrestrial food chains by several mechanisms, and it is likely that the levels of lead in most plants and animals, even at remote sites, are significantly higher than natural levels. The best available evidence suggests that the present level of lead in the human diet may be 2 orders of magnitude higher than natural levels. This estimate is highly tentative, and additional research on the question is needed.

Several independent lines of evidence indicate that natural levels of lead in pretechnological humans were between 100 and 1,000 times lower than those encountered in typical present-day Americans. The possible biological significance of the historical increase in human body burdens of lead is almost completely unknown. It is possible, however, that the "normal" body burden today is associated with significant effects on biochemical functions that cannot be detected because they are commonplace in the population. The implications of this perspective deserve sober consideration when attempts are made to define a "safe" level of lead in the body.

To improve understanding of the natural ecological cycling of lead, it is important to conduct some research at sites where perturbations by human activities have been minimal. A few such sites probably exist, most likely in remote regions of the Southern Hemisphere.

DECISION MAKING ON LEAD IN THE ENVIRONMENT

Uncertainties in scientific knowledge, noted above, have limited the ability to establish definitive, quantitative relationships between levels of lead in the environment and risks of adverse effects on human health. In order to set numerical standards for permissible environmental concentrations of lead, government agencies therefore have had to make arbitrary scientific judgments, as well as social, subjective decisions about how much risk and how much uncertainty are acceptable. Recent actions by Congress and the courts reflect a consensus that it is better to proceed with decisions in the face of uncertainty than to risk the consequences of inaction.

Up until the early 1970s, decisions to regulate exposure to lead were based on largely qualitative judgments. Recent decisions, however, have been founded on explicit, quantitative assumptions and conclusions about the relationships between exposure, risk to health, and needed degree of control. Although few of the assumptions made can be fully supported by scientific evidence, we believe the quantitative, explicit approach is a healthy development, because it makes arbitrary judgments obvious and draws attention to pivotal information needs.

Despite nearly a dozen recent or pending regulatory actions, the federal government presently does not have a coherent, consistent policy on the reduction of total human exposure to lead. The enabling laws assign responsibility for different parts of the problem to different agencies. Both the laws and the agencies' interpretations of them give different weight to important considerations, such as the costs and benefits of control measures, in different decisions. Communication and coordination among regulatory agencies with interests in lead have improved significantly in the last few years, especially since the formation of the Interagency Regulatory Liaison Group. Nevertheless, the fragmented approaches and inconsistencies of policies have not been fully resolved.

FEDERAL RESEARCH ON LEAD IN THE ENVIRONMENT

There has been a substantial recent federal research effort to improve the information base for policy decisions about lead and health. During fiscal years 1977 through 1979, the federal government supported $18 million worth of research on lead per se, and $63 million worth of additional research in which lead was one of several elements studied. Over the same 3-year period, total federal expenditures for environmental health research were about $1,700 million, and about $300 million was spent in support of studies on trace elements in environmental health.

Research that focused primarily on lead was supported by 15 federal agencies or sub-agencies, among which NIEHS, DOE, FDA, EPA, and HUD accounted for about 80 percent of total funding. More than 86 percent of the research concentrated on investigation of human exposures and biological effects of lead. The multi-element studies were supported chiefly by DOI, EPA, DOE, NIEHS, and FDA; topics investigated most heavily were environmental occurrence and biogeochemistry, analytical methods, biological effects, and control techniques. Very little research was supported that assessed the economic and technical implications of alternative approaches to the reduction of total exposure to lead; only one agency (HUD) supported a modest effort in this subject area. More balance in research and greater attention to other equally important topics are needed in future efforts.

There has been some recent effort to coordinate research planning among regulatory agencies with common information needs. Present coordination of research on lead could be improved, particularly by including nonregulatory agencies that conduct substantial amounts of research related to lead in the planning and coordination processes.

MAJOR CONCLUSIONS AND RECOMMENDATIONS

The Committee's major conclusions and recommendations are summarized here. Findings that support the recommendations, and details of the recommendations themselves, are presented in Chapter 4 and Chapter 5, respectively.

1. Scientific uncertainties can never be fully eliminated from assessments of the sources, extent, and severity of hazards associated with lead in the human environment. In regulatory decisions, judgments must be made, using the best scientific knowledge available at the time.

• *Efforts to control exposure to lead should proceed, with full acknowledgment of the necessary imprecision of estimates of the costs, risks, and benefits.*

2. Humans are exposed to lead from many environmental sources, and the proportional importance of different sources varies substantially among different specific populations. No one control strategy can adequately assure the protection of all populations.

• *Control strategies should be based on coordinated, integrated measures to reduce exposures from all significant sources.*

3. There has been a great deal of recent federal regulatory activity intended to reduce exposures to lead; however, federal programs are fragmented and disjointed.

• *Improved institutional mechanisms should be developed to permit a more systematic, consistent approach to the management of lead hazards.*

4. Further control of human exposures to lead is needed. Scientific evidence is persuasive that levels of lead in urban environments pose a

significant hazard to the health of some children. Other evidence suggests, less convincingly, that some risk of biological effects is associated with "normal" exposures to lead for some members of the general adult population.

● *Expanded and more concerted efforts should be made to identify children at risk and remove sources of lead from their environments. A serious effort should also be made to reduce the "background" level of exposure of the general population to lead. The most important elements in control strategies include population screening, lead paint removal, reduction of lead emissions from gasoline combustion, and reduction of lead levels in foods.*

5. Methods commonly used to measure levels of lead in environmental and biological samples are difficult and frequently subject to error, especially when very small amounts of lead must be measured.

● *Capabilities for reliable analysis for lead should be substantially upgraded, through dissemination of proper contamination control procedures, development of improved standard reference materials, and extensive interlaboratory comparison programs.*

6. The available scientific knowledge about lead and its biological effects is extensive, and the level of effort in federally supported research on lead is substantial. In order to improve the information base for decision making, further study is needed on the following topics:

● *Forms and amounts of lead in specific environmental pools to which humans may be exposed;*

● *The occurrence, statistical distribution, and trends over time of lead levels in people of all ages;*

● *Biological effects of lead in humans, especially the potential effects of typical present-day exposures;*

● *Factors that influence the absorption, distribution, and storage of lead in human tissues;*

● *Proportional contributions of lead from different sources to levels in people;*

● *Differences between natural and typical present-day levels of lead in the environment, in the food chain, and in people;*

● *Characteristics of individuals that contribute significantly to variability in the risks of excessive exposure to lead and of biological effects of exposure;*

● *Effectiveness and costs of control measures that have been implemented to date, especially in terms of contributions to reduced levels of lead in people; and*

• *Projections of costs and benefits of alternative strategies for further reduction of human exposures.*

7. The Department of Housing and Urban Development will have an appropriate role to play within a coordinated federal program of research on lead in the environment.

• *HUD's research should emphasize efforts to define more precisely the nature and magnitude of sources of lead in and around housing and assessments of innovative strategies for the control of exposure to lead from such sources.*

1 A Systematic Approach to Making Decisions about Lead in the Human Environment

INTRODUCTION

This report has two purposes. The first is to assess current knowledge about lead in the environment, hazards to human health associated with lead, and measures for reducing or eliminating those hazards. In the course of that assessment, critical gaps in knowledge will be identified. The second purpose is to recommend research priorities and management strategies for obtaining information needed to support rational decisions.

Accomplishing these purposes is made difficult by the number, diversity, and complexity of environmental problems related to lead and by the abundance of available scientific and technical information about them. This chapter, therefore, presents an organizational framework for the report. The structure chosen is a sequence of steps that might be followed in developing information to support government standards or regulations to protect the public health against adverse effects of lead.

The decision-oriented framework was chosen because it is comprehensive, requires systematic consideration of all aspects of problems, and shows the implications for public policy of both what is known and what is unknown. The approach used here is compatible with those used by several government agencies to assess toxic environmental agents, and by the National Research Council in previous comprehensive assessments of specific environmental pollutants, including an earlier report on lead (NRC 1972). Much has been written about the use of scientific information in making decisions about environmental hazards (Calabrese 1978; Kates

1978; Lowrance 1976; National Academy of Engineering 1972; National Research Council 1975a, 1975b, 1977a, 1977b). The approach developed here is drawn from that evolving discipline, and from the Committee's accumulated experience with issues related to lead and with efforts to organize information to support decision making.

The process followed here emphasizes both assessment of risk (a prominent concern of many earlier analyses) and assessment of alternative approaches to reducing or managing risk. At several pivotal points in the model process, explicitly subjective choices are required, such as the estimation of a "detrimental" degree of biological change. Such choices are in fact part of all decisions on environmental hazards, but they are frequently obscured in otherwise objective scientific summaries.

The model used here is focused on lead, but with minor modifications it could probably be applied to other toxic environmental hazards. The approach could be used both in cases where substantial knowledge exists (such as lead) and in cases where very little is known. When there is already a substantial base of knowledge, the order of steps in the process might vary, as long as each step is included.

The model decision process developed here is a somewhat abstract ideal, whose general features should be common to most regulatory activities on lead. Later in the report, this hypothetical ideal process will be compared with the actual basis of some recent regulatory decisions on lead in the environment (see Chapter 3).

DESCRIPTION OF THE MODEL

Decisions about chemicals in the environment require systematic appraisal of diverse scientific, social, and political information. Because knowledge is constantly evolving, the process followed in developing the basis for decisions ideally should permit new information to be easily incorporated at any step without repeating the entire process, and should give weight to information needs in terms of their likely impact on decisions. In addition, a systematic approach permits an explicit statement of the basis for the decision and of any uncertainties about it, and minimizes the selective use of information to support preconceived conclusions. These considerations underlie the model decision process developed here in reference to lead.

Prominent features of the model include primary concern for human health; systematic consideration of health hazards and aspects not related to health, such as environmental processes associated with exposure, and costs and benefits of alternative control measures; flexibility to permit the ready use of new information and new points of view; and an iterative nature that permits progressive advance from relatively superficial initial surveys to successively more detailed assessments of a problem.

The model consists of the following steps:

1. Identify sources of lead and pathways of environmental transfer.

2. Identify specific human populations with exposures to lead.

3. Estimate the level of exposure to lead by each environmental pathway for each specific population.

4. Establish the association between exposure to lead and the level of lead in the body for each specific population.

5. Establish the association between the level of lead in the body and biological change due to lead for each specific population.

6. Estimate the upper limit of non-detrimental biological change for each specific population and the level of lead in the body associated with that degree of biological change.

7. Identify and describe alternative control strategies.

8. Apply risk–benefit, cost–benefit, and other considerations, compare alternatives for control, and decide what is an acceptable level of lead in the environment for each specific population.

9. Evaluate the process and the decision.

KINDS OF INFORMATION

Three kinds of information are considered in the model decision process: scientific knowledge, values, and institutional factors. Uncertainties are associated with all three kinds of information.

Scientific knowledge includes both data and an understanding of scientific concepts, principles, and methods that permits meaningful interpretations of data. Data always have some uncertainty associated with them, related to limitations in the precision and accuracy of the scientific methods employed. Uncertainties in concepts result from gaps in knowledge about causal relationships. Examples in this case include estimates of biological changes associated with exposure to lead, or of changes in exposure that would result from particular control measures.

Values are subjective and social assessments of worth. Judgments about values underlie many disputes about lead-related policy questions, since the values and perceptions of decision makers may differ from those of other parts of society. In the context of this report, the term *values* includes both estimated dollar values assigned to direct and indirect consequences of environmental lead pollution or measures to control it, and less tangible costs and benefits, like the loss to society associated with possible slight mental retardation in children exposed to high-lead environments.

Subjective judgments in which values are weighed (explicitly or not) pervade decision processes, and are not restricted to steps that examine costs, risks, and benefits. For example, definitions of "good health" or "non-detrimental effects" require subjective judgments. Some of the judgments involve primarily moral questions, such as whether it is right, or equitable, for some individuals to bear a risk of adverse health effects caused by public or private decisions that are beyond their individual control, and whether different degrees of protection should be sought for some groups, such as children, than are sought for others, such as workers in lead industries.

Although it often makes the decision maker uncomfortable to attempt to quantify intangible values, every decision implicitly reflects them. The Committee believes that, where possible, it is essential to acknowledge and attempt to quantify values explicitly, and where this is less feasible, to recognize nonetheless that additional intangible values have been considered.

In this context, the term *institutional factors* refers to mechanisms of societal decision making. Components of this category include legislative authorities and mandates, the organization of government agencies, current or proposed standards and regulations pertaining to lead, and the procedures through which interested parties participate in the policy-making process. Uncertainties here include variable subjective estimates of the nature and importance of relevant political, economic, and social factors that affect the way institutions function.

All three kinds of information must be organized systematically to support rational decisions, but a model devised to ensure such organization often is a simplified representation of the whole process. Considered judgment is needed to distinguish the knowledge, values, and uncertainties that must be included from those factors that can be omitted without significant effects on the usefulness of the model.

The model used here also distinguishes between two kinds of activities. The first is primarily concerned with the assessment of scientific knowledge needed to identify problems related to lead and mechanisms for dealing with them. This activity requires gathering information and establishing associations. The second activity involves weighing values (costs and benefits), making subjective judgments, and choosing strategies. These processes require social choices and involve defining goals and making trade-offs.

The model described here resembles, in a general way, the decision-making processes of federal administrative agencies, such as EPA, OSHA, FDA, and HUD. Such agencies are the chief loci of federal decision making on lead in the environment; the administrators of the agencies, acting within the mandates and constraints of the legislation enacted by Congress, are legally empowered to assess scientific knowledge, identify values, and make trade-offs. Decisions about lead that are made in other contexts—such as legislatures, courts, and landlord–tenant contracts—might require only some of the same kinds of information, and a different series of analytical steps might be performed.

This report is not designed to answer all the questions that arise in carrying out the complicated systematic assessments conducted to support decisions. Instead, the report offers a summary of current knowledge and a structure of ideas that can serve as reference points for future efforts.

STEP-BY-STEP DESCRIPTION OF THE SYSTEMATIC APPROACH

Step 1: IDENTIFY SOURCES OF LEAD AND PATHWAYS OF ENVIRONMENTAL TRANSFER

Only a small fraction of the lead in the environment of modern industrialized societies is derived from natural geochemical sources; the remainder is released by technological activities. Figure 2.2 in Chapter 2 illustrates the environmental transfers of anthropogenic lead that can result in human exposures. Those complex processes require assessment in order to identify populations with real or potential exposures and to suggest strategies for controlling exposure.

Initially, qualitative understanding of potential sources and pathways of exposure is needed; subsequently, that knowledge must be expressed in quantitative terms (see Step 3). Once specific human populations with exposures have been identified (Step 2), it may be necessary and feasible to identify sources and pathways in much greater detail to obtain a complete description of exposure to lead. Thus there is an iterative interaction between Steps 1 and 2 as more specific information becomes necessary.

An examination of environmental transfers of lead will indicate some points at which lead accumulates. Some of these reservoirs (such as soils at certain sites) may be points of relatively permanent storage, and the lead accumulated there may seem unlikely to pose any hazards of human exposure. Nevertheless, it is important to identify such reservoirs, since future developments may release lead from these sites, shift human populations into greater proximity to them, or identify previously unsuspected environmental or biological effects of accumulation of lead.

Step 2: IDENTIFY SPECIFIC HUMAN POPULATIONS WITH EXPOSURE TO LEAD

Certain identifiable groups of people share common characteristics that influence their exposure to lead, and some groups may share characteristics that affect their susceptibility to lead-induced biological changes. Decisions about lead in the environment that apply to one population may therefore not apply to others. Consequently, it is essential that information be assembled and assessments conducted in terms of specific populations. Ultimately, it may be determined that some populations can be grouped into a common category for purposes of the final decision. However, unless the identity of each population considered is specified throughout the process, it may be difficult to establish that the information used to make the decision is appropriate to that population. Sometimes decisions are made with reference to a "critical" or most sensitive population; in such a case, some further assessment may be needed to determine whether all other population groups are also protected by decisions affecting the "critical" group.

In identifying specific populations for decisions related to lead, important characteristics include age, ethnic origin, socioeconomic status, and health status. Relevant components of health status include diet and nutrition, history of disease, and behavior, especially as they may affect exposure to lead or absorption of it, or influence other factors known to interact with lead. Some population groups can be identified in terms of the uniqueness of their exposure to lead. For instance, most children normally engage in mouthing objects in their early behavior, but a subset of children has pica, defined as the abnormal ingestion of non-food materials (which may include sources of lead). Another subset of the population may have inadequate nutrition and may suffer from related blood disorders. Thus three population groups—children with normal mouthing behavior, children with pica, and children with pica and nutritional anemia—may require three different degrees of protection from lead in their environment.

Many other specific populations, such as workers in lead industries, people who live near smelters, and people whose drinking water is stored in lead cisterns, can be identified in terms of their exposure to lead. Identification of such groups depends upon both an examination of the characteristics of populations and a precise definition of sources of lead and environmental transfer pathways that affect different groups.

While the emphasis of decision making usually is on identification of groups of people with the highest exposures to lead, it is also important to determine the exposures of other populations. Groups with intermediate exposure may be determined to be at risk in the future, and populations with very low exposures are of value as control groups for epidemiological studies of biological effects.

Step 3: ESTIMATE QUANTITATIVELY THE LEVEL OF EXPOSURE TO LEAD BY EACH PATHWAY THAT AFFECTS THE TARGET POPULATION

When a specific population has been identified, its exposure to lead needs to be estimated quantitatively. The assessment requires three kinds of information: (1) the amounts and chemical forms of lead in the environmental reservoirs to which the population is exposed, such as air, soil, water, paint, food, or cosmetics; (2) the amounts of air inhaled or water, food, soil, paint, or other materials ingested by members of the population; and (3) the duration of exposure and the distribution of exposure over time.

Adequately quantitative information of this sort is difficult to obtain for specific populations. While the concentrations of lead in various environmental media and dietary items are known in a general sense, lead levels vary widely. Specific, localized, elevated concentrations may be more important than ambient levels in causing exposure of specific populations. Also, individual humans exhibit great variations in dietary habits, amounts of water consumed, and the extent to which they ingest soil, dust, or paint. It would be extremely valuable to know the frequency distribution of individual exposures by all pathways, but it is generally impossible to obtain this information directly. For instance, it is ethically unacceptable to observe the behavior of children with pica without intervening to stop them from ingesting leaded soil or paint chips.

Because of the difficulty in obtaining satisfactory population-specific exposure data, other information, such as empirical relationships between levels of lead in environmental media and levels of lead in people, has sometimes been used in place of the data called for in Steps 3 and 4. The use of such relationships for establishing causality is subject to severe limitations, and provides a less satisfactory basis for decisions than verifiable estimates of exposures.

Step 4: ESTABLISH THE ASSOCIATION BETWEEN EXPOSURE AND LEAD IN THE BODY FOR THE SPECIFIC POPULATION

Defining the relationship between levels of exposure to lead and levels in people is a complex task. To do so conclusively would require determining the absorption of lead from each of several environmental media for each specific population considered, a goal that is impractical and perhaps unattainable. However, such knowledge of the relative contributions of specific sources to total lead absorbed is central to the decision process, and careful assessment of the best available information on the topic is vital.

The level of lead in specific organs or tissues of the body is a function of both exposure and physiological processes of absorption, distribution, storage, mobilization, and excretion of lead. These factors may differ among different populations. Because it is difficult to measure lead at all critical sites in the body, levels of lead in representative tissues (such as blood or teeth) are generally used to provide an index of body burden. The relevance of such indicators for assessments of effects of lead at specific sites of possible biological effects requires careful evaluation.

In general, scientific knowledge is insufficient to define very precisely the absorption and distribution of lead in the body with reference to specific exposures. However, a systematic effort to carry out this step focuses attention on numerous specific needs for better information.

The model decision process here emphasizes the accumulation of lead in humans, but storage of lead in plants and animals also is important, both because such accumulation may result in human exposure through the diet and because lead may be toxic to the organisms themselves. The state of knowledge about the associations between environmental levels of lead and levels in plants and animals is less precise than that pertaining to humans; nevertheless, a proper assessment must examine these questions.

Step 5: ESTABLISH THE ASSOCIATION BETWEEN LEAD IN THE BODY AND BIOLOGICAL CHANGE IN THE SPECIFIC POPULATION

The next step of the assessment process is to estimate the effects of lead on specific populations in terms of specific biological changes that can be attributed to different levels of lead in the body. The choice of specific health criteria is difficult, however, because some known effects of lead, such as neurobehavioral changes or anemia, can also be caused by other agents. For this reason, measurements of biological effects must be supported by measurements of lead in the body.

The objective of most government standard setting relating to lead is to provide assurance of protection from any of its adverse effects on health. Standard-setting agencies therefore are concerned with the minimal detectable biological changes that can be associated with specific amounts of lead in the body, using the most sensitive measurement methods available.

Determining what constitutes a detectable biological change is difficult, and requires careful statistical analysis to separate effects of lead from

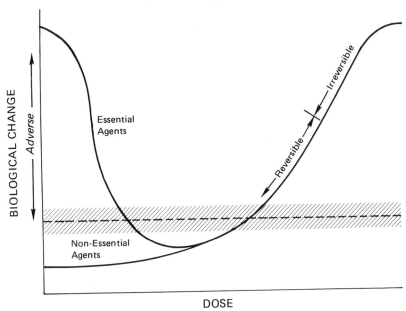

FIGURE 1.1   A generalized dose–effect relationship. At present, the curve for non-essential elements should apply to lead (see Chapter 2). This figure presents only a general qualitative form for the relationship; difficulties in determining a precise, quantitative dose-effect curve for lead-induced biological changes in humans are discussed in Chapter 2.

variations in the parameter measured that are typically found in presumably healthy populations. The definition of an effect depends on analytical tools susceptible to error, on subjective selection of a control population, and on imprecise and changing definitions of normality and criteria of biological significance.

The association between biological change and the level of lead in the body may be described as a dose–effect relationship. Figure 1.1 illustrates a hypothetical general relationship between dose and effect, and shows a zone of uncertainty around the boundary between adverse effects and presumably safe levels. At the present time lead is not known to be essential for any biological process. If such a role were to be established in the future, the multiphasic curve for essential agents shown in the figure would apply to the dose–effect relationship. Such a graph is an oversimplification, since biological changes require specific definitions of the nature, susceptibility, and severity of effects on specific organ systems and tissues.

To demonstrate a direct causal relationship, the dose should be meas-

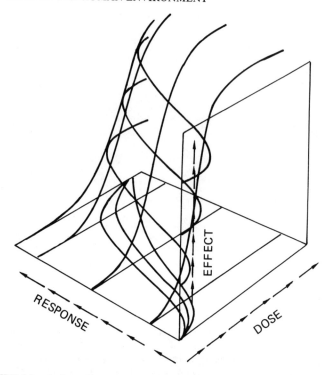

FIGURE 1.2 A three-dimensional representation of the interrelationships among dose, effect, and response. This figure shows the qualitative nature of the relationships; precise quantitative dose–response data on lead are very limited in extent, as discussed in Chapter 2.

ured as the amount of lead at the site where the effect occurs; however, the exact site of action of lead is not always known, and even if it is known, it may be impossible to obtain samples from that site for measurement. Dose, therefore, is frequently measured in some more available medium such as blood, serum, urine, feces, hair, or teeth. Great care must be used in determining how representative such measurements may be of likely levels of lead at the site of an effect when biological changes occur.

Although Figure 1.1 describes a simple, hypothetical, two-dimensional relationship between dose and effect, in reality multiple dose–effect relationships exist for different effects, and individuals within a population respond differently to the same dose. This variability within populations may be illustrated as a two-dimensional dose–response curve for a specific effect, but it is conceptually sounder to view the relationships as a three-dimensional surface, as portrayed in Figure 1.2.

A dose–response relationship for lead describes the fractions of a population that respond with a specific effect to different doses of lead. The distinction between dose–effect and dose–response relationships differentiates variations in magnitude and kind of effect from variations in numbers of individuals responding. To support environmental decisions, it is essential to know both the most sensitive effect of exposure to lead and the dose at which that effect is seen in only a small fraction of the population.

The model decision process described here is concerned almost exclusively with biological changes in humans. Similar biological changes may occur in plants and animals in association with accumulation of lead; and it is possible that such effects may have important ecological or economic consequences. It is useful, therefore, to examine potential effects of lead on nonhuman organisms, applying the same fundamental principles used to assess biological changes in humans. However, the weight given to human health hazards in decision making is greater by far than that given to any hazards to other species. Therefore, although the topic of effects of lead on wildlife and domestic species deserves serious attention in its own right, it is examined only briefly in this model decision process.

Step 6: ESTIMATE THE LIMIT OF NON-DETRIMENTAL BIOLOGICAL CHANGE DUE TO LEAD AND THE ASSOCIATED LEVEL OF LEAD IN THE BODY

When the relationships between lead in the body and various biological changes have been defined, the next step is to distinguish between those degrees of biological change that are considered adverse or detrimental effects and other degrees that are deemed non-detrimental. Since this distinction is critical for establishing the health-based goals that are the ultimate purpose of regulatory actions, the step is pivotal in the decision process.

Not every biological change is necessarily associated with damage to health, and opinions differ over whether some biological changes induced by lead should be considered harmless. This controversy is fueled by the fact that the ability to detect subtle biological changes—such as altered enzyme activity—has advanced more rapidly than the ability to interpret the physiological significance of such changes. Furthermore, lead is pervasively distributed in the environment and in people, and even if pollution were to cease immediately, it is likely that some detectable biological changes due to lead will continue to be observed, at least in some members of some populations, for many years. It is therefore essential to estimate how far biological changes can proceed before they should be considered detrimental.

A fundamental aspect of the concept of a non-detrimental level of biological change is the subjective judgment inherent in such definitions. There is no absolute standard for "safe" or "normal" or "healthy"; individual perceptions of the terms differ sharply. One school of thought holds that the body can compensate readily for low levels of biochemical or physiological changes induced by toxic agents, and that some threshold must be passed before an effect should be viewed as harmful. Others believe that the smallest detectable degrees of biological change should be considered the early stages of progressive disease, even if the changes may be reversible or compensated for by homeostatic mechanisms or reserve capacities. Currently available scientific knowledge cannot resolve these different views. Decision makers must exercise their own judgment on the question, and ideally should make explicit the criteria employed to arrive at the definition of detrimental biological change used in decisions.

When the upper limit of non-detrimental biological change has been defined, the level of lead in the body that corresponds to this degree of change can be estimated from the associations already established in Step 5 of this sequence. Dose–response data can be used to estimate the fraction of the population likely to exhibit a detrimental degree of change at a given average level of lead in people.

Figure 1.3 (A and B) illustrates in simplified, qualitative terms relationships that ideally would provide a basis for estimating a "safe" level of lead in the environment (relationships derived from Steps 3, 4, and 5). In some cases it may be possible to estimate a direct association between exposure and biological change without establishing the level of lead in the body. However, because of difficulties of measuring subtle biological changes and because there may be several different, significant sources of exposure, both associations shown in the figure generally will be useful.

Step 7: IDENTIFY AND DESCRIBE ALTERNATIVE CONTROL STRATEGIES

The previous step identified levels of lead in the environment that are considered to be associated only with non-detrimental biological effects in human populations. Step 7 examines whether or not such levels of environmental exposure can be attained, and if they can, how. In contrast to the emphasis on health that characterized the last three steps, the assessment here concentrates on technological and social methods for reducing exposure to lead, and on technical and economic evaluations of

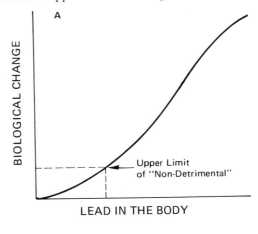

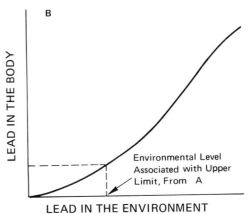

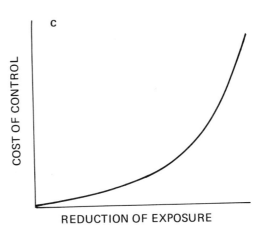

FIGURE 1.3 The general forms of some associations used for making decisions about lead in the environment. Although these associations may be conceived as abstract, qualitative relationships, the data needed to provide exact quantitative curves are seldom available (see Chapter 2).

the effectiveness and cost of alternative control measures and strategies. Ideally, the results of this step could be expressed in simple form as the association depicted in Figure 1.3 (C). In practical terms, however, this step, like the previous ones, is extremely complex and fraught with uncertainties.

Generally, the first step in an assessment of possible control strategies is to examine the sources of lead and routes of exposure that affect a specific human population and to identify all points at which intervention to reduce exposure is possible. Then, for each such control opportunity identified, information can be gathered to determine: (a) technical, social, or other methods that could be used to effect control; (b) the reduction of exposure to lead and associated reduction of risks to health that could be achieved by each method; (c) the technical and social feasibility of each method; (d) the economic cost of implementing each control measure; and (e) whether or not legal authority to implement control exists, and if it does, in which agencies the authority resides. Such an assessment is needed not only for specific control measures, but also for various combinations of measures and for different scenarios for the timing of controls.

In practice, this step also is iterative. An initial, relatively superficial survey of control possibilities can be made early in the information-gathering phase of decision making, and more detailed evaluations of promising alternatives can be conducted as the process moves closer to a decision.

The recognition and estimation, where possible, of costs and benefits of control measures is needed and should be an integral part of the assessment from its initial stages. Costs of control include both the direct costs of implementation (equipment, personnel, and administrative costs) and indirect costs, such as loss of benefits from uses of lead foregone, or changes in the structures of industries. Indirect costs and the economic benefits of control are generally more difficult to quantify than direct costs, because they comprise both monetary and nonmonetary measures of such things as improved health, reduced risk of illness, or lost amenities. The distribution of costs and benefits—who benefits from the use of lead, who bears risks of toxic effects, who benefits from control measures, and who bears the costs of control—is an important aspect of the needed information. Not only the distribution among societal groups, but also the distribution over time (i.e., hazards to future generations resulting from beneficial uses by present generations) must be considered. The results of attempts to estimate the costs and benefits of controls may be far from conclusive. Nevertheless, such analysis is valuable even if it does no more than emphasize critical gaps in knowledge.

Step 8: APPLY RISK–BENEFIT, COST–BENEFIT, AND OTHER CONSIDERA-
TIONS, COMPARE ALTERNATIVES, AND MAKE A DECISION

The previous steps required the systematic collection and assessment of
information needed to make decisions about lead in the human environment. At this step in the process, the various risks, benefits, and costs
identified earlier are compared and weighed and a decision is made about
the appropriate degree and manner of control.

Initially, an agency making a decision would need to define its goals
and the relevant decision–objective functions. For a national agency establishing standards for lead in the ambient environment, the objective
might be to balance the benefits of reduction in exposure to lead against
costs of achieving the reduction, and the critical decision would be the
definition of an "acceptable" level of exposure. For a local lead poisoning control program, the objective might be to eliminate all sources of
lead from the home environment of children with demonstrably unacceptable exposures, and the decision would be the selection of the most cost-
effective methods to achieve a predetermined degree of control. The
choice of an objective function has fundamental implications for the
kinds of information needed in the earlier steps of the process as well.

Regardless of the objective function chosen, however, several qualitative and quantitative comparisons are required at this point. Hazards
posed by lead in the environment must be compared to benefits that accrue from the production and use of lead. Similarly, benefits associated
with reduced risks of adverse effects must be weighed against costs of
lowering the risks. Different kinds of benefits and different trade-offs are
involved in each comparison.

It is important that such comparisons avoid attempting to base decisions on a rigidly defined cost–benefit ratio. In each case, some values
will be more readily estimated in quantitative terms than others, and it
may be difficult to express all considerations in a common metric that
makes direct comparisons possible. Nevertheless, it is desirable to quantify as many values as possible, and to include qualitative descriptions of
those less tangible factors that are more difficult to quantify. It is important that the subjective weight given to different kinds of values be
identified explicitly, so that the basis for trade-offs that are made is clear.

Risk considerations weighed at this point include definitions of detrimental and non-detrimental levels of biological change, dose–effect and
dose–response relationships that express the magnitude and probability of
occurrence of effects of various degrees, and characteristics of specific
populations and their exposures to lead that contribute to risks. If avail-

able, information about public perception of the risks associated with lead and the urgency of public demands for reduction of those risks may be an important consideration. Once this information has been assembled, the decision requires subjective judgments about the amounts of risk that may be acceptable for populations of greatest concern under various conditions. Cost and benefit considerations include both the magnitude of the values listed above and the distribution of the costs and benefits through time and among populations.

Even with the best available information in hand on the risks, costs, and benefits involved, decision makers, acting within legal mandates and constraints, must make subjective social choices. One such choice might be whether to tolerate a level of exposure to lead that carries a significant probability of inducing biological changes that are, by a conservative definition, detrimental. In a case where either the benefits of use of lead are irreplaceable or the costs of control are overwhelming, society might choose to bear the risk of exposure. Another social choice would involve the priority assigned to lead problems, where these and many other problems compete for shares of society's limited problem-solving resources. Still another difficult decision would be whether to take action in the face of uncertainties and risk making the wrong choice, or to wait for more information and risk incurring damages that might have been averted by prompter action.

Clearly, decisions on what to do about lead in the environment go beyond scientific and technical assessments. But the systematic approach described here is designed to present the best available information in a framework that projects the consequences of alternative courses of action.

When a decision has been made about permissible exposures to lead and required control measures have been identified, a strategy for implementation is required. Information on the feasibility of implementation (gathered in Step 7) provides a basis for development of timetables for achieving specified stages of control, detailed outlines of the steps necessary to meet specific goals, and provisions for evaluating the rate of progress and the effectiveness of the program. Since implementation often requires additional information, an agenda of specific data needs is an essential part of the plan. Insofar as possible, implementation plans should be flexible enough to allow for modifications of programs as the state of knowledge improves.

Step 9: EVALUATE THE PROCESS AND THE DECISION

At each step of the process it is essential to assess the validity of the procedures followed. To avoid repetition, examination of this aspect has been reserved until now; however, evaluative procedures should be incorporated in each stage of the process and not treated only as the final step in the sequence.

In the information-gathering steps, it is essential to determine whether available data are appropriate and adequate to provide answers to critical questions, and whether the sampling and analytical methods used to gather the data are accurate and reliable. The uncertainty inherent in estimates of critical variables must be assessed, and the influence of multiple uncertainties on the ultimate outcome of the assessment should be gauged. Where possible, gaps in knowledge that contribute to major uncertainties should be specified, and the feasibility of obtaining information that would reduce the uncertainties should be evaluated. The sensitivity of the ultimate decision to specific pieces of information can be estimated, and the results of an analysis to determine such sensitivity can be used to help establish research priorities. The structure of the assessment and decision-making process itself can be examined, and ways can be sought to improve the process.

Finally, it is important to evaluate the consequences of the decision. Will regulations or standards adopted achieve the goal of adequately protecting the populations they are intended to protect? Are other populations at risk also protected by the measures adopted? Such evaluations require continuing surveillance of problems once decisions have been made. Ideally, plans for such evaluation would be part of the procedures developed for implementing the decision. In many instances, there may be such serious gaps in knowledge that the correctness or usefulness of a decision cannot readily be determined. When this is so, research to improve the data base will generally have high priority.

CONCLUSIONS

The general approach to decision making described here provides a systematic framework for identifying critical questions and assembling and weighing the scientific and nonscientific information needed to support decisions. Ideally, the nine steps of the process represent procedures a standard-setting agency would follow in establishing permissible exposures to lead in the human environment. In practice, many of the questions raised at each step can be answered only crudely, if at all, with present-day knowledge. In addition, although the systematic approach supports the consideration of all relevant questions, care must be taken not to allow the actual process to become too cumbersome, or to substitute routine procedures for substantive assessments of issues. In subsequent chapters, the same nine-step framework is used to identify critical gaps in the scientific information base, and to examine the effects of those gaps on recent government decisions about lead.

REFERENCES

Calabrese, E.J. (1978) Methodological Approaches to Deriving Environmental and Occupational Health Standards. New York: Wiley-Interscience.

Kates, R.W. (1978) Risk Assessment of Environmental Hazard. SCOPE Report 8. New York: John Wiley & Sons.

Lowrance, W.W. (1976) Of Acceptable Risk: Science and the Determination of Safety. Los Altos, Calif.: William Kaufmann, Inc.

National Academy of Engineering (1972) Perspectives on Benefit–Risk Decision Making. Committee on Public Engineering Policy. Washington, D.C.: National Academy of Engineering.

National Research Council (1972) Lead: Airborne Lead in Perspective. Committee on Biologic Effects of Atmospheric Pollutants, Division of Medical Sciences. Washington, D.C.: National Academy of Sciences.

National Research Council (1975a) Decision Making for Regulating Chemicals in the Environment. Environmental Studies Board, Commission on Natural Resources. Washington, D.C.: National Academy of Sciences.

National Research Council (1975b) Principles for Evaluating Chemicals in the Environment. Environmental Studies Board and Committee on Toxicology. Washington, D.C.: National Academy of Sciences.

National Research Council (1977a) Decision Making in the Environmental Protection Agency. Volume II, Analytical Studies for the U.S. Environmental Protection Agency. Committee on Environmental Decision Making, Environmental Studies Board, Commission on Natural Resources. Washington, D.C.: National Academy of Sciences.

National Research Council (1977b) Research and Development in the Environmental Protection Agency. Volume III, Analytical Studies for the U.S. Environmental Protection Agency. Environmental Research Assessment Committee, Environmental Studies Board, Commission on Natural Resources. Washington, D.C.: National Academy of Sciences.

2

Application of the Systematic Approach to Specific Cases of Lead in the Human Environment

INTRODUCTION

In this section of the report, the systematic approach described in Chapter 1 is used to examine the base of information available to support policy decisions about lead in the human environment. Since one of the objectives of this study is to identify research needs to support rational decisions, the discussion here dwells more on what is not known about each topic than it does on what is known. Many areas also are identified in which there is considerable controversy over inferences that may be drawn from available information.

The information examined here is concerned almost exclusively with inorganic lead compounds. Some organic lead compounds are present in the environment, and exposure to them may pose some hazard to human health. However, because of the differing environmental chemistry and toxicologic properties of inorganic and organic forms of lead, it was impractical to consider both in this assessment. A recent, comprehensive review of environmental health aspects of organolead compounds is available elsewhere (Grandjean and Nielson 1979).

BASIS FOR CHOOSING EXAMPLES

The chapter consists of three examples in which the model decision process is applied to specific problems. The first example illustrates a hypothetical process of setting standards for lead in soils. The example was chosen because soil contributes to some degree to human absorption of lead, and the lead content of soils may eventually be regulated, as is lead in other environmental media. However, since no agency has proposed such action yet, the discussion here is only a hypothetical example of how the process would work. An agency setting standards for lead in soils would have to assess exposures from soil and other sources in an integrated manner, and the emphasis on soils merely provides a context in which all contributions to exposure may be examined.

At Step 2 of the first example, urban children are chosen as the primary target population, because of a greater likelihood of elevated exposure and a greater susceptibility to biological effects of lead among children less than 6 years old. Several government actions concerned with lead have emphasized protection of urban children, and several control strategies have been focused on special sources of exposure that affect this population. Although a standard-setting agency would undoubtedly assess the potential exposures of several different populations and appropriate control measures in each case, the initial illustration is confined primarily to urban children.

The second example presents a similar illustration of the decision process, with reference to the general adult population of the United States. In this case, exposure to lead in soils makes a small contribution to total exposures, and the assessment is more broadly focused on all possible sources of exposure and on potential biological effects of lead in average people. Whereas urban children in the United States clearly are at risk of elevated exposure to lead, the risk to a typical adult seems much lower in comparison. Only limited knowledge is available about biological effects of lead in adults at levels of exposure that occur in significant numbers of the population, in contrast to a considerably larger amount of data on effects of elevated exposure in children. In addition, if a decision is made that the exposure to lead of the general population should be reduced, control would need to be achieved through reduction of levels of lead in the ambient environment and in foods, rather than through more focused efforts of the sort required to protect urban children.

The third example presented examines the potential for human exposure to lead under natural, pretechnological conditions, and attempts to determine how much the average person's exposure to the metal has been increased by human uses of lead. Although current knowledge permits only crude quantitative estimates, it seems likely that natural levels of lead in people are much lower than typical present-day levels. However, the extent to which the historical increase in exposure to lead may pose a risk of significant biological effects in the general population is almost completely unknown.

Taken together, the three examples address all of the major concerns of the Committee. The first case examines a population at elevated risk, and probes for possible solutions to acknowledged, urgent public health problems. The second and third cases provide two different and complementary perspectives on the broader question of whether present-day levels of lead in the environment pose a hazard to the health of the general population. All three examples examine exposure to lead as an integrated, multisource problem, and each assessment is concerned especially with determining whether and how well the crucial questions for decision making can be answered with available knowledge.

CASE I: SETTING A STANDARD FOR LEAD IN SOILS TO PROTECT URBAN CHILDREN

Step 1: IDENTIFY SOURCES OF LEAD AND PATHWAYS OF ENVIRONMENTAL TRANSFER

Figure 2.1 illustrates the flow of lead in U.S. industry in 1976, and shows that a variety of end uses released about 600,000 tons of the element into the environment that year. Automotive emissions are the largest single source, and atmospheric emissions represent a much more mobile and widely dispersed form of lead than that in discarded battery casings, for example. Although the diagram does not indicate it, lead also is released into the environment at many points in mining, smelting, refining, and manufacturing processes in lead and other metals industries, and by the combustion of fossil fuels. The complex web of potential sources and pathways of human exposure to industrial lead is shown in Figure 2.2. The figure represents environmental transfers of anthropogenic lead; natural biogeochemical transfers of the element may be components of some of the potential exposures illustrated, but in most cases the natural component is believed to be a small fraction of the total (see Case III, later in this chapter). As the figure shows, the soil reservoir is a factor in several environmental transfers of lead that are linked to human exposure.

This initial step in the decision process requires only a semiquantitative understanding of the sources and pathways responsible for significant fractions of human exposures. (That picture must be refined and quantified, insofar as possible, in Step 3.) In general, although some unusual or minor sources of exposure may not have been identified, this initial state of knowledge currently exists for lead. People may be exposed to lead in inhaled air and in ingested water, foods, and such non-food items as dust, soil, paint, plaster, cosmetics, and occasionally other

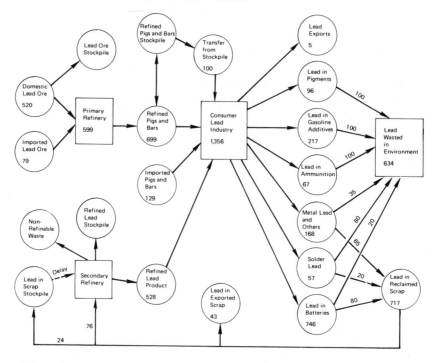

NOTE: Numbers in boxes are mass flows; those along arrows are percentages. Mass flows are in thousand metric tons.

FIGURE 2.1   Flow of lead in the U.S. lead industry in 1976. Source: Adapted from Ewing and Pearson (1974) in *Environmental Science & Technology,* Copyright by John Wiley & Sons, with 1976 data from Ryan and Hague (1977) and Ewing et al. (1979).

materials (WHO 1977, U.S. EPA 1977a). The difficulty of obtaining quantitative estimates of the contributions of each specific source is discussed in Step 3, below.

Step 2: IDENTIFY SPECIFIC HUMAN POPULATIONS WITH EXPOSURES TO LEAD

An agency developing the basis for standards for lead in soils would need to identify populations for whom exposure to lead in soils, either through direct ingestion or through the food chain, represented a significant incremental hazard to health. Human exposure to lead encompasses a wide range of variation, and the relative contribution of lead in soil to total ex-

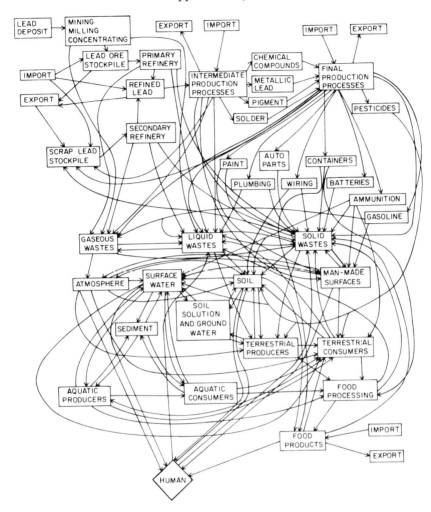

FIGURE 2.2 Sources and environmental pathways that can result in exposures of human populations to lead of anthropogenic origin. The figure suggests qualitative interrelationships and illustrates the complexity of the system. Quantitative estimates of transfers by the various pathways are subject to many uncertainties (see Step 3 for discussion). Source: Modified from Rolfe and Reinbold (1977).

posure is quite different for different groups within a total population. As Figure 2.2 indicates, people are exposed to lead in soil by several different kinds of environmental transfers. Some lead is absorbed from soil by plants or adheres to plant surfaces, and enters the human diet either in plant-derived foods or in products derived from animals that ingest lead in their diets. On the other hand, some people ingest soil directly, both accidentally and deliberately, and thereby ingest lead in proportion to its occurrence in the soil.

Figure 2.3 illustrates in a qualitative, schematic way the distribution of total exposure to lead within the population of the United States. The precise statistical features of the distribution are not yet well known (see Step 3, below); however, as a crude approximation, the function may be thought of roughly as a log-normal distribution. That is, the largest part of the population is exposed to levels of lead that are 1 or 2 standard deviations above or below the mean for the United States as a whole, but some groups within the entire population are exposed to much higher or much lower levels of the element.

The relative importance of soil lead in total exposure can be assessed for individuals at different points within the overall distribution. If the figure is taken to represent the present-day U.S. population, the very low exposures labeled "natural background" probably do not apply to any identifiable group (see Case III). For people within the low-to-typical portion of the range, exposures to lead are derived almost entirely from ambient levels of the element in the air, water, and foods. Since some of the lead in foods comes from soils, an agency setting standards for lead in soils might examine the effects of different amounts and forms of lead in various soils on uptake of the element by crops, and the contribution of this and subsequent food-chain transfers of soil lead to total human dietary exposure to the metal.

Some of the members of the total population who make up the high end of the distribution in Figure 2.3 may be exposed to unusually high levels of lead in the air, water, and foods, and some also are exposed to additional, occasionally intense, sources of lead. Such exposures are termed "special" in Figure 2.3, both because they represent special hazards to health and because special efforts and source-specific control measures are usually required to reduce such exposures. Some examples of subsets of the U.S. population that fall into the special exposure category are listed in the figure.

Soils that contain elevated amounts of lead can contribute substantially to some special exposures, especially in young children, who may ingest soil either inadvertently or deliberately. Elevated exposure by this environmental pathway has been demonstrated in children who live near

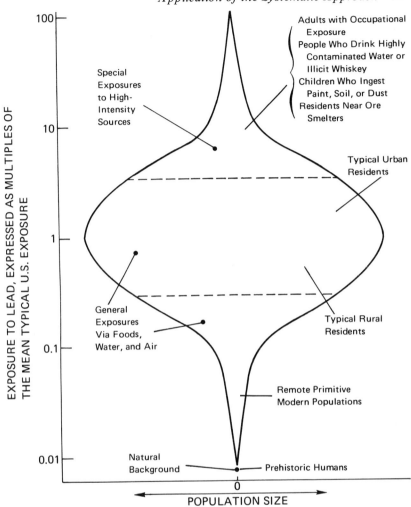

FIGURE 2.3   Schematic classification of populations according to level of exposure to lead. The actual distribution of exposures about the mean is not well documented quantitatively.

smelters (Landrigan et al. 1975) and in children in urban areas, where soils contain lead accumulated from automobile exhaust and from weathering of paint on building surfaces (U.S. EPA 1977a, 1979). Most adults also ingest soil occasionally in small, incidental amounts (from dirty hands, on unwashed vegetables), and some adults eat substantial amounts of soil intentionally (geophagia) (Layman et al. 1963).

Thus, the hypothetical standard-setting agency could identify several specific population groups for whom lead in soils might be a potential source of exposure. Two of those groups, children living near industrial sources and adults with geophagia, are relatively small populations, and the incidental ingestion of soil by adults probably makes a minimal contribution to total exposure (see Case II). While lead in soil may account for a significant fraction of the lead in or on foods, the exact contribution is uncertain (see Case III); and since soils at most sites contain relatively uniform small amounts of lead, the opportunity to achieve significant reductions of dietary exposure by establishing standards for lead in agricultural soils is limited. On the other hand, soils in urban areas much more frequently contain elevated levels of lead, and more than a million children under age 6 live in urban areas.

Aside from the likelihood that urban children may be exposed to and ingest soils that are high in lead, an agency would readily discern several other reasons to single out that population as a group at special risk. Children are generally more susceptible than adults to biological effects of lead because of the physiological stresses associated with rapid growth, and because the developing nervous system and associated intellectual, psychological, and behavioral development are especially vulnerable to perturbation by toxic agents. Children also may absorb and retain a higher percentage of ingested lead than adults do, and are more likely to ingest lead from some sources—especially paint, dust, and soils—than adults are. Furthermore, the urban environment exposes children to relatively higher levels of lead in the air, and possibly to a greater density of sources of lead-based paints in housing, than occur at most rural or suburban locations.

These considerations support the choice of urban children as a primary target population that could require protection from excessive exposure to lead in soils. A standard-setting agency would not necessarily disregard the other populations noted above, but its first priority would probably be to protect urban children from potential hazards associated with lead ingested in soil. The remainder of this first example, therefore, is focused on lead in the environment of urban children, and on an assessment of exposures from soil and other sources, as would be required to support protective measures. Later, in Cases II and III, the contributions of lead in soils to exposures to lead in other populations also are examined.

Subpopulations at Special Risk

The population of urban children is large, and in order to design effective protective measures it is necessary to identify more specific subsets of the population that may be at greater risk of excessive lead absorption than the average urban child. Two general approaches can be used to identify specific target populations. The first is to examine the health status of the larger population in order to identify subgroups of individuals with elevated body burdens or manifestations of biological changes due to lead. The second is to use a general qualitative understanding of sources and environmental pathways and of specific characteristics of individuals or groups that contribute to exposure to predict the risk to different subpopulations. The two approaches may be used in concert to define target populations as specifically as possible.

Epidemiological Approach   The EPA and the WHO reviewed available epidemiological data on levels of lead in the blood of various populations in recent criteria documents (U.S. EPA 1977a, 1979; WHO 1977). The available data show clearly that age is strongly correlated with blood lead levels; children in the 0-to-3-year-old group generally have higher blood lead levels than older children (McCabe 1979). However, even within specific age group, some children have much higher blood lead levels than others. In a recent report on blood lead levels of 1,929 children (ages 1 to 15 years), the mean blood lead level was 16.5 μg/100 ml, but 5.7 percent of the population had levels above 30 μg/100 ml (Mahaffey et al. 1979).

The high blood lead levels in some children are undoubtedly associated with exposure to particular sources of lead, and may also be associated with specific behavioral, health, or other characteristics of individual children. The number of possible contributing variables is large, and epidemiological evidence supports few satisfactory definitions of the relative importance of different factors. For instance, exposure to lead-based paints, exposure to soil containing more than 500 μg/g lead, an exaggerated tendency toward mouthing of objects in children, and a family setting in which supervision of a child's behavior is limited all exhibit positive correlations with elevated blood lead levels (U.S. EPA 1977a, Lepow et al. 1975, Chisolm and Kaplan 1968, Hunter 1977, McCusker 1979). However, it is still not possible to determine from epidemiological data the precise degree to which each of these factors (or others) contributes to elevated levels of lead in children, or to estimate the number of children for whom specific factors are significant.

About 60 urban areas of the United States now have blood lead screening programs, and a total of about 400,000 children are tested for blood lead levels annually (see Step 7, below). However, the data collected by such programs have not yet been used to any significant extent for epidemiological studies of factors that contribute to undue lead absorption. Screening programs are designed to prevent lead poisoning among a relatively narrowly defined target population: preschool children living in deteriorating housing in inner cities. The data therefore are insufficient for assessing the occurrence of lead in a broader population. Furthermore, the recording of blood lead measurements in such programs has rarely been accompanied by the collection of information about specific characteristics of individual children or their exposures to lead, since the objective of the programs is health protection, not epidemiological research.

In short, the available epidemiological data do not support a very precise definition of subsets of the total population of urban children who may require special attention in a standard-setting process concerned with lead in soils. The hypothetical agency in this example would therefore need to make effective use of predictive approaches, described in the next section.

Predictive Approaches   Prediction of subsets of the urban child population that are likely to be at greater risk requires at least qualitative knowledge of the ways in which children are exposed to lead and of factors within the population itself that contribute to risk. Figure 2.4 illustrates environmental transfers of lead that may occur in an urban child's environment. Airborne lead levels are likely to be elevated adjacent to heavy traffic and near stationary sources, such as secondary lead refineries; children who spend time at such sites may be exposed to relatively high doses of lead by inhalation or by ingestion of contaminated soil and dust. In some areas, leaded pipes in water distribution systems may be corroded by soft, acidic water, creating localized zones of high exposure by this pathway. The lead content of commercially processed foods is believed to be relatively uniform from site to site, because of homogeneous distribution of products, but locally grown foods from urban gardens may be high in lead in some cases. Children may ingest street dust, house dust, paint flakes, and soil through normal hand-to-mouth activity, pica, or contact with pets, toys, and other household objects. Occasionally children may be exposed to lead leached from improperly fired ceramics with lead-containing glazes, to lead-based cosmetics, to leaded inks on newspaper or magazine pages, to fragments of battery casings, and to other lead artifacts. All of these environmental sources of lead can be identified as potentially significant, and various combinations of them account for the total exposure to lead of different groups of children. For standard-setting purposes, however, the relative contributions of each to exposures of specific subpopulations need to be determined quantitatively as far as this is possible. That aspect of the process is examined in Step 3, below.

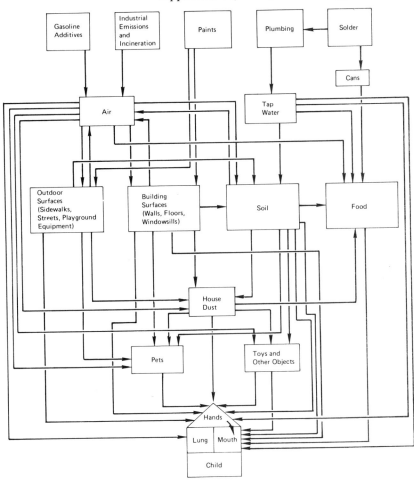

FIGURE 2.4 A schematic representation of sources and pathways of exposure to lead for urban children. The quantitative importance of different pathways varies substantially (see text).

Person Variables If there were no sources of lead in the child's environment, the numerous variables peculiar to individual humans that also contribute to lead hazards would be considerably less important. However, given the long-standing contamination of urban environments with lead, the question of why some individual children may be at above-average risk demands careful evaluation. The number of "person variables" and the complexity of interactions among them probably is even greater than the number of environmental variables just discussed.

As noted, age is one important factor. Children from infancy to 3 years of age are especially prone to elevated exposures to lead in dust, in soil, and from mouthing of objects, and also may absorb a greater fraction of ingested lead than older children or adults do (McCabe 1979). Ethnic, genetic, and cultural factors can affect exposure, for instance through dietary preferences, and may also be associated with differences in absorption of lead or susceptibility to toxic effects. Available data show that black children generally have higher blood lead levels than white or hispanic children (see Step 4, below). Socioeconomic status of families contributes to several risk-related variables, such as place of residence, access to medical information, and family life-style (Hunter 1977, 1978; Stark et al. 1978). The occupations of adults can result in added exposure of children to lead, for instance through contamination of the home with lead-laden dust borne on the clothing of adults who work in lead industries (Rice et al. 1978).

Characteristics of adults also can contribute indirectly to a child's exposure to lead; for instance, children whose families have inadequate resources to cope with multiple problems may be poorly supervised, and therefore more likely to ingest paint, dust, or soil without intervention by an adult (Chisolm and Kaplan 1968). Attendance at nursery school or a day-care center places a child under supervision, often in a different environment from the home, and may be associated with lowered exposure to lead (Stark et al. 1978). The marital status of parents, number of adults in the household, number and ages of children and the ordinal number of the individual child, cultural and individual variations in parent–child interactions, variations in household cleaning practices, length of time at a given place of residence, and characteristics of the residence (e.g., proximity to ground level, air conditioning) all may affect exposure to lead.

In addition, nutritional and health characteristics of individuals can have important implications for lead hazards. Dietary preferences such as the proportion of canned foods or home-grown vegetables in the diet may influence the amount of lead ingested, and the presence of adequate calcium, phosphate, or protein in the diet tends to reduce the absorption of lead from the intestine. Conversely, individuals whose diets are deficient in certain essential nutrients, especially calcium, iron, and zinc, may absorb more lead or be more sensitive to the effects of lead and other toxins (Mahaffey and Vanderveen 1979). Health conditions such as renal insufficiency or metabolic disorders that alter the mineral balance of the skeleton can influence the distribution of lead within the body, and may heighten susceptibility to biological effects.

Another critical factor in childhood exposure to lead is the behavior of children themselves. During their development most children exhibit a mouthing phase during which they are prone to lick their fingers, suck their thumbs, and place foreign objects in their mouths. The tendency is more pronounced and persistent in some children than in others. Pica, the abnormal and habitual ingestion of nonfood items such as dirt, paint, dust, cigarette butts, and many other substances, can be a critical factor in exposure to lead. While mouthing and oral exploration is part of normal pediatric development, pica that persists beyond age 3 is generally regarded by pediatric psychiatrists as abnormal behavior. The estimated incidence of pica among children varies with the definition used. Some studies suggest that pronounced mouthing activity may occur in up to 60 percent of children under age 3, and that it is encountered more frequently in blacks than in whites (Millican and Lourie 1970). Various investigators have suggested that nutritional, cultural, family, and emotional factors may be responsible for causing pica (Chisolm and Kaplan 1968, Layman et al. 1963, Millican and Lourie 1970). However, neither the precise causes of the behavior nor the incidence of pica in specific population groups are well understood. Without more precise knowledge, the relative contributions of both normal mouthing behavior and pica to the ingestion of lead by urban children cannot be accurately estimated.

Several epidemiological studies have established that social and personal variables are correlated with undue absorption of lead in urban children (Chaiklin et al. 1974, Stark et al. 1978). However, the knowledge required to move from this qualitative understanding to a more quantitative assessment of the specific causes of excessive lead absorption in specific populations does not exist. Research in this area could improve considerably the ability to identify target populations, and at the same time could suggest additional ways to protect those children from the hazards of lead in their environments.

Step 3: ESTIMATE QUANTITATIVELY THE LEVEL OF EXPOSURE TO LEAD BY EACH PATHWAY THAT AFFECTS THE TARGET POPULATION

Ideally, a decision to set standards for lead in the environment would be based on a quantitative assessment of actual contributions to total exposure to lead for each of the pathways shown in Figure 2.4 for each specific target population. An agency engaged in developing standards for lead in soils would like to know how much lead is in soil at a variety of sites that urban children may frequent, and how often and how much soil is ingested through pica or normal hand–mouth contact, contacts with pets or toys, or inhalation of re-entrained soil particles. The agency would also need to compare the exposure from soil with the amount of lead inhaled in air, or ingested in food, water, paint, and other materials.

In general, not enough is known about either the amounts of lead in the environment at specific sites or the rates of transfer along specific pathways to provide supportable quantitative estimates for specific populations of children. The best available estimates are based on more general knowledge, and the application of that information to specific populations frequently requires some relatively arbitrary, unproven assumptions (U.S. EPA 1977a, Drill et al. 1979). The state of knowledge is firmer for some pathways than it is for others; each is examined briefly below. Typical levels of lead in the air, water, and soil of urban areas in the United States are summarized in Table 2.1.

Exposure via Air

Extensive data are available on the levels of lead in urban atmospheres. Relationships between time and traffic patterns, proximity to traffic or industrial sources, and concentrations of lead particles in the air have been determined at some sites (U.S. EPA 1977a, Nriagu 1978a). Time-series data provided by the National Air Surveillance Network and certain other continuous long-term monitoring programs indicate recent downward trends in atmospheric lead concentrations in some, but not all, cities. The geometric mean annual average for all urban monitoring stations in the United States decreased from 0.99 μg/m^3 in 1970 to 0.75 μg/m^3 in 1974 (U.S. EPA 1977a). This trend coincides with a trend toward decreased consumption of leaded gasoline, but the exact nature of the relationship between the two trends is uncertain, in part because of simultaneous changes in other variables, such as traffic density (Provenzano 1978).

Several important aspects related to the contribution of inhaled airborne lead to the total exposure of urban children are not adequately understood. Most measurements of atmospheric lead are made from samples collected by filters that do not trap volatile organic lead compounds; yet organic lead may be from 1 to 15 percent of the total lead in some urban atmospheres (Harrison et al. 1975, Nriagu 1978a). There is insufficient information available on the particle-size distribution and chemical composition of lead in air; both of these factors influence mobility in the environment, solubility, and the likelihood that an inhaled particle will be retained and absorbed. While existing atmospheric transport models can provide adequate estimates of average atmospheric lead concentrations on a general areawide basis, lead levels may be very heterogeneously distributed on the more localized scale that is critical in determining exposures. For example, extreme variation in lead concentrations

TABLE 2.1 Typical Levels of Lead in Urban Environments

Medium	Range of Typical Lead Concentrations	Reference
Air (ambient) [a]	0.5-2 μg/m^3	U.S. EPA (1977a)
Air (near heavy traffic)	5-10 μg/m^3	U.S. EPA (1977a)
Water [b]	<1-20 μg/l	NRC (1977)
Typical foods [c]	0.1-0.5 μg/g	U.S. EPA (1977a)
Soil (upper few cm) [d]	<100->10,000 μg/g	U.S. EPA (1977a)
Street dust [e]	206-20,000 μg/g	Nriagu (1978b)
House dust [f]	279-11,000 μg/g	U.S. EPA (1977a)
	18-5,571 μg/g	Angle and McIntire (1979)
Paint [g]	<1->5 mg/cm^2	Billick and Gray (1978)

[a] Annual average data from 180 urban locations in the National Air Surveillance Network, 1966-1974. Averages for 83 percent of the station-years were between 0.5 and 1.9 μg/m^3; 8 percent were below 0.5 μg/m^3; 8 percent were between 2 and 3.9 μg/m^3; and 1 percent were above 4 μg/m^3.

[b] Up to 80 percent of samples in some surveys contained no detectable lead (<1 μg/l). Reported averages for large U.S. cities are 2-4 μg/l, and less than 2 percent of samples exceed 50 μg/l.

[c] Data are from U.S. FDA surveys of heavy metals in foods, summarized by the EPA (1977a:Table 10-1).

[d] Soil lead levels are highly variable from site to site. Most sites sampled in studies reviewed by EPA (1977a) generally had lead concentrations below 1,000 μg/g.

[e] The EPA (1979) cited one study of average lead values in street dusts from 77 midwestern U.S. cities. The average for dust from residential areas was 1,636 μg/g.

[f] The EPA (1977a) cites several studies with widely varying mean concentrations of lead in dust; the 11,000 μg/g figure was the *average* lead level reported in one study. A study by Angle and McIntire (1979) in Omaha, Nebraska, reported mean lead level of 337 μg/g, and 95 percent of samples were below 894 μg/g.

[g] Since there may be several layers of lead-based paint on a given surface, absolute concentration of lead in paint is less useful than mg/cm^2. Surveys by HUD in Pittsburgh showed that more than 70 percent of pre-1940 dwelling units and 20 percent of post-1960 dwelling units had at least one surface with more than 1.5 mg/cm^2 lead in paint.

because of the "canyon" effect of urban buildings has been reported (Cermak and Thompson 1977). Industrial point sources also can create local "hot spots" of high lead levels in air. The variation in vertical concentration gradients for airborne lead is inadequately understood; it is uncertain whether available monitoring data are representative of lead concentrations in the air at the height where young children breathe. Reentrainment of road dust appears to contribute approximately the same amount of lead to air near the surface of the ground that automotive emissions do, at some sites near roadways (Maxwell and Nelson 1978), but knowledge of the general importance of road dust as a source is relatively poor. Finally, the amount of air inhaled by children under various conditions, such as indoors and outdoors at different times of the day or year, is not well known.

Among these many information needs, the matter of the chemical and physical forms of lead in air deserves particular attention. In a recent study in Sydney, Australia, Mok and Smythe (1978) sampled air at street level 5 m from a busy highway. Their analysis showed an average of 2.76 $\mu g/m^3$ of particulate lead, and 18.2 $\mu g/m^3$ of "free vapor" lead. This result supported an earlier study (Robinson et al. 1975) that had reported very high levels of lead in vapor form (up to 200 $\mu g/m^3$ as lead) in some urban air samples. These reports raise more questions than they answer. It seems important to obtain better information on the chemical and physical characteristics of the vapor forms of lead, and on the environmental fate of such compounds, especially whether they persist in the air at distances from sources. The adequacy of sampling devices that collect lead in particulate forms may need re-evaluation, especially for estimating the total lead exposure of people who live and work near highways. The absorption characteristics and toxic properties of inhaled lead in vapor form also might need to be carefully examined, if environmental data suggest that significant exposures to these compounds are possible.

In summary, available knowledge can provide only a very rough estimate of the nature and degree of exposure of urban children to lead in inhaled air. General ambient air data, which were the focus of EPA's air quality criteria document, are inadequate for defining the exposures that some specific groups of urban children receive by inhaling lead, but more appropriate data are not yet available. Research using personal monitors (sampling devices worn on clothing that collect lead from the air at all sites where an individual spends time) might obtain valuable information on this question.

Exposure via Drinking Water

Most urban children drink water from public water supplies. The lead content of most urban water supplies is low; the median concentration of samples from the 100 largest U.S. cities was 3.7 $\mu g/l$ (Durfor and Becker 1964). However, water supplies are sampled infrequently, and usually at the treatment plant; fewer data are available on contaminant levels at the point of delivery to the consumer. This information gap is important, since the combination of corrosive water and lead pipes or solders in distribution systems can create localized zones of high lead concentrations in drinking water. Such conditions have been reported in several areas of the United States and in other countries, and strong positive correlations have been shown between the lead content of water supplies and the blood lead levels of populations that drink the water (U.S. EPA 1979, Drill et al. 1979). The combinations of circumstances that create significant exposures through drinking water are fairly uncommon, but in those cases water can be an important source of exposure. Additional efforts to determine where such exposures are likely are under way.

The importance of drinking water as a source of lead for the young urban child also depends on the volume of water ingested. Little specific information about the water consumption habits of children is available. The average liquid consumption by adults reported in nine surveys reviewed by the National Research Council (1977) was 1.63 l/day for adults, not including amounts used to prepare foods and beverages. However, individual variation may cover a range of approximately an order of magnitude on either side of the average. It seems likely that the water intake of typical children could range from less than 100 ml/day to at least 2 to 3 l. In addition, infants fed dried or condensed formulae obtain most of their total diet in water from the local supply. Therefore, while it is expected that the average urban child is probably exposed to less than 20 μg/day of lead from drinking water, the important exceptions to this general observation cannot be readily identified with current knowledge.

Exposure via Food

The diet is generally considered to be the largest component of background exposures to lead. The EPA reviewed available dietary surveys (U.S. EPA 1977a), and Mahaffey (1978) has assessed dietary sources of lead exposure for young children in particular. The FDA has surveyed the lead content of specific foods and of typical diets, including diets representative of the infant and toddler age groups (see Ewing et al. 1979). The FDA estimates that a child from birth to 2 years of age ingests on the average about 100 μg/day of lead in food and water, and that a child 2 to 3 years old ingests about 150 μg/day. The FDA attributed the lead in the diet to canned foods (about one-fifth) and unprocessed foods (four-fifths). Similar estimates can be obtained by multiplying the average lead content of typical foods (about 0.1 to 0.2 μg/g) by an assumed average intake of food of 500 to 1,000 g/day for a child of 0 to 3 years; this approach also suggests ingestion of about 50 to 200 μg of lead per day.

Several uncertainties limit the confidence that can be placed in current estimates of dietary exposures. There are significant questions about the representativeness of the "typical" diets that have been analyzed, especially as regards their applicability to urban children. The FDA is currently conducting research to develop more comprehensive information on dietary practices of different social groups (see Appendix B). Errors in the analytical measurement of levels of lead in foods seem likely, and the reliability of many reported data has been questioned (see Case III and Appendix D). Nevertheless, it appears that food is an important source of lead for the general population, and thus a major part of the baseline of exposure for urban children.

The lead in foods has several origins. Some is absorbed by plants from soil, or deposited on plants from the air, and transferred through the food chain to humans. Some vegetables absorb lead efficiently from cooking water (Moore 1979). Foods may also be contaminated with lead from air or water used in processing, dust and solders on processing machinery or cooking utensils, solder used to seal cans, and lead leached from storage containers. Depending on the dietary patterns and food-handling habits of individuals, different sources of lead in foods may be responsible for significant fractions of total exposure.

For instance, canned foods have generally been reported to contain about twice as much lead as fresh samples of the same foods (U.S. EPA 1977a, Ewing et al. 1979). However, Settle and Patterson (1979) reported that lead levels in tuna fish were increased 4,000-fold by canning. This result suggests that for certain foods that have extremely low lead levels when fresh, the relative increase caused by canning can be very great. Regardless of the relative magnitude of the increase, which undoubtedly varies with different foods, it is clear that a diet composed of canned foods to a greater-than-average degree will result in above-average exposure to lead.

The exact magnitude of additions of lead to foods by various processing or preparative steps has not been extensively documented. Because of the importance of dietary sources in the baseline of exposure for urban children and others, better information on this question is needed. Similarly, the origin of background levels of lead in unprocessed foods is not fully known, and estimates of the fractions of the lead in the food chain that come from soils and from deposition of aerosols are still subject to controversy. This topic and specific information needs related to it are discussed in some detail in Case III, later in this chapter.

In addition, more precise information is needed on the exposures of specific groups of urban children to lead in foods. The extent to which foods grown in urban gardens are lead-contaminated, and the amounts of such home-grown produce that are consumed, should be better documented. Differences in the fraction of the total diet that consists of canned foods, and especially the extent to which young children consume canned foods intended for adults, need better definition. The importance of variations in food consumption preferences in contributing to observed ethnic differences in blood lead levels deserves to be explored.

Exposure via Soil and Dust

An agency setting standards for lead in soils would need to know the amounts and chemical forms of lead in soils, the origins and residence time of lead in soils, how much lead-containing soil urban children ingest, and how they come to ingest it. Because these questions are highly similar in each case, outdoor soil, street dust, and house dust can be considered together at this point, although they are in fact different environmental reservoirs, and will be discussed separately when possible measures to reduce exposures are examined (Step 7, below).

The U.S. EPA (1977a) measured lead levels in surface soil samples from 17 U.S. cities, and found an average lead concentration of less than 500 ppm, but with very high variations (see Table 2.1). Solomon and Natusch (1977) reported that the lead content of soils in Urbana, Illinois, ranged from 132 to 11,760 ppm near houses, and from 240 to 6,640 ppm away from them. Nriagu (1978b) compiled reports of the lead content of urban soils in different cities of the United States; mean lead concentrations ranged from 99 to 1,088 $\mu g/g$. Street dusts are reported to contain 206 to 20,000 $\mu g/g$ of lead in samples from different cities (Nriagu 1978b); a survey of street dusts in 77 midwestern cities showed an average lead content of 1,636 $\mu g/g$ in residential neighborhoods and 2,413 $\mu g/g$ in commercial and industrial areas (NRC 1972). Nriagu (1978a) reports that lead accounts for 1 to 10 percent of the total mass of suspended particulate matter in urban atmospheres. House dust, which may be derived from atmospheric deposition, soil, and interior (paint) sources (Sayre and Katzel 1979), has been reported to contain 279 to 11,000 $\mu g/g$ of lead (U.S. EPA 1977a). Many site-specific factors influence lead concentrations in soils and dusts, and it is difficult to draw general conclusions about typical amounts of lead in these reservoirs. In addition, the chemical and physical forms of lead in soil and dust have been only sparsely investigated (Corrin and Natusch 1977).

The lead in outdoor or indoor dust and soil to which urban children are likely to be exposed may come from deposition of aerosols, from the weathering or removal of paint, from discarded artifacts, or from other sources (see Figure 2.4). In urban areas, "hot spots" of high concentrations of lead in soils may exist, for example, at sites where stormwater runoff from impervious surfaces is absorbed, or where previous industrial operations or demolition of buildings have left the soil contaminated. In general, there is a significant correlation between lead concentrations in street dust or roadside dirt and the proximity and density of traffic (Rolfe et al. 1977). Although high concentrations of lead in soils near buildings have been observed by many investigators, it has not been determined to what extent the lead comes from paint on the buildings, from wash-off of aerosol lead deposited on building surfaces, or from aerosol deposition enhanced by the aerodynamics of wind encountering barriers. A few studies have used isotopic ratios or other physical and chemical characteristics of lead in soils to try to identify the sources of the lead (Ter Haar and Aronow 1974), but the results have not been conclusive (U.S. EPA 1977a). More precise methods of determining the fractions of soil lead that originate from different sources are needed.

Similar questions exist about the sources of lead in house dust. It is not known to what extent lead enters houses by tracking in of outdoor soil and street dust, by re-entrainment and wind transport, or through building ventilation. Contributions from dust on clothing of adults with occupational exposures to high levels of lead have been reported (Rice et al. 1978), but the magnitude of this transfer is not well understood. The fraction that comes from paint as a result of damage, weathering, or dust remaining from prior removal is also undetermined.

The question of how much lead from soil and dust is ingested or inhaled by children and how significant these modes of exposure are in total exposure to lead has been the subject of a number of recent studies, summarized by the U.S. EPA (1977a). Most of the studies compared levels of lead in children's blood with concentrations of the element in soil or dust; a few studies (Lepow et al. 1975, Sayre 1978) also measured lead on children's hands. Correlations have been demonstrated between lead in soil, lead on hands, and lead in blood. It seems well established that children who play in dust and soil, especially in urban areas or on sites polluted by long-term fallout from smelter emissions, ingest lead in soil because of behavior noted earlier, i.e., handling foods, mouthing fingers, thumb-sucking, oral contact with toys and other objects, or pica. The relative amount of lead that children may ingest in each of these ways is not well defined, and further research to try to quantify these exposures is needed.

Exposure via Paint and Other Building Materials

Lead paint poisoning in children was identified and described in the medical literature nearly a century ago (Gibson et al. 1892). As early as 1904, it was recognized that accidental ingestion of paint dust and flakes, associated with mouthing of hands, posed a serious health hazard to young children (Gibson 1904). Pica for paint chips was identified as a major contributor to exposure early in this century (Strong 1920, Ruddock 1924). Although this clinical picture was well established by the mid-1920s, the problem of prevention proved intractable, and the use of lead pigments in paints was not banned until 1971. In the intervening half-century, thousands of children were identified with clinical lead poisoning attributed to paint (Guinee 1972).

Although paints sold today must, by law, contain less than 0.06 percent lead (see Appendix C), many buildings, especially those built before 1950, still contain lead-based paints on interior and exterior walls, window sills, and other surfaces accessible to children. Some plasters and putties also contain lead. Even if covered by subsequent coats of low-lead paints, old lead-based paints represent a very large reservoir of lead in the child's environment.

Exposure of children to lead in paints remains a public health problem of serious magnitude today. However, knowledge has grown concerning other sources of lead that also affect children, and it is clear that some individual children who have elevated levels of lead in their bodies may be exposed to lead primarily or entirely by other pathways, such as ingestion of soil and dust and inhalation of air near traffic. In such cases, determining the relative contributions of paint, gasoline, diet, and other sources to exposures and absorption of lead is far more difficult than in clear-cut cases of pica with exposure to paint sources.

Cases at both ends of the spectrum, and at various points in between, are all parts of the problem of childhood exposure to lead today, and a multisource strategy is clearly needed to guide preventive measures. In order to know which elements of a control strategy will have the greatest protective effects, it would be desirable to know how many children are affected primarily by ingested paint, and how many are victims of more general contamination of the urban environment with lead.

While it is clear that a child who ingests lead-based paint chips directly is at demonstrable risk, the questions above cannot be answered well with current knowledge. It is not known, for example, what fraction of the housing in the country contains significant amounts of lead-based paints, or what fraction of that paint is in deteriorating condition that would enhance the likelihood of a child's exposure. Very little is known of the likely ingestion of lead by children with different mouthing habits who are exposed to such paint sources; and, as noted in Step 2, the fraction of children with mouthing behavior that might constitute a risk in the presence of a paint hazard is very poorly known.

Some limited evidence on these topics is available. For instance, two analyses of data from childhood lead poisoning prevention projects concluded that in 32 to 45 percent of cases of children with elevated blood lead levels, no source of lead paint exposure was detected by the methods used in inspection of the home environment (Billick and Gray 1978, Kennedy 1978). One study showed a correlation between children's blood lead levels and the age of the dwelling in which the children lived, but showed no correlation between the level of lead paint on dwelling surfaces and blood lead levels (Urban 1976). However, some inspections may fail to detect lead paint that is present; and since many families in lower socioeconomic brackets move frequently, lead in a child's blood may reflect exposure in previous housing (Stark et al. 1978).

The failure to demonstrate a correlation does not mean that no exposure to lead paint exists. It is apparent, however, that the precise contribution that paint makes to total exposure to lead has not been determined for most children, and the conclusion seems justified that other sources are responsible for a significant fraction of the lead in the bodies of at least some part of the urban child population.

HUD has conducted some research on the occurrence of lead paint hazards in housing. A survey in Pittsburgh found that 73 percent of houses built before 1940 had leaded paint (containing 1.5 mg/cm^2 of lead or more) on at least one surface; and 22 percent of houses built *after* 1960 contained such lead-painted surfaces. About 14 percent of the 2,730 randomly selected homes contained lead paint that was peeling, flaking, or otherwise deteriorating and thus was judged a hazard to children (Shier and Hall 1977). These results cannot be extrapolated to other urban areas, although similar findings have been reported on a smaller scale in Washington, D.C. (Billick and Gray 1978).

Instruments developed through HUD-sponsored research have recently become available for determining the amount of lead paint on walls *in situ*, which makes it possible to gather additional information about the extent and condition of lead paints in the environments of urban children. More data of this sort are needed, and continued improvement in instruments for detecting lead paint is desirable, because paint containing less lead than the limit of sensitivity of present instruments could be an important source of exposure if ingested repeatedly by children. In addition to measurements of the amount of lead present, information on the chemical and physical forms of the lead in paint would be valuable. Different pigments used in paints and particles of different sizes may have differing toxic properties, and knowledge of the precise chemical identity of lead in paints could help trace the sources of lead ingested by children.

The greatest area of uncertainty in assessing exposures to lead-based paints is in estimating how much lead from paint is actually ingested by children. It is not known what fraction of children may ingest paint chips or what factors predispose a child to pica. The rate of transfer of lead from paint to soil and dust reservoirs by weathering or other processes is also unknown, and the extent to which the lead ingested by children from such pools is derived from paint has not been determined.

Contributions to Total Exposure

The uncertainties associated with estimates of exposure to lead from each of the sources discussed are such that the fractional contributions of each to the total exposure of an average child have not been conclusively determined. It is clear that the importance of specific sources varies widely from one individual to the next, and the attempt to define an "average" case may be inappropriate. However, precise estimates of exposures to critical sources of lead are equally difficult to obtain for more narrowly defined subsets of the urban child population.

The qualitative conclusion that air, diet, dust, soil, paint, and occasionally water all contribute to total exposure is firmly established. Because of the difficulty of measuring specific source contributions directly, various modeling techniques have been used to assess the relationships between lead in particular environmental pools and lead in people's bodies. Such models require considering the absorption of lead from various sources as well as exposure, and will be discussed in Step 4.

Step 4: ESTABLISH THE ASSOCIATION BETWEEN EXPOSURE AND LEAD IN THE BODY FOR THE SPECIFIC POPULATION

The standard-setting agency in this hypothetical example would next need to establish the relationships between environmental levels of lead and the amount of lead in the bodies of urban children. To determine the contribution of soil lead to body burden, the agency would need to examine the total amount of lead absorbed by all routes of exposure that affect children.

The amount of lead in the body at any one time is the product of dynamic interactions of partially offsetting processes of absorption, distribution, storage, mobilization, and excretion. Some lead that is inhaled or ingested passes out of the body before being absorbed; and some lead that is absorbed from the lungs or the gastrointestinal tract is removed from the blood and excreted, primarily through the kidneys. The level of lead in one tissue (e.g., blood) responds to many internal and external factors (including exposures to lead) in ways that are not yet fully understood.

Ideally, to demonstrate a causal relationship between lead in the body and a biological change (Step 5, below), one would like to know the amount of lead present at the site and time of the effect. For instance, if lead is suspected of inducing neurophysiological changes, it would be desirable to measure the level of lead present in nerve cells when the changes occurred. It is rarely possible, however, to measure lead levels at such sites in living humans, and data obtained at necropsy cannot reveal the variations in exposure experienced over the life of the individual. Consequently, surrogate measures, such as the level of lead in blood, are commonly used to indicate body burden, and much of the understanding of the distribution of lead in the body is based on qualitative inferences from animal studies.

Absorption of Lead from Different Sources

The primary sites of absorption of lead are the large surfaces of the lung and the intestinal tract. Some organic lead compounds also are absorbed through the skin, but this is associated with occupational exposure for the most part, and is not believed to be pertinent to the urban child population (WHO 1977).

The amount of lead absorbed into blood depends both on the amount inhaled or ingested (i.e., the exposure) and on many other variables, including the chemical and physical form of the lead, the presence of other factors (pollutants, dietary constituents), and the age, nutritional and physiological status, health, and perhaps ethnic origin and genetic characteristics of the individual human. For instance, in animal studies the presence of calcium, phosphate, or certain other mineral nutrients in the intestine has been shown to decrease absorption of lead, while fat and iron deficiency have been reported to increase absorption (U.S. EPA 1979, Mahaffey 1978). Few quantitative data are available to indicate how important or widespread these factors are in humans.

Current knowledge of the absorption of lead from ingested paint, dust, soil, foods, water, and inhaled particles is relatively poor. Some data on absorption from the intestine show that children under 3 years old may absorb 40 to 50 percent of ingested lead (Alexander et al. 1973, Ziegler et al. 1978). Adults have generally been reported to absorb, on the average, only 8 to 10 percent of ingested lead (WHO 1977, U.S. EPA 1979), but recent studies (Barltrop 1978, Moore et al. 1979) have shown absorption rates as high as 40 percent in some individuals. The assumed differences between children and adults therefore demand further evaluation, and the range of human variation in this regard, in individuals of all ages, needs to be more clearly defined.

Improved understanding of absorption of different forms of lead from specific materials under different conditions can be obtained through animal studies. Although the results of such research could not be applied directly to humans, the qualitative information gained would be valuable for assessing the relative hazards of different sources of lead in the child's environment.

The absorption of lead from soil would be of special concern to the hypothetical standard-setting agency in this example. Drill et al. (1979) reviewed the literature and concluded that no definitive studies on absorption of lead in soil or dust are available; they estimated from available data on the chemical and physical characteristics of soil lead that about 30 percent of lead ingested from this source might be absorbed from the gastrointestinal tracts of young children.

Statistical Approaches

In order to determine the sources of lead in blood convincingly, an enormous amount of information is needed. Either the exact amount of exposure to lead and the amount of absorption into the body must be measured for all routes of exposure for individuals, or statistical data on each of these parameters must be gathered for populations. At present, only limited information of either sort exists. What is known has been thoroughly reviewed in several recent summary documents (U.S. EPA 1977a, 1979; WHO 1977; Jaworski 1979).

In the absence of more detailed knowledge of specific exposures and absorption rates, empirical statistical regressions have been used to estimate the influence of individual sources of lead on lead in blood. Such regressions have been calculated for relationships between blood lead and lead in the ambient air (U.S. EPA 1977a), the air of the workplace (U.S. OSHA 1978), drinking water (U.S. EPA 1979), soil (U.S. EPA 1977a), and gasoline (Billick et al. 1979). Each of the calculated regressions is derived from a small number of studies, and some of the data (those on occupational exposures and drinking water in particular) apply chiefly to adults.

The statistical associations obtained in this manner provide useful qualitative insights, but quantitative conclusions based on them can be misleading. Instead of correlations between single environmental factors and blood lead, a multiple regression analysis of the simultaneous influence on blood lead of lead in air, water, dust, soil, paint, foods, and gasoline would be much more meaningful. A few recent studies have used this approach to test two or three simultaneous variables (Angle and McIntire 1979, Johnson et al. 1978, Sayre 1978), but none have been ambitious enough to include all the known important sources of lead. Such research might require a massive and costly data-gathering effort, but the results would have great potential value.

In order to provide results general enough to apply to urban children everywhere, the multifactorial correlation studies just described would probably need to be replicated for several different populations. Even if such studies suggested strongly the relative contributions of specific sources, confirming evidence (precise data on exposures and absorption) would also be needed. However, the statistical approach could both narrow the scope of required measurements and greatly enhance the value of a few precise data.

Integrated Models of Source Contributions

Despite uncertainties about exposure to and absorption of lead, two recent attempts have been made to assign quantitative fractions of the total lead in children to specific sources. In its air quality criteria document, the EPA (1977a) estimated that at a lead concentration of 1.5 $\mu g/m^3$ in ambient air, one-fifth of the average level of lead in the blood of urban children would be derived from airborne lead. The EPA included all lead emitted to the atmosphere, whether inhaled or ultimately ingested in soil or dust, in that fraction. The remainder (80 percent) of the average urban child's body burden was assumed to come from diet, drinking water, paint, and other sources. This assignment of relative contributions was based on little conclusive scientific evidence; it was a necessary but arbitrary assumption, essential for standard setting, but subject to modification through future research (see Chapter 3 for discussion).

More recently, EPA's Office of Drinking Water sponsored a study to develop a more detailed model for estimating the relative contributions of air, water, and other sources of lead to total exposure for several hypothetical populations under assumed sets of environmental conditions (Drill et al. 1979). The study considered exposures of urban children with and without pica, rural children in both groups, and adults of both sexes without occupational exposures. Numerous assumptions were made about the amounts of air inhaled, amounts of food, water, soil/dust, and paint ingested by each population, and the degree of absorption of lead from each source. The model was used to project effects of different levels of lead in air, drinking water, and soil on total absorption. The same model can be used to examine the relative contributions of different sources of lead for a great number of other hypothetical situations, simply by varying the assumptions.

The results of such modeling cannot be accepted as exactly correct; some assumptions that went into the model may be wrong, and important variables may have been left out. Nevertheless, the approach is a valuable contribution to methodology. Modeling techniques offer tools for examining the possible importance of specific exposure factors for specific populations under variable conditions. Continued research to develop and validate a general model for the contributions of different sources to total exposure to lead is needed, and efforts should be focused on obtaining better data to use in modeling studies. Modeling is no substitute for measurements of real exposures by specific pathways for well-defined populations, but it can greatly enhance the meaning that can be drawn from good measurements.

The exposure and absorption model developed by Drill et al. (1979) is used in each case in this chapter as a method for producing a hypothetical result that can then be examined in light of other evidence. The assumptions used to select input values for the model are our own, and not necessarily those used by Drill and colleagues.

Table 2.2 shows estimates of the relative contributions of different sources of lead in the environment to total absorption for urban children with and without pica, derived by this modeling approach. It must be emphasized that the cases shown in the table are *hypothetical*. Both the exposure factors and the absorption factors are values selected from a range that may be typical of urban children and their environments. Changing the values of any variables, such as the concentration of lead in paint or the amount of soil ingested, could markedly affect the apparent relative importance of specific sources. It is uncertain whether the examples in Table 2.2 apply to any specific populations of real children. Nevertheless, the model provides a valuable framework into which better estimates for the critical variables can be inserted as data become available.

Distribution of Lead in the Body

Lead that is absorbed into the blood may be transported to virtually all of the organs and tissues of the body. The level of lead at any one site and time is determined by complex, dynamic interchanges among the various tissues and fluids of the body. At present, the pharmacodynamic behavior of lead in the human body is understood only in relatively general qualitative terms; the WHO (1977), the EPA (1979), and Drill et al. (1979) have reviewed available data.

Absorbed lead is removed from the body by several routes. About 95 percent of excretion is in the urine, but lead is also excreted in bile, sweat, and milk,. and stored in tissues that are later shed, such as deciduous teeth, hair, and nails. A small amount of lead also is passed from the blood through the intestinal wall into the gut and eliminated with the feces.

Lead that remains in the body can be divided conceptually into three pools, depending on whether it is in the blood, in soft tissues, or in the skeleton (see Figure 2.5). The largest pool is skeletal lead, which accounts for about 94 to 95 percent of the total body burden in adults, and about 70 percent in young children (Barry 1978, Drill et al. 1979). Lead in the skeleton is believed to be relatively inactive physiologically; it is lead in soft tissues and blood that is most likely to be associated with bio-

TABLE 2.2 Two Hypothetical Estimates of Contributions of Specific Routes of Exposure to the Total Absorption of Lead by Populations of Urban Children[a]

Route of Exposure	Concentration of Lead in Environment	Amount Inhaled or Ingested Per Day	Absorption Factor	Amount of Lead Absorbed (μg/day)	Percent of Total Lead Absorbed
Case I: Children With Pica and an Accessible Source of Lead-Based Paint					
Air	0.75 μg/m³	10 m³	0.4	3	0.5
Water	10 μg/l	1.4 l	0.5	7	1.3
Food	0.1 μg/g	1,000 g	0.5	50	9.1
Soil/dust	500 μg/g[b]	1 g	0.3	150	27.3
Paint	10,000 μg/g	0.2 g	0.17	340	61.8
TOTAL				550	100
Case II: Children Without Pica and Without Accessible Paint					
Air	0.75 μg/m³	10 m³	0.4	3	4
Water	10 μg/l	1.4 l	0.5	7	9
Food	0.1 μg/g	1,000 g	0.5	50	67
Soil/dust	500 μg/g[b]	0.1 g	0.3	15	20
Paint	—	—	—		
TOTAL				75	100

[a] Follows the method developed by Drill et al. (1979), with values for specific variables chosen to suit the needs of this example. For references to sources of estimated environmental levels, see Table 2.1. References and discussion of the basis for absorption factors can be found in Drill et al. (1979).

[b] Lead levels given for soil/dust are typical of outdoor soils in urban areas. Levels in dust inside a house and in soil near exterior walls would be expected to be higher in the presence of lead paint in deteriorating condition; however, a quantitative estimate of the difference is difficult to justify from available data.

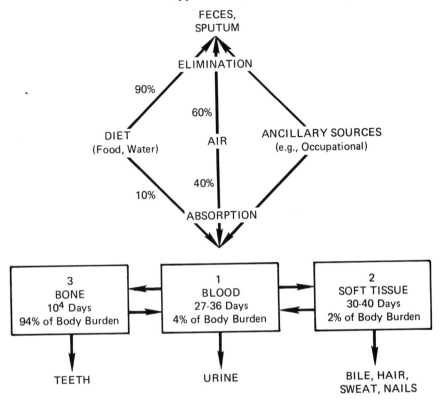

FIGURE 2.5 A simple three-compartment model for absorption, retention, and elimination of lead in humans. Quantitative estimates apply to adult males. Source: Modified from Drill et al. (1979); derived from Rabinowitz et al. (1975).

logical effects. However, lead may be released from the skeleton into the blood under some conditions of stress (see below).

Barry (1978) compiled an exhaustive summary of data on levels of lead in human tissues from adults and children, and Holtzman (1978) reviewed knowledge of the pharmacodynamics of lead in humans that was gained through studies using isotopic tracers. The latter research has been performed almost exclusively on adult male volunteers, and far less is known of lead metabolism in women or children. In addition to the human data, additional information is available from studies on animals; however, the implications for humans of pharmacodynamic evidence from other species are qualitative at best.

Current knowledge of the dynamics of lead in humans is relatively crude, but some important qualitative aspects are well understood. For instance, it is known that lead in blood and soft tissue pools is turned over rapidly in comparison to lead in the skeleton. As Figure 2.5 shows, the residence time of lead in blood and soft tissue is about 4 to 6 weeks, while the residence time of lead in bones appears to be about 3 decades (Rabinowitz et al. 1975, Barry 1978). (Residence time is the average interval between input and removal for the lead in a specific physiological reservoir.) Lead is being both added to and removed from each pool at the same time, however, and in theory under some conditions some of the pools of lead will reach a steady state, where inputs equal outputs and concentration is relatively constant.

In a dynamic equilibrium, a change in one variable, such as absorption of lead from the environment, will shift the balance to a new steady state. The relatively short turnover times for lead in blood and soft tissues suggest that steady states in lead levels in these tissues reflect primarily recent exposures, while the long turnover time for lead in bone makes the amount of lead in that tissue a reasonable indicator of the cumulative exposure to lead over a lifetime, especially in children. Although blood lead has been reported to reach an apparent steady state in adults within 60 to 100 days following an increase in exposure, the exact role of the skeletal reservoir in the equilibration process is not fully understood (U.S. EPA 1979, Drill et al. 1979). When exposure ceases or is reduced, some lead is released from the skeleton, so that the decline in blood lead levels and excretion rates is less than would be predicted from the amount absorbed. The time required for a steady state between the blood and skeletal pools to be attained is uncertain, but it may be very long (U.S. EPA 1979).

Research is under way to improve the level of resolution of pharmacodynamic models for body burdens of metals and other toxic substances. Improved knowledge of the concentrations at specific sites of likely effects (including intracellular sites) and quantitative estimates of the transfer coefficients among reservoirs of lead in the body would be very useful. Information is also needed about the physiological mechanisms of homeostatic processes that affect the distribution of lead in the body. In this regard, a recent study by Gonick (1978) identified a lead-binding protein in human blood. Further exploration of the role of such phenomena in regulating the distribution and physiological activity of lead in human tissues is an important need, as this question is closely tied to the evaluation of the potential for biological effects. (See Case III for additional discussion.)

Additional information is also needed on factors that can modify specific internal transfers of lead. For instance, under certain conditions such as chelation therapy, dietary deficiencies, hormonal imbalances, some metabolic diseases, and possibly pregnancy, considerable demineralization of the skeleton may occur, and substantial amounts of lead might be released. The extent of and reasons for this elevated lead release are not fully known. Research on this topic could increase understanding of when a given skeletal burden of lead might be a hazard, and might indicate whether children, in whom skeletal metabolism is relatively active because of growth, are different from adults in terms of the mobility of lead in the skeletal pool.

Measuring Lead in the Body

Only a limited number of tissues and bodily fluids can be readily sampled to provide some indication of the amount of lead in the body. These include blood, sweat, urine, saliva, deciduous teeth, hair, and nails. Lead levels in these tissues exhibit some correlations with exposure for various populations. The level of lead in blood is neither an exact measure of exposure (because of the intervening processes of storage and mobilization in the body) nor a direct indicator of lead levels at critical sites in the various organs and tissues. Nevertheless, because blood is obtained easily and relatively harmlessly, and because no other tissues are free of the same shortcomings, lead in blood has been most widely used as an index of exposure.

As noted above, blood lead levels are believed to reflect primarily the recent exposure history of an individual. In a case (such as a retrospective epidemiological survey) where past exposures also were important, another indicator, such as lead content of deciduous teeth (which are believed to record total exposure over the life of the tooth) might be more suitable. Analyses of shed teeth have shown good correlations between tooth lead and both blood lead and free erythrocyte protoporphyrin (FEP) concentrations in children, and techniques are being developed for measurement of tooth lead concentrations *in situ* (Shapiro et al. 1978). Knowledge of the relationships between lead levels in hair, nails, or other readily sampled biological materials and the history of lead exposure or body burden of individuals is generally insufficient to make such materials reliable quantitative markers, but they are useful as confirming indices of exposure (Grandjean 1979).

Certain biochemical tests also have been used to estimate body burdens of lead, including measurement of delta aminolevulinic acid in urine (ALAU), assays for the activity of the enzyme delta aminolevulinic acid dehydratase (ALAD) in blood, or measurements of concentrations of FEP or zinc protoporphyrin (ZPP) in blood. These are measures of biological effects of lead, and have been reported to show close correlations with specific symptoms of toxic effects (Grandjean 1978, Lilis et al. 1977). As such, these biochemical indices are valuable confirming evidence in clinical assessments, but they are no substitute for measurements of lead per se. In some cases, moreover, interpretation of such a bioassay may be complicated by other factors. For instance, iron deficiency also elevates FEP levels, and if both iron deficiency and lead exposure are present, the usefulness of the FEP index may be compromised unless care is taken to assess this confounding factor.

Two recent reports have reviewed the advantages and disadvantages of the various available indices of lead in the body (U.S. EPA 1977a, Jaworski 1979). It is clear that neither blood lead nor any other available indicator is a fully suitable marker for most purposes that require information on lead in the body. Blood lead levels are generally regarded as the best alternative now available, but an augmented arsenal of methods for estimating critical aspects of body burden might flow from future research on pharmacodynamics of lead in humans.

Epidemiological Data on Urban Children

As discussed in Step 2, above, some 400,000 urban children are screened each year by local lead poisoning control programs. According to the Center for Disease Control (CDC) of the U.S. Department of Health, Education, and Welfare, from 3 to 20 percent of the children tested who live in lead-contaminated environments are found to have undue lead absorption. (CDC's criteria for classifying children according to degrees of risk of lead poisoning are summarized in Table 2.3.) Between 1973 and 1978, 2,380,942 children were screened by CDC-supported programs, and 162,580 (6.8 percent) were found to have undue lead absorption. Chelation therapy was administered in 20,994 cases (0.9 percent).

The data summarized by CDC are obtained from screening programs designed to locate children at special risk. The recent national Health and Nutrition Examination Survey (HANES II) provided blood lead data on a more representative sample of the general population of the United States. Mahaffey et al. (1979) reported on a preliminary analysis of data from 1,354 infants and young children (age 6 months to 6 years) examined in HANES II. Mean blood lead levels were 13.4 μg/100 ml for infants, 18.5 μg/100 ml for children 1 to 3 years old, and 17.2 μg/100 ml for the group 4 to 6 years old. Among the entire age group 1 to 15 years old, the fractions with blood lead levels exceeding 30, 40, and 50 μg/100 ml were 5.7, 1.3, and 0.66 percent, respectively.

Since CDC's screening programs reported that in recent years about 6.8

TABLE 2.3   Definitions Used by the Center for Disease Control for Classification of Children Examined in Blood Lead Screening Programs

Lead poisoning is defined as existing whenever a child has any one or more of the following:

1. Two successive blood lead levels equal to or greater than 70 μg/dl with or without symptoms.
2. EP level equal to or greater than 250 μg/dl whole blood and a confirmed elevated blood lead level equal to or greater than 50 Gg/dl with or without symptoms.
3. EP level greater than 109 μg/dl associated with a confirmed elevated blood lead level ($\geqslant$30 Gg/dl) with compatible symptoms.
4. Confirmed blood lead level greater than 49 μg/dl with compatible symptoms and evidence of toxicity (e.g., abnormal EP, calcium disodium EDTA mobilization test, urinary aminolevulinic acid excretion or urinary coproporphyrin excretion).

Lead toxicity is defined as biochemical [e.g., erythrocyte protoporphyrin* (EP) equal to or greater than ($\geqslant$) 50 μg/dl] or functional derangements caused by lead.

Undue lead absorption refers to excess lead in the blood with evidence of biochemical derangement in the absence of clinical symptoms. It is defined by confirmed blood lead levels of 30-69 μg/dl associated with EP levels of 50-249 μg/dl whole blood.

Elevated blood lead level is defined as a confirmed blood lead 30 μg/dl or greater.

SOURCE: CDC (1978).

percent of children examined have had blood lead levels over 30 μg/100 ml, the HANES II data suggest that the incidence of elevated lead levels in some "high-risk" populations may not be greatly different from that in children in general. However, many of the data reported by CDC were obtained in cities that have had active educational and abatement programs for many years, and probably represent populations that have felt some effects of control programs. Data from cities where lead poisoning prevention programs are relatively new or have not yet been established show that as many as 25 percent of high-risk children examined may have elevated blood lead levels ($\geq$ 30 μg/100 ml) (Mahaffey et al. 1979). Exact interpretation of the available information is limited by differences in sampling strategies and other features of the data base. Further work to develop more precise estimates of the size of the primary risk categories is needed.

Several studies have shown that selected groups of children have blood lead levels that are markedly higher than the population mean. McCusker (1979) found that age (less than 3 years) and/or exposure to sources of paint or plaster were factors most strongly associated with blood lead levels above 35 μg/100 ml in children in New York City. In a population living near a lead smelter, 70 percent of children under 4 years old had blood lead levels above 40 μg/100 ml (Landrigan et al. 1975). In New York City, the geometric mean blood lead levels for a sample of 3-year-old children were 23 μg/100 ml in whites, 25 μg/100 ml in hispanics, and 30 μg/100 ml in blacks (Billick et al. 1979). Guinee (1972) reported a much higher incidence of severely elevated blood lead levels (> 60 μg/100 ml) in black than in hispanic children in New York; presumably both groups lived in essentially similar housing, and no explanation for the difference was available. There are still relatively few data on ethnic differences in blood lead levels, and this topic deserves further study.

Some individual children also have been reported with far higher blood lead levels, i.e., above 100 μg/100 ml. Blood lead levels this high are usually associated with clinical lead poisoning, but have occasionally been reported in asymptomatic children (NRC 1972). Exact estimates are not available on the number of children who may fall into this high-risk category, but blood lead levels above 100 μg/100 ml appear to be quite rare in children.

The data that exist are difficult to interpret, for a number of reasons. Despite the large number of individual children screened, the typical distribution of blood lead levels in urban children is still not known quantitatively, and the fraction of the population that may be at significant risk of excessive absorption cannot be estimated with much confidence. Relatively few sets of data on specific populations have been analyzed statistically to indicate a geometric mean and geometric standard deviation. (These measures are essential to predict the effects of changes in average blood lead levels on the number of children with levels above a particular value, such as 30 μg/100 ml [see Chapter 3, Step 4].)

The question of whether average blood lead levels of populations of urban children have declined in response to control measures is critical to the assessment of further protective steps (see Step 7, below). Few available data are suitable for answering the question. The data gathered in childhood lead poisoning prevention programs have seldom been analyzed to determine general trends in children's blood lead levels. Such an analysis would be difficult, because measurement methods and criteria for classifying children screened for blood lead have changed with time (see Chapter 3), and no continuous, uniform data base exists. One study sponsored by CDC showed that more than 70 percent of children whom screening identified as having undue lead absorption showed improvement (lower blood levels) when subsequently tested (Kennedy 1978); but this finding applies only to a subset of the population for whom special protective measures were initiated. Two recent studies by HUD have shown downward trends in blood lead levels in children in New York City and in Louisville, Kentucky, over intervals of 7 and 4 years, respectively (see Figure 2.6). The changes in blood lead levels show significant correlations with changes in amounts of leaded gasoline sold in the two cities and their environs. However, other measures to control exposure to lead have also been pursued over the same period, including population screening, removal of some lead paint and other hazards, and public education. Aside from the studies noted, little research has compared available blood lead data with indices of control measures, or sought correlations between changes in the levels of lead in the environment and levels in children's bodies.

Step 5: ESTABLISH THE ASSOCIATION BETWEEN LEAD IN THE BODY AND BIOLOGICAL CHANGE IN THE SPECIFIC POPULATION

The primary goal of most government standard-setting activities related to lead is to protect against adverse effects on the health of the target population. Consequently, attempts to describe or establish dose–effect and dose–response relationships have been a central concern of several recent criteria documents (U.S. EPA 1977a, 1979; WHO 1977; NIOSH 1978). An agency setting standards for lead in soil would need to show that levels of lead in the bodies of urban children, estimated in the previous step, were associated with specific biological changes.

Toxic effects of lead have been extensively documented in both humans and laboratory animals. Lead is a general metabolic poison that affects a great many organs and organ systems. The most extensively studied effects have been relatively severe forms of toxicity associated with exposure levels that are higher than those likely to be experienced by an urban child today, e.g., occupational exposures of adults, or high doses administered to test animals. There is a substantial body of knowledge of the effects of lead in children, and concern about pediatric lead poisoning has stimulated research on both clinical effects and subclinical changes associated with lead in young children.

For standard-setting purposes, an agency would need to know the lowest exposures to lead that have produced detectable effects on biological functions of humans. Exposures that produce obvious clinical illness would be above the critical range for decisions; however, knowledge of effects of higher exposures provides useful inferences about target organs or systems and the nature of effects of smaller doses. Most effects that are relevant to standard setting would be present in asymptomatic children, and could be detected only through specific functional or biochemical tests. Many of the effects fall in the gray zone between "normality" and clearly adverse conditions.

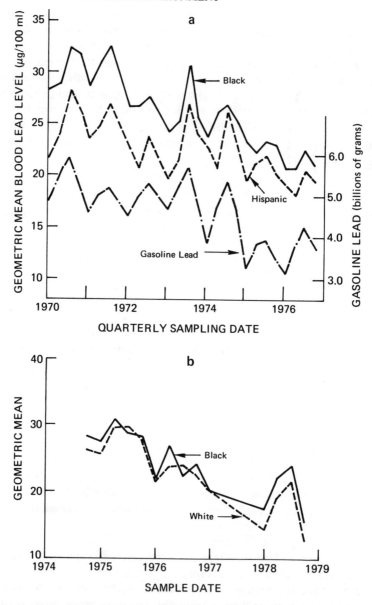

FIGURE 2.6   Recent trends in blood lead levels for specific populations of urban children. A. New York City, composite geometric mean blood lead values for all children tested by race. Quarterly sales of leaded gasoline shown for comparison. Source: Billick et al. 1979. B. Louisville, Ky., blood lead values for 3-year-old children, showing racial differences. Source: I. H. Billick, Department of Housing and Urban Development, personal communication, 1979.

TABLE 2.4   Summary of Lowest Blood Lead Levels
Associated with Specific Biological Changes in Children[a]

Blood Lead Level (μg Pb/100 ml)	Effect
10	ALAD inhibition
15-20	Erythrocyte protoporphyrin elevation
40	Increased urinary ALA excretion
40	Anemia (lowered hemoglobin count)
40	Coproporphyrin elevation
50-60	Cognitive (CNS) deficits
50-60	Peripheral neuropathies
80-100	Encephalopathic symptoms

[a] SOURCE: Modified from U.S. EPA (1979).

The four criteria documents cited above contain extensive reviews and assessments of present knowledge of the biological effects of lead on several human populations and on animals. The lower limits of levels of lead in the body that have been associated with a number of specific effects are summarized in Table 2.4.

Target Organs and Systems

Lead is known to affect the nervous system, the hematopoietic (blood-forming) system, the kidneys, the reproductive system, and behavior; however, relatively good dose–effect and dose–response data specific to children exist only for effects on heme synthesis. Some evidence is also available, but in amounts insufficient to support well-defined dose–effect relationships, for effects on the developing embryo, the immune and endocrine systems, cardiovascular functions, the liver, and the gastrointestinal system. Animal data suggest that lead may be carcinogenic, but studies on human populations have shown no clear or significant effects of lead exposure on the risk of cancer mortality (see Step 5 of Case II, later in this chapter).

As Table 2.4 demonstrates, some biochemical processes and organ systems appear to respond to lower levels of lead than others. Since the decision process is focused on the lower limits of biological change associated with lead, this discussion will concentrate on two systems believed to be most sensitive to lead in children: the hematopoietic system, particularly the biosynthesis of heme; and the developing nervous system and behavior. (Effects on other organs and systems are discussed in Case II.)

Throughout the discussion here, the common measure of lead in the body is the blood lead level, with a few noted exceptions. As explained in Step 4 above, blood lead levels do not necessarily accurately represent the actual amount of lead present at the time and specific site of a biological effect. However, empirical associations between blood lead and specific biological changes provide the basis for the criteria for health effects of lead adopted by EPA, NIOSH, and the WHO.

Effects on Heme Synthesis

As Table 2.4 shows, effects on certain enzymes involved in heme synthesis have been observed in association with lower blood lead levels than those that produce effects on any other system. For this reason, EPA has identified effects on heme synthesis as the "critical effects" for standard-setting purposes (U.S. EPA 1977a, 1979).

A word of caution about the concept of "critical effects" is required at this point. There is no *a priori* reason to assume that the biochemical processes of heme synthesis are inherently more sensitive to effects of lead than are other human biochemical functions. Studies on laboratory preparations suggest that many biological molecules are also affected by comparably low concentrations of lead (U.S. EPA 1977a, Jaworski 1979). The fact that effects are observed in erythrocytes at lower levels of lead in the body than those at which they are observed in other tissues might be explained either by a lesser concentration of lead in tissues other than blood, by an inability to measure effects in other tissues as readily as in erythrocytes, or by a lack of efforts to date to identify other specific sensitive markers of biochemical change. Thus, the designation of heme synthesis as the critical effect may reflect primarily the limits of observation, and not a lack of concern for other potential effects.

Several detailed reviews of dose–effect and dose–response data for effects of lead on human hematopoietic functions are available (e.g., Zielhuis 1975a, U.S. EPA 1977a, WHO 1977, Chisolm 1978, Posner et al. 1978, Jaworski 1979). Relatively high blood lead levels (about 60 μg/100 ml or more) have been associated with shortened lifespan of erythrocytes, and anemia is a common symptom of clinical lead poisoning. At blood lead levels above about 20 to 25 μg/100 ml, inhibitory effects of lead on the activity of enzymes partially block the synthesis of heme. As a result of that inhibition, precursors of heme, including delta aminolevulinic acid (ALA), coproporphyrin (CP), and protoporphyrin IX or free erythrocyte protoporphyrin (FEP) can accumulate to elevated levels in the blood. (As noted in Step 4, an elevated FEP level may also occur because of iron deficiency.) The elevation of ALA and CP is also frequently measured in urine, as these molecules are readily excreted. Zielhuis (1975a) reports

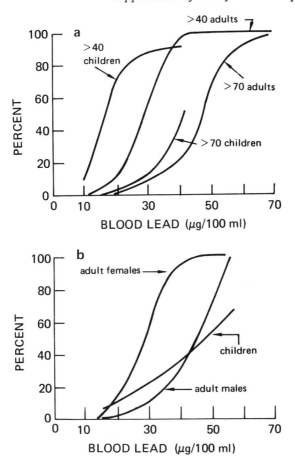

FIGURE 2.7 Dose–response curves for effects of lead on heme synthesis in adults and children. A. Percentage of population with 40 percent and 70 percent inhibition of ALAD in relation to lead in blood. B. Percentage of population with increased FEP in relation to lead in blood. Source: Zielhuis (1975a).

that the fraction of children with 40 percent reduction of activity of delta aminolevulinic acid dehydratase (ALAD) increases from about 10 to about 90 percent as blood lead rises from 10 to 30 μg/100 ml; and the fraction of children with elevated FEP rises from about 5 percent at 10 μg/100 ml lead in blood to about 70 percent at 44 μg/100 ml (Figure 2.7).

The dose–response curves shown in Figure 2.7 are crude "best fit" averages based on several studies, and the lower portions of the curves are largely extrapolated, with a wide margin of uncertainty. The reported measurable inhibition of ALAD and elevation of FEP at blood lead levels as low as 15 μg/100 ml rests on a very small data base; most studies have observed no significant effects on heme synthesis at blood lead levels below 25 to 30 μg/100 ml. (See U.S. EPA [1977a], Chisolm 1978, and Jaworski [1979] for detailed critical reviews of the literature.) It is apparent that human biological responses to lead are variable, and that the levels of lead in blood associated with observable changes in heme synthesis in different individuals may span a considerable range, perhaps 15 to 30 μg/100 ml. As future research provides more detailed understanding of the nature and causes of variability in this response, a basis may emerge for a more precise definition of the amount of lead associated with the onset of detectable biochemical changes.

The health significance of the effects of low levels of lead in blood on heme synthesis is currently unknown. Obvious anemia, indicated by significantly low hemoglobin levels, has not been associated with blood lead levels below 40 to 50 μg/100 ml. The U.S. EPA (1977a) concluded that elevation of FEP probably has greater physiological significance than the inhibition of ALAD, because the former may indicate an impairment of mitochondrial function and cellular respiration. That conclusion has been questioned by the Lead Industries Association, which presented arguments that elevated EP may be due to several nonlead causes, and that another mitochondrial step, ALA synthesis, is unimpaired by lead (Jandl 1978). Regardless of the question of whether the mitochondria per se are impaired, it is clearly important that further research be pursued to determine the ultimate physiological significance of the observed changes in heme synthesis. In addition, recent research suggests that the accumulation of precursors of heme may also have toxic consequences; specifically, ALA may have toxic effects on neuromuscular functions (Moore and Meredith 1976, Silbergeld 1979). The evidence available at present is primarily derived from *in vitro* and animal studies using relatively high doses of ALA, but this question also demands further examination.

Neurological and Behavioral Effects

Effects on the central and peripheral nervous systems are notable symptoms of clinical lead poisoning in children and adults, and behavioral changes and impaired learning ability have long been recognized as common sequelae of childhood lead poisoning. The extensive literature on neurological and behavioral effects of lead in humans and animals has recently been reviewed in detail by the EPA (1977a), Jaworski (1979), and

Repko and Corum (1979). The most critical unresolved question at present is whether effects that have been unequivocally linked with unusually high exposures to lead may also occur in some members of the general population, especially children with levels of lead in their bodies typical of the range observed in urban areas (see Step 4).

Epidemiological Evidence Byers and Lord (1943) reported that children who had been clinically ill with lead poisoning as infants later exhibited impaired learning ability, characterized by poor sensorimotor control, short attention span, impulsive behavior, and hyperactivity. Perlstein and Attala (1966) observed mental retardation in 24 percent of children who had been clinically lead poisoned, and in 9 percent of a group that had had elevated body burdens of lead without toxic symptoms. Since that time, research has emphasized subclinical effects on behavior and learning ability. More than a dozen studies have shown higher blood lead levels in retarded children than in control groups (see Jaworski 1979). David et al. (1972) measured blood lead levels of 26 to 30 μg/100 ml in hyperactive children, and 22 μg/100 ml in controls. De la Burde and Choate (1972, 1975) found performance deficits on motor functions and behavioral tests in children with blood lead levels of 40 to 100 μg/100 ml (mean: 58), and Perino and Ernhart (1974) reported impaired cognitive and perceptual performance in preschool children with blood lead levels of 40 to 70 μg/100 ml. Landrigan et al. (1975) measured an 8-point deficit in performance IQ, but no differences in verbal IQ, behavior, or hyperactivity, in a population of children with a mean blood lead level of 48 μg/100 ml. A few studies have found no differences in mental abilities associated with differences in lead burdens at blood lead levels of 50 μg/100 ml or less (see Jaworski 1979).

Current epidemiological evidence cannot provide conclusive proof that lead causes intellectual deficits, even in children with blood lead levels of more than 40 μg/100 ml. The statistical associations that have been observed cannot demonstrate a causal relationship, and it is plausible that mental retardation and hyperactivity could contribute to excessive lead burdens, rather than the reverse. However, Beattie et al. (1975) reported a strong association between high levels of lead in household water supplies used during pregnancy and mental retardation in children born to mothers using such water. Blood samples obtained a few days after birth showed lead levels of 25.4 $\pm$ 12.1 μg/100 ml in the retarded children, and 17.8 $\pm$ 4.9 μg/100 ml in a control group. In this case, the children's lead exposure cannot be explained by their behavior, and the inference that lead is a causal factor in impaired intellectual development is more strongly supported.

More serious limitations on the epidemiological evidence are related to several fundamental methodological issues. A majority of published studies deal with unusual populations of children, such as students in schools for the retarded; as a result, it is uncertain whether findings of such studies can be applied to "average" children. Virtually all of the studies relied on blood lead as a marker of body burden. The serious deficiencies of blood lead as an indicator of exposure during critical periods of neurological development were discussed in Step 4. The various studies used different measures of outcomes, making comparisons difficult, and raising the question of which tests are most appropriate for measuring possible neurobehavioral effects of lead. Finally, with few exceptions, the earlier studies failed to incorporate satisfactory controls for numerous nonlead variables that also may affect the intellectual development and behavior of children, such as parental IQ, nutrition, and socioeconomic status.

A recent study by Needleman et al. (1979) specifically addressed each of these methodological problems in its study design. The authors used lead levels in deciduous teeth as the marker of exposure (see discussion in Step 4), and obtained teeth from 2,335 children, 70 percent of the total population of first and second graders in the community during the study. Children whose tooth lead levels fell below the 10th percentile of the entire sample served as the control group, and those whose tooth lead values were above the 90th percentile were the primary group studied for possible effects of lead. A battery of tests of neuropsychological functions was administered to the high-lead and low-lead groups. Subjective evaluations by teachers on 11 indices of classroom performance were also obtained for 2,146 of the children. Data were gathered on 39 nonlead variables that might affect learning ability and behavior, and a statistical analysis was performed to assess the effects of differences in those confounding variables and differences in lead exposure on the intellectual development of the two groups of children. The high-lead group exhibited statistically significant performance deficits on several of the neuropsychological tests, including verbal intelligence, verbal and auditory processing, attention span, and full-scale IQ. The high-lead group also scored significantly lower on 9 of the 11 indices of classroom performance rated by teachers; the teachers' evaluations showed consistent dose–response relationships between lead levels and proportion of negative ratings, across the full range of exposure in the population. The statistical analysis shows that, when the influence of confounding variables was taken into account, a significant difference in performance associated with lead remained. Although the difference in IQ between the high-lead and low-lead groups was small (4.5 points), the authors concluded that such a deficit, and the behavioral differences observed in the classroom, could result in significant impairments of the social adjustment of the high-lead children.

The study by Needleman and colleagues was largely successful in overcoming the methodological deficiencies of earlier studies, and is a major contribution to knowledge of the possible hazards of childhood exposure to lead. A number of criticisms of the study design have been published (Barr et al. 1979, Cole 1979, Coplan 1979, Graham 1979, Hall 1979, Kramer 1979, Lynam 1979). The authors of the study have answered most of the criticisms (Needleman 1979, Needleman and Leviton 1979), but opportunities still exist to improve the methodology for such studies. It is important that the advantages and disadvantages of the use of tooth lead as a marker of exposure be further examined, and continuing attention is needed to development of additional sensitive tests to detect subtle neurological effects. More elaborate statistical procedures might be applied to test an even larger number of potential confounding variables. However, it must be recognized that no epidemiological study, no matter how elegant and elaborate its design, can entirely eliminate uncertainties about causal factors. Given that fundamental limitation, the epidemiological evidence now available includes significant evidence that some "average" children may be at risk of impaired neurobehavioral development because of their exposure to lead.

Evidence from Animal Studies   Substantial knowledge of neurological and behavioral effects of lead has been obtained through animal experiments; the EPA (1977a) and Jaworski (1979) have reviewed the literature in detail. Animal studies permit direct tests of hypotheses about causality, but face substantial methodological problems related to the choice and measurement of outcomes and the control of confounding variables. A more fundamental limitation is the difficulty in translating dose–response data from animal studies into implications for human health; it is generally agreed that such evidence supports, at best, qualitative inferences.

Nevertheless, the evidence now available from animal studies indicates clearly that prenatal or perinatal exposure to lead impairs neurological development, learning ability, and behavior in rats, mice, dogs, sheep, and monkeys. One recent study showed that delays in maturation of the cerebral cortex, associated with delayed expression of exploratory and locomotor behavior, occur in rat pups exposed *in utero* to lead levels of 32 μg/100 ml in maternal blood (Bull et al. 1979). Although the dose–effect data cannot be extrapolated to humans, present evidence from animal studies suggests strongly that amounts of lead that produce no overt toxic effects can impair neurobehavioral development if exposure occurs during critical periods before or shortly after birth.

Neurochemical Evidence A third important line of evidence related to possible effects on the central nervous system comes from recent studies of biochemical changes that occur in brain cells in the presence of lead. Lead has been shown to inhibit enzymes involved in energy metabolism and other fundamental cellular functions in brain tissues (see Jaworski [1979] for a detailed discussion). Concentrations of lead as low as 0.02 ppm (2 μg/100 ml) affect the biochemical balance of transmission and inhibition of nerve impulses (Silbergeld and Adler 1978, Silbergeld 1979). Evidence that very small amounts of lead interfere with neurochemical functions is already persuasive, and is growing.

As is true for other kinds of evidence, knowledge of neurochemical effects of lead supports only limited inferences. The fundamental question of whether effects observed *in vitro* occur in humans at typical levels of lead in the body cannot yet be answered, because of the inability to estimate lead levels in brain cells (see Step 4). In addition, relationships between the observed neurochemical changes and specific effects on behavior or learning have not yet been established, and the possibility that compensatory mechanisms in the intact organism may ameliorate the consequences of neurochemical effects cannot be assessed. Nevertheless, in the absence of more precise knowledge, it is appropriate to assume as a working hypothesis that the neurochemical effects of lead suggest possible mechanisms for the toxic effects observed by other methods. Evidence that very low levels of lead can interfere with sensitive biochemical processes in the brain adds significant additional weight to the qualitative assessment of potential neurobehavioral effects, but as yet cannot be translated into dose–response terms.

Conclusions None of the three kinds of evidence reviewed here provides definitive proof that lead causes, or is a primary contributing cause of, the impaired intellectual development that afflicts some children. Significant methodological issues limit the inferences that can be drawn from any one approach. Nevertheless, the evidence from epidemiological studies, animal experiments, and neurochemical studies is consistent and well integrated. Taken as a whole, the evidence provides strong support for the inference that a causal relationship probably exists.

The critical issue, then, is the dose–response relationship. It seems well established that levels of lead in the body associated with blood lead levels above 50 μg/100 ml represent hazards to neurological development (Zielhuis 1975b; U.S. EPA 1977a, 1979; WHO 1977). The best evidence now available strongly suggests that some fraction of children with more typical exposures to lead may also be at risk of potential effects on behavior and learning ability. However, present knowledge cannot define the exact magnitude of the risk, the fraction of the population potentially affected, or the level of lead in the body below which such effects would not be expected to occur.

Research to provide better answers to these questions is an obvious and important need. Epidemiological studies are needed to corroborate and refine the results reported by Needleman et al. (1979), and further improvements in study design should be a continuing focus of such research. Animal studies are needed, in particular, to examine the questions of timing of doses and the most critical developmental periods in which exposure may produce deficits. Neurochemical research is needed to pursue relationships between the subcellular effects observed in brain cells and the functional and behavioral effects that occur in intact organisms. In addition, sensitive methods are needed to determine whether neurochemical effects observed in the laboratory occur in humans at typical levels of lead in the body.

Effects on Other Organs and Systems

There are relatively few data to suggest that effects on other organs or systems in children are associated with levels of exposure to lead below those that produce clinical lead poisoning. Most of the evidence of toxic effects other than those on heme synthesis or neurobehavioral functions has come from studies of occupationally exposed adults, or from experiments with animals. Discussion of potential effects on reproduction and potential chromosome damage, carcinogenic, and teratogenic effects of lead will be reserved until Case II later in this chapter.

Reports of toxic effects of lead on the kidney in children and adults have been reviewed by the EPA (1977a) and the WHO (1977). Both short-term, apparently reversible damage to renal tubules associated with acute lead poisoning and a progressive loss of renal function characteristic of chronic elevated exposures have been demonstrated. Acute aminoaciduria was observed in 8 of 43 children with blood lead values of 40 to 120 μg/100 ml (Pueschel et al. 1972); chronic renal insufficiency appears to require prolonged high exposure, perhaps exceeding 70 μg/100 ml, and has not been shown to occur in children. Although long-term studies in Australia suggest that childhood exposures to lead could result in effects on renal function later in life, other studies have shown no such effects, and the question is still unresolved (WHO 1977).

Experimental studies in animals suggest that lead may affect some functions of the liver. In particular, the metabolic breakdown by the liver of some pharmacologically active substances (e.g., drugs, pesticides) depends on the availability of a hemoprotein, cytochrome P-450. Inhibition of heme synthesis reduces subsequent synthesis of cytochrome P-450, and thus might impair the detoxification capabilities of the liver. Only a few studies have sought to identify such effects in humans; to date none have been demonstrated in either children or adults (U.S. EPA 1977a).

Colic, constipation, and other gastrointestinal effects may occur with other symptoms of clinical lead intoxication in children and adults, but dose–response relationships have not been defined from the available information (WHO 1977). Some children with clinical lead poisoning have been reported to have associated myocarditis (inflammation of the heart), but the evidence is too limited to support firm conclusions about the role of lead or the dose involved (U.S. EPA 1977a). Animal experiments have revealed that exposure to lead increases susceptibility to infection; apparently only one study on a small group of children has looked for effects on the human immune system, and it failed to detect any (U.S. EPA 1977a).

In contrast to knowledge of effects of lead on heme synthesis and on neurobehavioral functions, evidence of effects on other systems in children is quite sparse, and at present the possibility of such effects seems unlikely to carry much weight in environmental standard-setting decisions.

Factors That Affect Susceptibility

In Step 2 above it was noted that different humans are differentially susceptible to toxic effects of lead, and some of the dietary, genetic, physiological, disease, and other environmental factors that contribute to such differences were mentioned. It is clear in a qualitative way that the distribution of such variables within human populations has significant implications for the form of dose–response curves for effects of lead. Current information, however, cannot provide quantitative definitions of the effects of any one of these factors or of their combined influence on lead toxicity in children.

While research on this topic will surely be valuable as a source of information about subpopulations that require special attention, it seems improbable that multivariable interactions of this complexity will ever be fully understood. Furthermore, regulatory standards rarely seek a delicate balance between "health" and "disease" that would place some individuals at significant risk because of these ancillary factors. Instead, environmental regulations must generally afford protection to the most sensitive subpopulations that can be identified, and ideally should allow some margin for error on the basis of incomplete knowledge.

Summary Assessment of Knowledge of Biological Effects

Dose–response data using blood lead as an indicator of lead in the body provide evidence of significant inhibition of the biosynthesis of heme at levels of 15 to 30 μg Pb/100 ml of blood. The full health implications of these effects are uncertain.

Recent research on effects on behavior and intellectual development of children has not produced conclusive evidence of perturbations of normal function at blood lead levels below about 50 μg/100 ml, but blood lead is a poor marker of exposure in terms of the etiology of such effects. Recent studies relying on lead in teeth, as well as numerous developmental, behavioral, and neurochemical studies in animals, suggest that exposures typically encountered by at least some urban children may be associated with adverse effects on mental functions. Although it is not readily measurable, the biological and social significance of such effects could be profound.

Present knowledge does not suggest that effects occur in other organs and systems in children at levels of exposure as low as those that affect heme synthesis, but knowledge is incomplete and inconclusive, and the possibility of more general toxic effects cannot be ruled out.

Future research on effects of low-level exposure to lead on the health of children will need to consider that some of the effects now being studied are likely to occur in "typical" urban children. The blood lead levels associated with elevated FEP levels fall within the range of "normal" blood lead values for urban children, i.e., 15 to 30 μg/100 ml. In the study by Needleman et al. (1979), the "high lead" group had concentrations of lead in dentine that were only a factor of four greater than those of the "low lead" group.

These observations indicate that studies that attempt to measure biological effects of typical exposures in urban children must take great care to demonstrate that "control" populations were exposed to significantly less lead than "exposed" populations, and suggest that research may be nearing the limits of observable effects of lead in this population. Nevertheless, there is a possibility that biological effects might occur at or below levels of exposure to lead that typify "control" populations. That issue is discussed in Case III, the last section of this chapter.

Step 6: ESTIMATE THE LIMIT OF NON-DETRIMENTAL BIOLOGICAL CHANGE DUE TO LEAD AND THE ASSOCIATED LEVEL OF LEAD IN THE BODY

Using the dose–effect relationships identified in the previous step, a standard-setting agency would next need to define a harmful degree of biological change. As explained in Chapter 1, this is primarily a subjective judgment. Scientific knowledge is too incomplete to define all of the steps in sequential processes that result in toxic effects of lead in humans. It therefore has not been determined conclusively whether some effects, such as impaired heme synthesis, are ultimately detrimental to the organism as a whole.

Some largely scientific questions arise at this stage of the decision process, but present knowledge is inadequate to answer them, and the estimation of a detrimental degree of change must be for all practical purposes an arbitrary one. For instance, scientific criteria that might be used to distinguish detrimental from non-detrimental effects include reversibility, and whether biological changes overstress the homeostatic mechanisms or functional reserve capacity of the body. However, insufficient information is available to determine whether even these broad criteria are met for most effects of lead on children. For example, although most clinicians believe that effects of lead on learning ability are irreversible, especially in cases of encephalopathy (e.g., Byers and Lord 1943), some studies have failed to detect lasting effects (Sachs 1978), and the question cannot be considered fully resolved. In addition, the fundamental question of whether there is a "threshold" for toxic effects of lead (or other substances) is controversial. The latter controversy is examined in more detail in Case III.

Most biological effects of lead in humans involve continuums of change, in which subtle biochemical or physiological changes are precursors of more obvious symptoms of illness. For instance, mild inhibition of heme synthesis and elevation of erythrocyte protoporphyrin in blood are observed at lower levels of lead in the body than those that produce frank anemia, but all are part of a continuous spectrum of interference with the hematopoietic system. The disease process can be divided into arbitrary stages, as follows: (1) no observed biological changes; (2) biochemical or physiological changes of uncertain significance; (3) physiological changes of a pathological but compensable nature, unaccompanied by overt symptoms of impaired health; and (4) overt illness. There are no sharp boundaries between the stages of the process, and a given level of lead in the body can produce different degrees of change in different individuals. Standard-setting agencies have become increasingly concerned with preventing measurable biological changes that may be the first early indicators of more serious damage to health in the future (see Chapter 3). Thus, the definition of a non-detrimental degree of biological change often involves an attempt to define the boundary between stages (2) and (3) of the disease process just described, for the specific population examined.

Most of the issues that must be confronted at this step have a philosophical content, as well as a scientific one. For example, if the body is able to compensate in some way for damage done by low-level lead exposure, is the effect still detrimental? When a biological change can be shown to occur, but its health significance is unknown, where should the burden of proof lie? For policy-making purposes, should it be assumed that all changes are non-detrimental until proven otherwise, or the reverse? These are questions on which no clear consensus now exists, but an agency setting a standard for lead in the environment would need to address them explicitly.

Once the agency in this hypothetical example had made its judgment of the upper limit of non-detrimental biological change due to lead, it could review the information assembled in Step 5 and estimate the level of lead in the body that corresponds to non-detrimental biological change. Given the major gaps in knowledge discussed in the previous step, there could be a large uncertainty in this estimate. The dose–response relationships described in Step 5 then could be used to estimate the fraction of the population (urban children) that would exhibit a response—in this case, a detrimental degree of biological change—at any particular average level of lead in the body. Such an estimate is needed to define an "acceptable" degree of risk of biological change, at Step 8 of the process.

Several government agencies have had to make subjective decisions about the limits of non-detrimental biological change during the last 2 years. Specific cases involving the establishment of standards for lead in ambient air, drinking water, and workplace environments, and criteria for childhood blood lead screening programs are discussed in Chapter 3.

Step 7: IDENTIFY AND DESCRIBE ALTERNATIVE CONTROL STRATEGIES

It is possible that an agency would conclude at the end of Step 6 that no detrimental biological changes were likely to occur in a target population as a result of present or likely exposure to lead, and that no reduction in exposure was needed. When the population under discussion is urban children, however, a reasonable definition of detrimental biological change will show that current levels of lead in the body are excessive for at least some children, and that some measures still need to be taken to reduce exposures.

An agency setting standards for lead in soils would have estimated the contribution of soil to total exposure and uptake of lead in urban children (see Steps 3 and 4, above). That information would indicate how much reduction of lead in children's bodies could be achieved by limiting the ingestion of lead in soils. It would then be necessary for the agency to identify alternative methods either for reducing lead inputs to soils or for limiting the amount or probability of ingestion of leaded soils by children. Each method identified would need to be described in terms of effectiveness, feasibility, costs, and benefits, in sufficient detail to select preferred methods (at Step 8).

However, as previous steps have made clear, soil is only one source of exposure to lead, and the most effective ways to protect urban children from excessive exposures would likely involve combinations of many kinds of measures to reduce lead intake by several pathways. The task therefore requires determining the relative feasibility, effectiveness, costs, and benefits of alternative combinations of measures that affect exposure from air, water, diet, soils, dust, paint, gasoline, and incidental sources.

Basic Approaches to Control

Innumerable actions of many kinds taken by government, industry, or individuals can affect the exposure of urban children to lead. Most of the variables that affect exposure, listed in Step 2, might potentially be changed in ways that could reduce risk. Both actions undertaken specifically to reduce exposure to lead and measures adopted for reasons unrelated to lead can contribute to reduced hazards. A complete list of possible opportunities for control would be very long. A number of general approaches and examples of each are listed in Table 2.5.

Regulatory actions, including many of those listed in the table, have already been taken by federal, state, and local governments (see Chapter 3 and Appendix C). For an agency concerned specifically with exposures to lead in soils, regulatory opportunities might include limits on the allowable lead content of soils, or restrictions on certain uses of sites with high lead levels in the soil. For instance, the use of lead-contaminated sites for schools, playgrounds, parks, or residences might be prohibited to prevent exposure of children to the leaded soils. Effective control over the lead content of soils would also require controls of atmospheric emissions, paints on exterior surfaces, lead-contaminated sludges, solid wastes, and other sources of lead in soils.

Urban planning measures are undertaken for many reasons, among which environmental considerations much broader than exposure to lead

Table 2.5   Fundamental Approaches to the Control of Exposure of Urban Children to Lead, with Examples of Possible Actions in Each Case

Regulatory Actions
  Limitations on permissible amounts of lead in air, water, soils, foods, paint, gasoline, or other sources of exposure
  Limitations on emissions of lead to the air, discharge into waters, or disposal on soils
  Requirements for the removal or rendering inaccessible of lead paints on building surfaces
  Restrictions or bans on the sale of specific products that contain lead
  Regulation of land use to reduce exposure of populations to lead
Urban Planning Measures
  Rerouting of traffic away from residential areas, improving traffic flow through densely traveled areas, provision of mass transit systems
  Design of the geometry of buildings and densely built areas to permit meteorological dilution of lead emissions
  Provision of green belts and buffer zones between traffic or industrial sources and population centers
  Increased frequency of street cleaning
Basic Changes in Technology
  Replacement of lead-based paints and leaded gasoline with unleaded varieties
  Replacement of lead-soldered cans with unsoldered containers
  Increased use of recycled lead
  Improved recovery of lead from process wastes, mine spoils, and other materials
Population Screening and Hazard Abatement
  Screening to identify individuals with elevated levels of lead in their bodies
  Screening to identify individuals with traits or environs likely to contribute to excessive exposure to lead
  Identification and abatement of sources of exposure to lead in the environments of children with undue lead absorption
  Follow-up by health professionals to assist in management of children with undue lead absorption
Information Programs
  General education about the nature of lead toxicity, sources of exposure, and possible corrective measures
  Information programs directed toward families with children in high-risk categories, such as tenants in housing that contains lead-based paints
  General information programs about proper health care, nutrition, and other aspects related to lead hazards
Social Welfare Programs
  Provision of decent housing at reasonable cost for low-income families
  Provision of adequate medical care, sound nutrition, and mental health care
  Job training
  Family counseling services

sometimes are important. The possible value of planning measures in managing exposure to lead has generally been overlooked, and deserves more attention (Cermak and Thompson 1977).

Some technological changes that affect exposure to lead may be results of government actions, while others come about because of their own intrinsic worth. Technological changes can reduce exposure to lead directly, by eliminating uses or environmental releases of the metal, and indirectly, by decreasing demand for lead and the level of activities in the lead mining, smelting, and manufacturing industries. The substitution of other materials for some uses of lead might reduce exposure to the metal, but the technological, economic, and environmental consequences of such changes would require careful evaluation, since some of the alternatives might be more hazardous than lead.

The population screening and abatement approach has been used widely, especially in programs to prevent lead-based paint poisoning (see Appendix C). About 60 cities currently have screening programs operated by state or local governments, and roughly 400,000 children are screened annually. The programs include public education, inspection and hazard removal, and health follow-up elements designed to reduce exposure and provide medical surveillance for children found to have elevated blood lead levels.

Information programs may be integral parts of control efforts, although they are generally insufficient by themselves to eliminate exposures to lead. The social welfare programs listed in Table 2.5 all are undertaken for their own value, and seldom with specific intent to alleviate lead problems. However, insofar as poverty contributes to risk of exposure to lead (see Step 2), measures that help families cope with the stresses of urban living may also mitigate lead hazards.

In addition to the positive acts of government or others listed in Table 2.5, some unforeseen events can affect exposure to lead. For example, fuel shortages, rising gasoline prices, and severe winter weather all contribute to reduced consumption of gasoline and reduced emissions of lead. Earthquakes, tornadoes, arson, or other natural or human-instigated disasters can accelerate the replacement of old housing that contains lead paints. The list of factors that reduce the exposure of urban children to lead should include an element of serendipity.

Current Status of Control Efforts

All of the approaches listed in Table 2.5 have been implemented to some extent by the federal government, states, local authorities, or industries. Before the need for additional measures can be determined, it is necessary to assess the net effects of actions taken to date.

Reduced Incidence of Lead Poisoning   There is a consensus among experienced clinical workers that the incidence of cases of clinical lead poisoning has declined substantially during the last decade. The number of observed cases has dropped most notably in cities that have had population screening, education, and abatement programs in effect for a number of years. However, the evidence is largely anecdotal; lead poisoning is not classified as a reportable disease by the National Center for Health Statistics, and no national data base exists that permits a precise assessment of improvements.

Progress in preventing undue absorption of lead without clinical evidence of illness is even less readily estimated. Although CDC reports on the incidence of cases in each risk category (Table 2.3) each year, the available data are not suitable for estimating trends, because of changes in the population screened, changing definitions of the degrees of risk, and problems with the reliability of blood lead analyses in the early years. There is no consistent long-term data base that permits a satisfactory estimate either of changes in the status of the high-risk population (inner city children less than 6 years old) or of trends in the exposure to and absorption of lead by other populations.

Control Programs in Effect   Appendix C describes a variety of federal programs enacted to reduce exposure to lead; most of the measures affect potential exposures of urban children. HUD has promulgated regulations forbidding the use of lead-based paints in federally owned housing, requirements for removal of deteriorating lead paint with a change in occupants in housing associated with HUD funding, and informational programs about lead paint poisoning for tenants in such housing. CDC supports the local population screening programs described previously, and spent $10.25 million in fiscal year 1979 to support population screening. This amount represented about half of the total cost, with the remainder coming from state and local funds.

Since 1973, EPA has required the use of lead-free gasoline in vehicles equipped with catalytic emission control devices, established a timetable for the phased reduction of lead in gasoline, promulgated a national primary ambient air quality standard for lead and an interim national primary drinking water standard, and enacted limitations on emissions of particulate matter (including lead) from some stationary sources. The agency is currently developing final drinking water standards, effluent limitations for several industrial categories that discharge lead wastes, air emission limitations for additional categories of stationary sources, and limitations on heavy metals in solid wastes and sludges (see Appendix C). The FDA enacted limitations on the allowable lead content of glazes on ceramic products and of certain silver and pewter wares in the early 1970s, and is currently preparing to propose limits on lead in foods. In

1978, and pewter wares in the early 1970s, and is currently and banned the use of lead-based paints on toys and other objects that may be accessible to children.

Technological Changes   Lead pigments in paints were gradually replaced by other, less toxic compounds over a period of decades, before legislation (in 1971) imposed limits on their use. As Figure 2.1 shows, about 40 percent of the lead used in the United States is recycled scrap, and up to 80 percent of the lead in some products is recycled. Extruded (aluminum) cans have taken over a significant fraction of the container market formerly filled by cans sealed with lead solders, especially in the beverage industry (Ewing et al. 1979).

Other Measures   There has been little attention to urban planning as an approach to controlling lead exposure, and the extent to which measures that have been adopted by local and state governments may have affected children's exposure to lead has not been determined. It is similarly difficult to estimate the extent to which the extensive social welfare programs implemented during the last 2 decades may have helped families with children at risk of undue exposure to lead cope with that problem. The effects of accidental or serendipitous events are even less amenable to an assessment. While it is evident that many regulatory and social programs that have been carried out could affect some variables that influence exposure to lead, no concerted effort has been made to identify and measure such effects.

Summary   It seems evident that the incidence of severe overexposure of children to lead has declined in at least some cities, but the exact degree of improvement is not readily estimated, and the contributions of different control measures to the observed changes cannot be identified. It seems likely that blood lead screening programs and abatement programs directed at lead paint hazards have had a significant effect, especially where they have operated for 8 to 10 years. The removal of lead from gasoline has reduced current (1979) emissions to about half of the 1975 level, and in some cases the decline in sales of leaded fuels exhibits a correlation with a decline in children's blood lead levels (see Figure 2.6 and discussion in Step 4, above). Most other environmental regulations either were adopted relatively recently or are still pending, and there has been insufficient opportunity to determine their effects on exposure. While there is no simple way to assess the effects of informational efforts and general programs to alleviate poverty, these also have been in operation for more than a decade, and may have contributed significantly to observed progress.

The actions taken to date have substantially reduced the amounts of lead newly introduced into the environments of urban children each year, but have made relatively little headway toward eliminating the large reservoirs of lead accumulated in paints, plumbing, soils, and dusts in urban areas. Because high-intensity exposures are frequently attributable to the lead in these reservoirs (see Step 4), it is unlikely that the measures adopted to date will prevent the occurrence of elevated levels of lead in some urban children. It therefore is reasonable to conclude that further and more effective control measures are still needed.

Opportunities for Further Control

Assessments of the need for further controls of exposure of urban children to lead begin with major uncertainties about how much progress has already been made. Nevertheless, both the current incidence of elevated levels of lead in children and the reasonable expectation that health research will continue to produce evidence of potential health hazards at lower levels of exposure support a conclusion that there will be a continuing need for control efforts. It is therefore appropriate to examine opportunities for further control, even if the ultimate goals of control efforts cannot be sharply defined.

Opportunities to reduce the exposure of urban children to lead include both controls of special, high-dose sources and reductions in the general baseline of exposure through ambient air, drinking water, and foods. Control opportunities of many kinds can be identified, involving all of the approaches listed in Table 2.5. When an initial survey has determined the nature of various opportunities to exert control, it is necessary to determine their potential effectiveness in terms of reduced exposure, their technical and administrative feasibility, and their potential costs.

Ewing et al. (1979) recently assessed the needs and opportunities for additional regulatory measures to control lead in the environment. The assessment presented here is broader and more systematic, and is therefore necessarily relatively superficial. It is not intended as a basis for choosing whether or not to pursue any of the opportunities identified, but rather as a starting point for more detailed iterative assessments to narrow the range of choices. The chief result of this survey is a list of information needs related to such decisions.

Opportunities for further control of exposure to lead can be divided into three general categories: those that focus on sources of lead in the child's environment, those that begin with the children themselves, and those that emphasize eliminating potentially hazardous uses of lead. Ultimately, the design of effective control strategies requires integrated assessment of the possible value of many different approaches in all three categories. The last section in this step will consider such integrated strategies, after components of the system are examined individually.

Environmental Control Opportunities   Opportunities to reduce levels of lead in the urban environment may involve application of regulations, new technology, or planning measures to control sources of lead in the air, water, soils, paints, dust, gasoline, solid wastes, foods, or other media of exposure. Lead levels in foods, the largest source of baseline exposures, and soils, a source of more intense exposures for some urban children, currently are not subject to direct regulations. The other sources listed are now controlled to some degree, and further control would involve either increasing the stringency of current limitations or extending regulations to new categories of sources.

Control of Exposure to Lead in Soil and Dust   Because soils and dusts in urban areas may contain very high levels of lead (see Step 3), control over these sources might contribute significantly to reduced exposure in urban children. Lead in soils tends to remain in place for many years (see Case III), and reductions in the rates of addition of lead to soils by deposition from the atmosphere or weathering of paint would do little to reduce the reservoirs of lead accumulated in urban soils over recent decades. On the other hand, street dust is removed over relatively short periods by street cleaning, precipitation runoff, and wind, and it seems likely that reduction in emissions of lead from motor vehicles will reduce the amounts of lead in this environmental pool, although current knowledge cannot provide a quantitative estimate of the rate of change.

The most effective methods of reducing exposure to lead in soils probably rely on preventing ingestion, either by prohibiting uses of lead-contaminated areas that would allow children to be exposed to soils, by covering soils with uncontaminated sod, topsoil, or pavement, or by turning under or removing the leaded surface soil layer. However, unless controls were also implemented to reduce deposition of lead from the air or from paint, decontaminated sites would be subject to gradual recontamination with lead. In addition, since many if not most exposures to lead in soil and dust occur on private property, the limits of government authority to take corrective action may be quite narrow. In many cases, educational efforts may be the most effective form of government intervention that is socially acceptable. When contaminated soils are present in parks, schoolyards, and along roadways, control measures of this sort would be a more appropriate government function.

House dust, like street dust, would appear to have a relatively short turnover time. It is likely therefore that control of atmospheric deposition (either by reduction of emissions or by filtering indoor air) and reduction of other contributions (e.g., flaking paint, tracked-in street dust) could significantly reduce the amount of lead in dust. Quantitative data are needed to support this intuitive judgment. House cleaning habits of families affect the amount of dust available for ingestion by children, but there are few precise data on the influence of this variable (Solomon and Natusch 1977). Control could be approached through educational efforts about the importance of dust as a potential source of lead, with emphasis on the need for frequent cleaning. In theory, ingestion of soil and dust as a result of either pica or normal play and oral exploratory behavior might also be decreased by more effective supervision, keeping children indoors, or other forms of intervention by adults. However, the effectiveness of efforts to alert adults to possible hazards to children of lead in soils and dusts has not been determined, and these theoretical approaches may be impractical or socially unacceptable as policy options.

Control of Exposure to Lead in Paint   The limitation on the lead content of paints, adopted by the CPSC in 1978 (see Appendix C), should substantially reduce the hazard of clinical lead poisoning from paints sold in the future. However, as noted above, there is still a large reservoir of lead-based paint on building surfaces, much of it containing 100 or more times the amount of lead now permitted. Preventing children from ingesting some of that paint remains a critical element in the control of exposure of urban children to lead.

There are three basic approaches to the control of lead paint hazards: remove paint from the environs of children, cover painted surfaces with impervious barriers, or modify the behavior of children who might ingest paint. The technical feasibility and costs of numerous paint removal techniques and barrier methods have been relatively thoroughly evaluated (Billick and Gray 1978; Chapman and Kowalski 1979a, 1979b). Demonstration projects have provided information about methods and costs to "de-lead" typical homes. Some research also has investigated behavioral approaches, such as the application of a bitter-tasting substance to painted surfaces (Billick and Gray 1978).

HUD presently administers programs and regulations that effect the removal of lead paint hazards within broader programs that are intended to improve the general quality of the urban housing stock (see Appendix C). From the narrower perspective of protecting children from paint hazards, HUD's broader approach appears to give too little emphasis to the abatement of a health hazard. It would be proper to continue discussions and evaluations of the priority that should be given to lead paint abatement programs. However, in our judgment, the approach that treats lead paint removal as but one part of a fundamental need to provide decent housing is sound and appropriate.

The greatest information needs related to control of exposure to lead paint hazards are estimates of the costs and benefits of alternative strategies for dealing with the problem. Several different degrees of government effort can be described, ranging from the complete removal of all lead paint from all surfaces, to removal of some lead paint under some conditions, to simply informing the public and leaving hazard abatement efforts to individual homeowners. Using data from a few demonstration projects and various sets of assumptions about the degree of removal of lead paint hazards that might be attempted, HUD estimated that the costs of alternative strategies for control of paint sources might be from $2.1 to $55 billion (Billick and Gray 1978). Research on additional techniques for removing paint from surfaces might improve the cost-effectiveness of hazard abatement, but the removal or covering of paints in housing is a labor-intensive process, and further technological changes seem unlikely to reduce the basic cost of abatement substantially.

The major uncertainties about the extent to which lead from paints is ingested and absorbed by children, discussed in Steps 3 and 4, above, make it difficult to determine how effective efforts to control paint sources would be, regardless of their cost. The greatest research need for assessing control opportunities related to paint is therefore to obtain more exact information on the routes and rates of transfer of lead from paints into children's bodies.

As noted in the discussion of control of exposure to lead in soil and dust, increased awareness on the part of adults of the forms of behavior that can result in exposures of young children to lead in paints may contribute to better supervision of children. Informational programs therefore will remain a valuable part of the effort to reduce exposure to lead in paints.

Social programs, such as the provision of day-care facilities that allow removal of the child from some sources of lead and the replacement of old, deteriorating housing with newer units that are free of leaded paints, also may be beneficial. Such programs are undertaken for broader reasons than the prevention of exposure to lead, but where they are being implemented they may reduce lead hazards.

Control of Lead in Air   To reduce exposure to lead in the air or in atmospheric fallout already implemented measures—including the ambient air quality standard, emission standards for industrial sources of lead particles, and limits on the lead content of gasoline—could be made more stringent, the timetables for achieving existing limits could be accelerated, or both. Current knowledge of control techniques for reducing emissions of lead is extensive (U.S. EPA 1977b), and the effects of current regulations on emissions have been estimated. On a national scale, emissions of lead from automobiles are currently about half of their level in 1975, and should be reduced by about 80 to 95 percent by the late 1980s (Provenzano 1978). Local effects of stationary sources on ambient air quality probably will be curbed by the mid-1980s, as measures are implemented to comply with the national ambient air quality standard (U.S. EPA 1978); however, EPA acknowledges that compliance will be costly to industry, and perhaps difficult to attain at some sites. To the extent that the expected controls are achieved, significant reductions in exposure by inhalation and in the accumulation of lead in soils and dusts will also be attained. Because of the uncertainties discussed in Steps 3 and 4, above, the effect of these changes on lead levels in children's bodies is difficult to predict.

Even though emissions of lead from motor vehicles are declining, dense traffic in urban centers still can create zones of unusually high levels of lead. Such situations might be alleviated by planning measures, either to improve the flow of traffic or to prevent children from being exposed. Information is needed on the effects such measures might have on amounts of lead in areas where children live or play.

Possible changes in the technology of automobile engines could either increase emissions of lead (if engines that can meet current emission standards and still use leaded fuels account for an increased fraction of sales) or decrease them (if diesel engines, which use unleaded fuel, become more common). Some research would be valuable to forecast possible technological trends in the auto industry and to examine the implications in terms of lead emissions of different engine designs and changes in average fuel economy over the next decade. Similarly, the projected impacts of the future oil supply situation on the availability of leaded and unleaded fuels, the kinds of automobiles sold, and the driving patterns of the public would be useful knowledge.

Relatively detailed estimates of the costs of controls of lead emissions are available (U.S. EPA 1977b). However, so many variables have changed simultaneously, including the fuel economy of vehicles and the prices of fuels, that even recent economic assessments may no longer be valid. Continuing efforts to develop more definitive information on the costs of removing lead from gasoline are needed.

Control of Exposure via Drinking Water The EPA has established an interim drinking water standard for lead of 50 μg/l (see Appendix C). Most water supplies contain little lead (0 to 10 μg/l); exceptions occur chiefly where "aggressive" (corrosive) water supplies leach lead from pipes or solder in the distribution system. Controls of point-source discharges into waterways and water treatment measures to remove lead at central facilities therefore probably cannot accomplish significant reductions in exposure. Approaches that may be effective include removal and replacement of lead plumbing, corrosion control measures to reduce the amount of lead transferred to the water, use of small-scale purification systems in individual dwelling units, and public education.

Inadequate information is available at present to determine how many dwellings with lead plumbing are served by sufficiently corrosive water supplies to create a hazard. Efforts are needed to identify such hazards, and to determine the long-term costs and feasibility of removal and replacement of lead pipes. Corrosion control can be effected by several methods at central treatment facilities, without specific knowledge of the location of leaded plumbing, and can be effective in reducing lead concentrations (Patterson and O'Brien 1979). At present there is insufficient experience with this approach to allow a definitive assessment of its costs or potential side effects. Home water purifiers, which are generally available now, remove some lead along with other cations (Hanes et al. 1979). However, the costs of purchase, installation, and maintenance of such devices would likely make them too expensive to be used exclusively to achieve a small reduction in total exposure to lead, in the absence of other reasons for their use.

Public education cannot reduce excessive levels of lead in water, but informational programs may have supplementary value. Corrosive water that stands in pipes overnight absorbs more lead (and other metals) from the distribution system than does water flowing through the pipes, and "first flush" samples of tap water taken in the morning commonly have much higher trace metal levels than samples taken later in the day (NRC 1977, Drill et al. 1979). Increased public awareness of the value of letting water run for a few minutes to flush the pipes before drawing water for drinking or cooking could result in significant reduction of exposures from this source.

Control of Lead in Foods Sources of lead in foods, discussed in Step 3, above, include absorption into the food chain from the soil; deposition of aerosol and soil lead on surfaces of plants; contamination during food processing, especially canning; and contamination during home preparation, cooking, and storage.

The most direct approach to reduce levels of dietary exposure to lead is to establish limitations on the lead content of foods, an action the FDA has now begun to implement (see Appendix C). In order to estimate the potential effects of such regulations, improved information is needed on the relative importance of each of the sources of lead in various foodstuffs and on the effectiveness and costs of methods that could prevent or reduce lead contamination by each route of entry.

The origins of lead in unprocessed foods have not been precisely determined (see Case III). Until better knowledge is available about the extent to which edible parts of plants take up lead from various soils and about the degree to which lead deposited from the atmosphere is absorbed into the food chain, the feasibility of reducing the baseline level of exposure to lead in the diet will be uncertain. Information is needed to determine what effect the decrease in atmospheric emissions of lead noted earlier has had or will have on the lead content of foods. Although it appears that most of the lead added to soils in fertilizers, sludges, and other materials is relatively immobile and not likely to be taken up by plants (Council for Agricultural Science and Technology 1976), some soil conditions favor more uptake than others (Koeppe et al. 1977). Conceivably, regulations might limit the addition of lead-containing materials to soils where conditions could result in added human exposure through the diet. More precise information about factors that make uptake likely and the extent of the resulting dietary exposure would be needed to support such action.

The lead content of some foods grown in urban gardens, especially leafy vegetables, may be much higher than that of produce grown in rural areas (Preer and Rosen 1977). It seems likely that atmospheric deposition is the primary source of the elevated lead levels in urban-grown foods (see Case III). To reduce this exposure, requirements might be enacted that urban gardens be located away from heavy traffic or on relatively uncontaminated soils, but public education about the problem might also be an effective approach.

Ewing et al. (1979) reviewed the use of solder-sealed containers by the food and beverage industries, and described several alternatives to present containers. They concluded that technical characteristics or costs of the alternatives currently limit their availability or appeal for widespread use by the food industries. However, regulatory action by the FDA probably will stimulate more rapid adoption of new container technologies. Ewing et al. also concluded that close attention to "good manufacturing practices" produced more than a 40 percent reduction in the lead content of 10 representative canned foods between 1974 and 1976. Those authors suggested that if such practices could be adopted uniformly throughout the food industries, a substantial reduction in exposure could be achieved almost immediately, without excessive costs.

Other additions of lead to foods during processing have been less well documented. Better information is needed on the contributions of lead in air or water used in processing and of dust and solder on food processing machinery to the lead in the diet, and on the most effective methods for reducing these contributions. The potential for exposure to lead from ceramic glazes has been reduced by regulations (see Appendix C) and public information programs. However, the possibility exists of exposure to lead from other cooking utensils, such as electric tea kettles (Wigle and Charlebois 1978), and additional research to identify products that can contaminate foods with lead would be valuable.

In summary, it is evident that a great many opportunities exist to reduce exposures to lead in foods. Systematic assessments of the origins of lead in foods, the numerous points at which intervention could reduce exposure, and the effectiveness and costs of such interventions will be needed to support regulations now being developed.

Control of Exposure to Other Lead Hazards   Few of the numerous additional ways in which children may be exposed to incidental ingestion of lead are amenable to effective control. Some sources, such as cosmetics with high lead content, might be banned by government action. In other cases, such as magazine pages with lead-based inks, ammunition, fishing sinkers, battery fragments, or other lead artifacts, the most effective preventive approach probably is for adults to be alert to such hazards and to keep those objects out of the reach of children. The most appropriate action government might take to prevent such incidents appears to be to inform the public about them.

Population-Oriented Approaches   In Step 2, above, it was emphasized that characteristics of individuals, including behavior, nutrition, health, family structure, and socioeconomic status all can influence exposure to lead and the likelihood of excessive absorption of the element. Although the sources of lead in the child's environment that are the primary cause of excessive exposure must be the major targets of protective measures, the fact that some individuals are clearly much more likely to be affected than others also has important implications for control measures. This is especially true in urban areas, where the cost of complete removal of the lead accumulated in various reservoirs of the system may be prohibitive. Population screening programs, which in effect allow children to serve as monitors, can focus source abatement efforts on cases where they are most needed and likely to be effective. Information programs that increase public awareness of lead hazards and social welfare measures that improve the health, nutrition, housing, family stability, or emotional well-being of poor families also may help somewhat to alleviate lead hazards, without directly affecting the sources of lead in the environment.

Screening Programs Programs to screen urban children in order to identify individuals with elevated blood lead levels have been mentioned in Steps 2 and 4 above. Local lead poisoning prevention programs attempt to determine the sources of exposure for children with elevated levels in their blood, and to take appropriate abatement action. Most programs also include medical follow-up and subsequent blood lead measurements.

A report prepared for the CDC has evaluated the effectiveness of selected childhood screening programs (Kennedy 1978). The study found that more than 75 percent of children with undue lead absorption and more than 80 percent of children with lead poisoning as defined by the CDC (see Table 2.3) showed improvement (reduced blood lead levels) as a result of the programs. The study was unable to define the precise contributions that source abatement, medical surveillance, or educational programs made to the improvements that occurred, but the combined impact was clearly effective. An analysis of another program concluded that intensive follow-up by a health practitioner combined with effective abatement of sources resulted in a marked improvement of blood lead levels in children, but when source abatement could not be carried out other forms of intervention were ineffective (Klein and Schlageter 1975).

The available evidence suggests that population screening combined with abatement of specific sources is an effective strategy for reducing excessive exposure to lead in individual urban children who are prone to such exposure. Further information on the reasons for failure to observe improvement in 20 to 25 percent of the cases studied (Kennedy 1978) could suggest ways to improve the effectiveness of programs.

Current screening programs are aimed primarily at children under 6 years old who live in deteriorating inner-city areas; there are an estimated 1.5 million such children in the United States, and about 15 million children in the total under-6 age group. Current programs examine less than 30 percent of the targeted high-risk group each year, and less than 3 percent of all children under 6. The epidemiological data discussed in Step 4 indicate that excessive levels of lead in children are not restricted to the inner-city poor, but occur to some degree in all sectors of the population. The expansion of blood lead screening programs to include a larger fraction of the general population of children under 6 years old therefore could make it possible to identify additional children at risk and to initiate measures to reduce their exposures to lead. The federal government currently spends about $25 per child screened, and local authorities provide nearly an equal amount of funds. If 15 million children were screened each year, the annual cost might be almost $750 million.

Information about blood lead levels is only one valuable result that can be obtained by population screening. In fact, some health authorities believe that routine monitoring of populations for numerous health and nutritional conditions is needed, and a few programs (such as the HANES II survey discussed in Step 4) have applied that principle on a limited scale. Ideally, blood lead screening would be best conducted within broader health and nutrition screening programs, which could also provide other information of value in assessing appropriate responses in cases of elevated blood lead levels. General health outreach programs are more costly than single-purpose screening for blood lead, but provide needed information on many aspects of health.

At present there are relatively few comprehensive health and nutrition screening programs. However, several of the existing programs have begun to incorporate blood lead/FEP screening as part of the examination services they provide. Lead screening is now included in the Early and Periodic Screening, Diagnosis, and Treatment programs supported by the Health Care Financing Administration (Medicaid) of the Department of HEW. HEW's Bureau of Community Health Services (U.S. BCHS) encourages all programs it supports to conduct at least a pilot screening project, to determine whether there is a signficant incidence of undue lead absorption in the population served (U.S. BCHS and CDC 1979). The Food and Nutrition Service of the U.S. Department of Agriculture, through its Women, Infants, and Children Program, also supports erythrocyte protoporphyrin screening, as of July 1979 (Vernon N. Houk, CDC, personal communication, 1979). As such general health screening programs become more commonplace in the future, it should be possible to decrease the emphasis on categorical programs to find children with elevated blood lead levels, and increasingly to integrate that concern into comprehensive public health surveillance efforts.

Other Population-Oriented Measures　Most social measures that can affect the "person variables" listed in Step 2 either are undertaken for reasons other than preventing exposure to lead or are single elements in multifaceted programs, and their influence alone cannot be estimated. In order to determine how important they may be in controlling exposure to lead, research is needed to examine the relationships between levels of lead in children's bodies and such measures as information programs about lead hazards, information programs dealing with general health and nutrition, nutritional supplementation programs, provision of day care for preschool children, family counseling services, job training, and other social welfare programs. Better information is also needed on the extent to which general renovation of urban housing has eliminated sources of lead paints (or failed to do so), independent of lead paint poisoning prevention programs.

Opportunities Based on New Technology   Several opportunities for control of exposure to lead that were identified in earlier sections involve the development of new technology, especially substitution of other materials for current uses of lead. An example is phasing out the use of lead-soldered cans as food containers. It is likely that many other opportunities exist to eliminate uses of lead that result in human exposures, and a systematic assessment of the end uses of the metal would be valuable for identifying such opportunities. The needed information includes a survey of current uses and a forecast of future uses of lead; an assessment of the suitability of alternative materials for the same uses; and examination of the possible consequences of substitutions, including changes in exposure to lead, effects on industries and on the availability and costs of products, and hazards of the alternatives. A related information need is an analysis of opportunities within the lead mining, smelting, refining, manufacturing, and consuming industries for process changes that could either curb releases of lead to the environment or reduce demand for lead. An examination of the value of such changes to industrial production and the potential effects of government regulations in stimulating or inhibiting such innovations would also be useful.

Integrated Assessments of Control Strategies

Information needs have been identified in relation to each of the many potential measures that could contribute to controlling exposures of urban children to lead. The most important information needs, however, are concerned with identifying the most effective overall strategies. That is, given all of the measures now in effect and all of the possible additional steps that could be taken, what combinations of actions would result in the greatest improvements for a specific population of urban children? What elements in an overall strategy would have the greatest beneficial effects, and therefore might be pursued first? What are the costs of different combinations of measures? What are the benefits to health and other positive consequences associated with reduced exposure to lead in each case?

Because the number of potential elements in control strategies is large, interactions among variables are complex, and information needs are abundant, definitive assessments of alternative strategies employing different combinations of measures have not yet been achieved. However, it seems likely that useful results could be produced if such assessments were attempted.

Most analyses of control strategies undertaken by government agencies to date have been relatively narrowly focused on single sources of exposure, and often on an unduly limited number of approaches to control of the sources (see Chapter 3). Under existing laws, no single agency has broad enough responsibility that it can implement measures to deal with all important routes of exposure to lead. The development of an effective strategy to protect urban children against excessive exposure therefore requires cooperation among agencies in the collection of information, the development of goals, and the assessment of alternative combinations of control measures. At present, control programs are fragmented, and agencies rarely have carried out systematic assessments of alternative control strategies for reducing total exposure to lead. Two recent efforts along these lines, both supported by the EPA, are summarized in Appendix A (Drill et al. 1979, Ewing et al. 1979).

Costs and Benefits   The information needed in descriptions of control strategies includes not only assessments of the physical effects of control measures (reduced levels of lead in the environment or in children), but also estimates of the economic and social values associated with those effects. (The process of measuring or estimating costs and benefits is a technical and scientific one, and should be kept separate from the comparison of values and weighing of trade-offs, a largely social and political process that occurs in Step 8.)

Various estimates of the costs of individual control measures were described in the earlier sections of Step 7. Many of the available estimates are relatively crude, and no estimates at all are available for the costs of several of the control approaches discussed. In cases where measures that affect exposure to lead have other purposes as well (such as renovation of housing or control of multiple toxic substances in wastes) only a fraction of the total cost might reasonably be assigned to lead control efforts.

Estimates of the benefits of control measures are doubly difficult to obtain. First, the values derived from reduced exposure to lead are seldom readily expressed in quantitative terms; there is no simple way to measure the value of reduced risk of subtle effects on intellectual development or of reduced frequency of impaired heme synthesis. Second, the lack of precise information on exposures and effects of lead in urban children, discussed in Steps 3, 4, and 5 of the process, prevents exact prediction of the reduction in risk associated with control measures. Nevertheless, a few crude estimates of the value of controlling exposure to lead are available. Kennedy (1978) estimated that moderate to serious permanent brain damage in children would cost society about $27,000 for institutional care and remedial education for each child affected. Provenzano (1979) used the study by Needleman et al. (1979) as a basis for projecting the possible incidence of learning disabilities and neurobehavioral effects in all urban children in the United States, and calculated that medical care and remedial education programs costing between $300 and $700 million per year might be required to compensate for effects of lead. Both of these estimates are tenuous and speculative; however, despite the crude nature of the analysis, they suggest that the benefits of preventing exposure to lead could be substantial.

Detailed, definitive estimates of all of the possible economic ramifications of alternative control strategies for reducing exposure to lead are not possible, because of the great number of variables and the numerous uncertainties about causal relationships, discussed throughout this chapter. However, some useful economic assessments of different combinations of approaches are feasible, and even rough approximations can be of great value for decision making. The current lack of knowledge on this topic does not appear to have come about because such rough estimates cannot be made, but rather because there has been a dearth of economic and decision-oriented research that attempts to describe and estimate the risks and benefits of lead in the environment and the costs of controlling it.

Step 8: APPLY RISK–BENEFIT, COST–BENEFIT, AND OTHER CONSIDERATIONS, COMPARE ALTERNATIVES, AND MAKE A DECISION

At this step, the hypothetical agency would draw together the conclusions developed in previous steps, apply its own weighting system to the risks associated with lead and the costs and benefits of controlling lead hazards, and decide what action should be taken. It is not the role of this report to make such a decision, and this account stops short of making the value choices a real agency would have to face. This discussion summarizes and reviews each of the critical issues an agency would have to address if it were setting a standard for lead in soil.

Risk Considerations

The assessment of risks associated with lead in the environment draws together information assembled in Steps 1 through 6 of the decision process. An agency setting standards for lead in soils would recognize automobile emissions, industrial emissions, lead paint from building surfaces, solid wastes, and other materials as sources of lead in soils, particularly in urban areas. The agency would choose urban children as the primary population of concern, because of the inherent sensitivity of children and the likelihood that children will ingest lead-contaminated soil. Factors such as pica, which would place specific subsets of the larger population at greater risk, could be identified only qualitatively. Only limited data are available on the concentrations of lead in urban soils and street dusts, and less is known about the amount of soil ingested by children of different ages, or about the probability that it will be ingested either through pica or through normal oral contact with dirty hands or toys. The agency, therefore, could determine exposures of children to lead in soil and the relative importance of soil compared to other sources of lead in children in only semiquantitative ways. In addition, because the extent of absorption of lead from soil is almost entirely unknown, the fraction of the lead in the bodies of urban children that is attributable to lead in soil could not be precisely estimated.

From available blood lead data and knowledge of the biological effects of lead in children, the agency would conclude that levels of lead in the bodies of some urban children almost certainly cause changes in the biochemical process of heme synthesis. The agency might also determine that it is possible that typical exposures to lead produce behavioral and learning dysfunctions in at least some children. Given its interpretation of available dose–effect and dose–response data, the agency would then have to determine whether the effects of low levels of lead in the body are detrimental to children's health, and, if so, how many children are at risk of harm at current levels of exposure.

In considering what weight to attach to the risk of effects of lead on the health of urban children, the agency might find it valuable to consider public perception of the risk, and to compare the risk associated with lead to other, similar hazards of the urban environment in assessing the urgency of remedial measures.

Control Considerations

When it examined the need for control measures to reduce exposure to lead in soil, the agency would be unable to determine exactly how much the existing controls of lead in gasoline, emission standards for industrial sources, efforts to abate lead paint hazards, and childhood screening and source abatement programs have already reduced the amount of lead in children's bodies. It would be unable to specify the further reduction that would follow if soil were eliminated as a source. The search for useful control techniques could identify numerous technical and nontechnical ways to prevent children from ingesting soil that contains lead, but could provide little basis for definitive estimates of their effectiveness or costs. Some of the potential control measures could be implemented by the federal government, but for other approaches actions would be taken by state or local governments. Information programs to educate and motivate parents also could be important aspects of control programs.

Risk–Cost–Benefit Comparisons

Because of the numerous unknowns cited above, it is difficult to conduct a definitive assessment of the costs and benefits of alternative strategies to reduce risks associated with lead in soils. Nevertheless, such an analysis might be attempted, if the responsible agency were willing to make a number of explicitly arbitrary assumptions. There would be value in the attempt, since it could show which assumptions carried the most weight, and where the need for better information was greatest (see Chapter 3), and even a less-than-definitive assessment may provide some policy guidance.

The risk associated with exposure to lead in soil can be expressed as a fraction (with a wide range of uncertainty) of the aggregate risk of lead in the total environment of urban children. That risk is borne by current and future generations of children who are or will be exposed to lead in soils, and by their families and communities. The benefits that would accrue from reduced exposure to lead in soil (in terms of decreased health damage and other, less tangible gains) would be distributed among the same populations. The costs of various measures to remove, cover, or fence off lead-contaminated soils might be estimated rather directly, but the value of loss of potential playgrounds or parks in inner-city neighborhoods would be more difficult to assess. In general, benefits from the uses of lead that ultimately resulted in contamination of soils (e.g., the manufacture, sale, and use of lead alkyl fuel additives or lead-based paints over a period of several decades) would be included only peripherally in this calculation, since control over those uses has not been based primarily on avoiding contamination of soils.

While an agency setting standards for lead in soils would probably concentrate on comparing the risks, costs, and benefits associated with that particular action, a broader assessment would also be extremely valuable. Similar comparisons of risks, costs, and benefits associated with controlling lead in the air, water, diet, gasoline, and paints in housing might be undertaken using the same methods, to provide a comparison of the reduction in exposure that could be achieved for a given cost by control of different sources or pathways of exposure. However, as noted earlier (Step 7), definitive assessments of multimedia strategies have not been effectively achieved to date.

The Decision-Making Step

In the example used here, an agency might decide that there is too little information to support action, and decide to take no steps other than to pursue the needed data. However, as noted in Chapter 1, decisions will always be made on the basis of less-than-perfect knowledge, and an agency might reasonably determine that standards for lead in soil should be set, using stated assumptions and "best-guess" estimates for critical variables where knowledge is weak. Given its assumptions, the agency would then have to apply its subjective value judgments to choose objectives and establish a standard.

In reaching its decision, the agency would have to determine in at least a rudimentary way the acceptable level of risk on the one hand, and the acceptable cost of control on the other. To define acceptable risk requires subjective judgments of the degree of biological change considered detrimental in an individual child (from Step 6) and of the fraction of all urban children that should be protected against that degree of biological change. The agency would then need to make arbitrary assumptions to define the level of lead in soil associated with likely detrimental effects in an acceptably small fraction of the population. Because of incomplete data on the distribution of lead concentrations in urban soils, the number of instances in which abatement measures would be needed and the costs of abatement would also be estimated rather arbitrarily. The agency would then have to decide whether such costs were acceptable to society.

If such a standard-setting process were followed to completion and regulations were adopted, implementation would probably be carried out almost entirely at the local level, perhaps within existing programs established to prevent childhood lead poisoning. A major part of the implementation effort would be to identify sites where soil lead levels exceeded acceptable limits for intended uses, and to accumulate information on the cost-effectiveness of different abatement techniques. Research to obtain better answers to many questions identified earlier in this section would make it both possible and necessary to reexamine the basis for the standards periodically.

Step 9: EVALUATE THE PROCESS AND THE DECISION

Evaluation of the quality of the data base and of the adequacy of available information for supporting judgments that must be made has been an essential element at each step of the process up to this point. Innumerable examples were discussed where data are not available, where the available data are of questionable accuracy or limited applicability to the specific questions posed, or where basic knowledge of causal relationships is insufficient to support firm inferences from the data. As explained in Chapter 1, an agency developing the basis for standards would need to include such evaluations in its assessment of existing knowledge.

Methods also exist for examining the effects of gaps in knowledge and uncertainties on decisions. Decision analysis and sensitivity analysis can estimate the degree of uncertainty inherent in specific assumptions, show the combined effects of multiple uncertainties on the ultimate decision, and identify the variables and uncertainties that have the greatest impact on the decision. This example of a hypothetical decision process for setting standards on lead in soils is a crude, qualitative analysis of that type. An agency faced with an actual decision might benefit greatly from a more formal, quantitative decision analysis that ranked uncertainties and information needs in priority order in terms of their effects on a specific policy choice. Such assessments may have been conducted within agencies that have recently set standards for lead in the environment; if so, the results have not been published, probably for reasons of political expediency (see Chapter 3). Ideally, analyses of this kind would be valuable both at the outset of information-gathering steps and at the time decisions were rendered.

The need to evaluate the consequences of a decision was also stressed in Chapter 1. Ideally, evaluative steps would be part of the plan for implementing a decision, and the plan would be flexible enough to be guided by subsequent evaluations. Evaluation of the effectiveness of a standard for lead in soils would require the collection and analysis of considerable information about the levels of lead in soils at specific sites, changes with time in those levels, the number of sites at which soil had been rendered inaccessible to children, changes with time in the levels of lead in children's bodies, and the associations between actions taken to reduce hazards of lead in soils and improvements in the health status of children. In order to evaluate the effectiveness of the limitations on soil lead, the agency would need the same kinds of information about the effectiveness of other control measures that simultaneously influence the exposures of urban children to lead, such as reduction of atmospheric emissions of lead, paint hazard abatement measures, changes in levels of lead in foods, public health surveillance programs, and many of the other factors examined in Step 7. Finally, the agency would need to estimate the economic and social consequences of governmental programs and responses of the private sector to requirements to comply with standards that were established.

In Step 7 of this example, the attempt to assess the current status of efforts to protect urban children from lead in their environments reached a very uncertain conclusion. A post-decision evaluation of a standard for lead in soils would confront the same uncertainties. Because of the complexity of the problem and the many gaps in information, it has not yet been possible to determine the consequences of specific decisions with much accuracy. In addition, decision-making agencies generally are pressed to apply their analytical resources to support pending decisions, and concerted efforts to evaluate past decisions have not been practical (see Chapter 3). Nevertheless, information of this sort is extremely useful, both to permit corrections (if needed) in existing standards or regulations and to provide a more precise definition of the starting point for future decisions.

CASE II: LEAD IN THE ENVIRONMENT AND THE GENERAL ADULT POPULATION

Policy decisions that set limits for permissible levels of exposure to lead are concerned initially with protecting the population groups judged most likely to be at risk; thus, Case I was focused on urban children. At the same time, however, standard-setting agencies need to determine whether one standard can protect all populations with exposures, and usually examine potential hazards of lead to the "average" person.

This second example, therefore, is concerned with exposures to lead that are the result of normal, everyday contact with air, water, foods, soil, dust, and (for some) tobacco. Unusual or special exposures for which special control measures might be needed are excluded. If it should be determined that average exposures are unacceptably high, general reductions in the amount of lead in air, foods, or other media of exposure would be required, rather than measures aimed at specific populations. Although the general exposure category includes both children and adults, this example will concentrate on adults. Young children, who are both more prone to exposures of some types and more likely to be sensitive to toxic effects of lead, were discussed as a special case in the previous example.

Step 1: IDENTIFY SOURCES OF LEAD AND PATHWAYS OF ENVIRONMENTAL TRANSFER

The qualitative description of sources and environmental pathways of exposure to lead for the general adult population is similar to that described for urban children in the previous case (see Figures 2.2 and 2.4). One major difference is that adults are less likely to ingest significant amounts of soil, dust, or paint than children are. In addition, tobacco may contribute to lead absorption for those who smoke. Current understanding of the quantitative contributions of lead in air, water, foods, soil, dust, and tobacco to exposures and blood lead levels of average adults will be examined in Steps 3 and 4, below. In general, typical contributions from each source can be relatively accurately estimated.

Step 2: IDENTIFY SPECIFIC HUMAN POPULATIONS WITH EXPOSURES TO LEAD

This example was chosen to be relatively nonspecific, since it is concerned with "average" exposures. Thus, groups of adults who work in industrial environments that involve high exposures to lead or who drink "moonshine" whiskey that may be contaminated with lead would be considered special cases, meriting special control measures, and excluded from this illustration.

However, the general population with "average" exposures is not entirely homogeneous. Typical exposures span a broad range (see Figure 2.3), and exposures are significantly higher for some groups, such as urban residents and smokers, than for others, such as rural residents and nonsmokers. Other characteristics of population groups, such as age, sex, socioeconomic status, or cultural and ethnic background can contribute to different degrees of exposure to lead (WHO 1977), and some individuals with several such predisposing characteristics may experience exposures that are far above average.

In addition, specific traits of some subpopulations may make them more susceptible to potential biological effects of typical exposures to lead than the average person. For instance, persons with kidney disease that reduces ability to excrete lead or individuals whose diets are deficient in calcium, iron, or zinc might be hypersusceptible to lead toxicity. The fetus is known to be more sensitive than an adult or child to effects of many environmental toxins, and the exposure of pregnant women to typical levels of lead in the environment is therefore a matter of special concern. At any one time there are about 2 million pregnant women in the United States (U.S. EPA 1977a).

Present knowledge of the factors that differentiate subsets of the general population in terms of likelihood of hazardous exposure to lead is largely qualitative. In general, understanding of the importance of "person variables" that may be significant for typical adults is more rudimentary than it is for children. The relatively few epidemiological studies of nonoccupationally exposed adult populations provide an insufficient data base to estimate precisely the extent to which specific characteristics of subsets of the general population enhance the risks associated with exposure to lead.

Step 3: ESTIMATE QUANTITATIVELY THE LEVEL OF EXPOSURE TO LEAD BY EACH PATHWAY THAT AFFECTS THE TARGET POPULATION

Exposure to lead in different environmental media depends on both the concentration of lead in the medium (air, water, food, tobacco smoke, etc.) and the amount inhaled or ingested. The amount of lead in the body also depends on the amount absorbed from each source of exposure (see Step 4, below). Several recent summary documents have reviewed what is known of typical exposures of adults to lead (U.S. EPA 1977a, 1979; WHO 1977; Mahaffey 1978; Drill et al. 1979). Table 2.1, earlier in this chapter, summarized the typical levels of lead in various environmental media to which urban children might be exposed. The general exposure category includes both urban adults, for whom levels of lead in the environment would be much the same as for urban children, and populations in suburban or rural areas, whose exposures to some sources are significantly lower.

Exposure via Air

Abundant information is available about the amount of lead in ambient air at many locations, and typical exposures by this route are reasonably well understood. Annual average lead concentrations in most urban areas fall between 0.5 and 2 $\mu g/m^3$; the mean value for all urban stations in 1974 was 0.75 $\mu g/m^3$, and only 3 percent of the stations exceeded 2 $\mu g/m^3$ for that year (U.S. EPA 1977a). Annual average lead concentrations at nonurban stations in the National Air Surveillance Network (NASN) from 1966 to 1974 ranged from less than 0.03 $\mu g/m^3$ to 0.45 $\mu g/m^3$, with 88 percent of the sites below 0.2 $\mu g/m^3$ as of 1974 (U.S. EPA 1977a). In remote mountain areas of North America, recorded air lead levels average about 0.01 $\mu g/m^3$, and levels below 0.001 $\mu g/m^3$ have been measured in the Southern Hemisphere (see Case III). This information indicates that even in many rural areas the air is significantly contaminated by lead of anthropogenic origin (Nriagu 1978a).

The chief sources of lead in the atmosphere are automobile emissions, incineration of wastes, smelting of ores and secondary smelting of nonferrous metals, and combustion of coal. (An inventory of sources is presented in Case III.) The automobile accounts for 95 percent or more of lead emissions in most urban areas. Concentrations of lead in the atmosphere may be considerably higher near a source of heavy traffic (or near a point source) than the average ambient levels summarized above. Short-term peak values of 25 to 50 $\mu g/m^3$ have been recorded near freeways, in tunnels, and where urban buildings produce a "canyon" effect (U.S. EPA

1977a). Under more open conditions, lead concentrations within a few meters of a heavily traveled highway may be in the range of 5 to 10 $\mu g/m^3$, but the level declines rapidly with increasing distance from the road, and approaches ambient concentrations within a few hundred meters (NRC 1972, U.S. EPA 1977a, Nriagu 1978a).

While the relationship between traffic sources and levels of lead in air nearby is relatively well known, less is understood of the impact of regional traffic patterns on concentrations of lead in the atmosphere at distances of more than a few kilometers. Current models for long-range transport of particles generally can provide only semiquantitative predictions, and present knowledge of the chemical and physical transformations that affect suspended lead-containing particles is inadequate. The deposition of larger lead particles near roadways has been studied rather extensively, but much less is known about the rate of removal of smaller particles from the air during long-distance dispersal. The relative roles of wet and dry deposition and the influence of vegetation in removal processes have generally been studied less intensively.

Additional significant gaps in knowledge concern the concentrations of lead in indoor atmospheres, the size distribution and chemical composition of lead-containing particles in indoor air, and the relationships between indoor and outdoor ambient lead levels. The majority of adults spend more time indoors than outdoors, but virtually all of the available air monitoring data apply only to outdoor air.

Time trends in lead concentrations in the atmosphere are also difficult to quantify. Tepper and Levin (1972) showed that annual geometric mean lead concentrations in the air of Los Angeles, Cincinnati, and Philadelphia increased by from 20 to 56 percent between 1961 and 1969, while concentrations in other cities showed little or no change. Decreasing use of leaded gasoline since 1973 is expected to lower the levels of lead in the atmosphere (Provenzano 1978), and the mean annual average concentration of lead for NASN urban stations declined from 0.99 to 0.75 $\mu g/m^3$ between 1970 and 1974 (U.S. EPA 1977a). However, there has been insufficient analysis of recent monitoring data to indicate quantitatively the extent to which general exposures to lead in air may have decreased during the last few years.

Estimates of the amount of air inhaled range from about 4 m^3/day for a 1-year-old child to from 20 to 25 m^3/day for adults (Task Group on the Reference Man 1975). Assuming an average adult respiratory volume of 20 m^3 and mean lead concentrations of 0.75 $\mu g/m^3$ at urban sites and 0.083 $\mu g/m^3$ at nonurban stations (U.S. EPA 1977a), it can be calculated that the average urban adult inhales about 15 $\mu g/day$ of lead, and the average rural adult inhales about 1.7 $\mu g/day$ of lead. In addition to the difference in absolute amount inhaled, the particle size and chemical form of the lead in each case may be different as well.

Exposure via Drinking Water

Most adults are exposed to the same water supplies discussed in the urban child example, earlier in this chapter. Available surveys suggest that only 1 to 2 percent of samples of both central water supplies and tap water obtained in residences exceed the present national interim primary drinking water standard for lead of 50 $\mu g/l$ (U.S. EPA 1979, NRC 1977). Where corrosive water supplies act on lead pipes, storage vessels, or solders, concentrations above 50 $\mu g/l$, and occasionally as high as 800 to 1,000 $\mu g/l$ have been reported (Drill et al. 1979). Water supplies that exceed the 50 $\mu g/l$ standard constitute special cases of exposures, for which special control efforts are warranted.

Published surveys suggest that the drinking water used by the average urban resident contains lead concentrations that range from below the limit of detection of methods employed (<1 $\mu g/l$) to about 20 $\mu g/l$. Fewer data are available on rural water supplies than on urban supplies, and less is known of the concentrations in tap water than concentrations at treatment plants. Since most water supplies are low in lead, and since water that contains less than 50 $\mu g/l$ is believed to contribute little to total exposure in comparison to dietary sources (see below), relatively little information has been gathered on the variation in exposure from water supplies that meet current standards.

This gap in information may be significant in some cases. It is known that average water consumption varies greatly from one individual to another. A standard assumption is that the "average" adult ingests 1 to 2 l of water per day, including amounts used to prepare foods and beverages (see Case I). However, definitive information is not available on the distribution of average individual water intakes around that theoretical mean. Some subsets of the general adult population can be identified whose average daily intake is clearly much higher than 2 l. For instance, people who perform heavy manual labor in hot environments may need to replace 1 to 2 l of lost body fluids per hour (Environmental Defense Fund 1975); and some diseases, such as uncontrolled diabetes mellitus or some forms of kidney disease, are characterized by high fluid intake and excretion. Some people also habitually consume several liters of beer or other water-based beverages each day. It is not unreasonable to assume that some fraction of the total population consumes up to 10 l of fluid per day. If that water should contain lead concentrations in the upper portion of the currently permissible range (i.e., 25 to 50 $\mu g/l$), ingestion of lead in water could equal or exceed that from other sources for individuals with high water intake.

The number of people in this category is uncertain. There are an estimated 5 million diabetics in the United States (Environmental Defense Fund 1975), and about 4 percent of the adult population is believed to have identifiable kidney disease (Hine et al. 1978). The fraction of each group that consumes abnormally large quantities of water is unknown, but even if it is only a few percent, the number of individuals would be large. The number of adults with occupationally related excessive thirst is unknown, but may also be large. It seems possible that at least a few percent of the total population may habitually consume well above average amounts of water. In order to estimate the lead exposure of such subpopulations accurately, it would be necessary to have better information about both the range of variation of normal human water intake and the distribution of concentrations of lead in water supplies to which the general population is exposed.

Exposure via Food

Sources of lead in foods were discussed in Steps 3 and 7 of Case I. The diet appears to be the most important general source of exposure to lead for the adult population. As Table 2.1 indicated, samples of typical foods analyzed by the FDA contained lead concentrations of about 0.1 to 0.5 μg/g. An extensive recent review of exposure to lead (Ewing et al. 1979) summarized survey data on lead in many kinds of foods and beverages.

Several methods have been used to estimate the average exposure to lead in the diet of a typical adult. One approach is to measure the lead content of typical foods and beverages, to estimate typical consumption patterns, and to calculate the theoretical lead content of an average diet. Another is to analyze food samples that duplicate the meals actually eaten by specific individuals. A third method involves analysis of feces, and correction for the amounts absorbed to estimate the amounts of lead ingested. These approaches have been used to estimate dietary exposure to lead for more than 3 decades.

Mahaffey (1978) and Ewing et al. (1979) have reviewed published estimates of typical dietary ingestion of lead by adults. Estimates of average ingestion arrived at by different methods are in relatively close agreement; most fall between 200 and 300 μg/day, and the range is from less than 100 to more than 500 μg/day. Estimates have been available for more than 30 years, but differences in methodology over that time preclude determining trends in exposure.

Although there is relative agreement among various estimates of dietary exposure to lead, several important unknowns and uncertainties remain. For instance, chemical analysis for lead in foods is often subject to error (see Appendix D), and the accuracy of available data is open to question in many cases (Patterson and Settle 1976; also, see Case III). Published information shows substantial variation in the amounts of lead in different samples of the same foods, as well as in different kinds of foods (Ewing et al. 1979). It is well established that canned foods contain more lead on the average than fresh samples of the same foods (U.S. EPA 1977a). Individual dietary preferences, including the fraction of the diet made up of canned foods or other items likely to be relatively high in lead, vary greatly among individuals, among ethnic groups, and among geographic regions of the country. The total food consumption of the average adult has been estimated at from less than 1 to more than 3 kg/day, excluding beverages (Ewing et al. 1979); again, a range of individual variation about the mean can be assumed.

The range of variation that occurs in normal dietary exposure of adults to lead because of combinations of these variables is unknown. The National Research Council (1972) estimated that typical American adults' exposures to lead via foods may be from 100–2,000 μg/day. This range seems reasonable, but there are few measurements from large populations to support it. Since individuals who ingest as much as 1,000 to 2,000 μg/day of lead in foods would be at significantly greater risk than the rest of the population, it would be useful to determine the statistical distribution of typical dietary exposures, the number of individuals with high intakes, and the personal characteristics that contribute to excessive exposure.

Some recent trends also add uncertainty to estimates of average dietary ingestion of lead. Many families now plant vegetable gardens, and urban gardening has enjoyed a significant increase in popularity. Neither the fraction of the year's diet that is home-grown nor the lead content of typical home-grown foods has been determined. However, some vegetables from urban gardens have been reported to contain significantly elevated levels of heavy metals (Preer and Rosen 1977), and it seems likely that produce from urban gardens could be more contaminated by lead from the air or soil than produce imported from rural areas. On the other hand, lead emissions from combustion of gasoline have been declining for several years, and some measures taken by food processors have lowered the lead content of some canned foods (see Step 7 of Case I). The impact of either of these trends on the amount of lead in foods consumed by the general population has not yet been determined.

Another recent development raises additional questions. Schutz (1979) measured lead in typical diets of present-day Swedish adults, and estimated average exposure to be about 30 μg/day, a result that is 5 to 10 times lower than the accepted range of dietary exposures in the United States and other countries. Schutz initially assumed an error on his part, and repeated the study several times, with no change in the result. Schutz cited similarly low measurements of fecal excretion of lead, lead in blood, and lead in bones and teeth of Scandinavian people, reported by other investigators (e.g., Grandjean et al. 1979), which add support to the validity of his estimates. If confirmed, this finding suggests either that typical dietary exposure to lead has heretofore been systematically overestimated or that some present-day populations, even in industrialized countries, are exposed to almost an order of magnitude less dietary lead than Americans are.

The argument that poor analytical capabilities have led to systematic overestimation of lead concentrations in fresh foods, made by Settle and Patterson (1979) and Patterson and Settle (1976), might support the former explanation. If commonly used analytical techniques have consistently overestimated lead levels in biological samples, dietary exposures to lead may not yet have been properly measured. Further discussion on this point and a wider evaluation of the adequacy of analytical techniques for lead in foods are essential. On the other hand, if measurements are approximately accurate and Swedish adults are in fact exposed to an order of magnitude less lead in foods than Americans are, the reasons for this difference require careful study. The answers could shed considerable light on the relative contributions of soil, air, processing, and canning to lead in the U.S. diet, and might suggest an achievable degree of reduction of dietary exposure.

Appendix C describes preparations now under way within the FDA to regulate the lead content of foods. In developing regulations, the FDA will need better information than is currently available about the lead content of foods, the dietary preferences of individuals, the range of typical intake of lead in the diet for adults, children, and infants, the variation of dietary exposure over time, and the contributions of different sources to the lead in foods. Development of improved analytical methods and standard reference materials for measuring the lead content of foods will be an important element of the information-gathering effort.

Exposure via Dust, Soil, and Paint

The behavior patterns that make soil, dust, and paint potentially critical sources of exposure for young children (i.e., crawling, oral contact with dirty hands, pica) are generally not present in adults; consequently, ingestion of lead from these sources is usually minimal among the adult population. Some adults have been reported to ingest nonfood items; for instance, clay-eating (geophagia) is relatively common among some ethnic groups in the southeastern United States (Layman et al. 1963). Recently, a case of clinical lead poisoning in an adult who habitually ingested contaminated garden soil was reported (Wedeen et al. 1978). Like children with pica, adults with geophagia constitute a subpopulation at special risk. There is only sparse information at present to estimate the size of this population, and efforts would be justified to explore the extent of this mode of exposure.

The most common form of exposure of adults to lead in soil and dust is through incidental contamination of foods and dishes. No data are available to estimate quantitatively the exposure by this route; but it seems unlikely that the amount of lead ingested could exceed 10 μg/day. Ingestion of lead-based paints can safely be assumed to be nil for the average adult (excluding those with pica).

Exposure via Tobacco

Tobacco, like other plants, contains some lead absorbed from the soil, and may also contain lead deposited on the surface of the leaves. The widespread use of lead arsenate as a pesticide on tobacco crops in the past contaminated tobacco products with both lead and arsenic. Since the late 1940s, lead arsenate has gradually been replaced by organic pesticides, and by 1975 no domestic production or use of this compound was reported (U.S. EPA 1977b). However, residual lead in the soil from past applications and from atmospheric deposition remains a potential source of lead in domestic tobacco products.

Relatively few data have been published on the amounts of lead in tobacco, and the effects of decreased use of lead arsenate on lead levels in tobacco products cannot be precisely estimated. Patterson (1965) inferred from published data on the arsenic content of tobacco that lead in tobacco had decreased from about 130 μg/g in the early 1950s to about 20 μg/g in the mid-1960s. The WHO (1977) cited measured values of 21 to 84 μg of lead per cigarette (19 to 80 μg/g) in a study published in 1957, and 10 to 12 μg per cigarette in unpublished data collected in the early 1970s. Results of 10 studies on exposure to radioactive lead-210 in cigarette smoke, published between 1964 and 1974, showed no discernible trend in lead-210 levels in American cigarettes (Holtzman 1978); however, it is not certain that lead-210 is an appropriate surrogate for total lead in tobacco. On the basis of a small number of available measurements, the WHO (1977) has estimated that the current lead content of tobacco may be between 2.5 and 12.2 μg per cigarette.

Estimates of the fraction of lead in tobacco that is transferred to mainstream smoke and might be inhaled when a cigarette is smoked have been reviewed by the WHO (1977). The few estimates derived from studies of the lead concentration of smoke fall between 2 and 6 percent. A third study estimated lead in the total smoke from eight brands of cigarettes, and concluded that an average of 19 percent of the lead content before smoking was transferred to smoke. The authors of the WHO document inferred from this study that most of the lead was lost in sidestream smoke (that is, the smoke that drifts from the burning tip of the cigarette between puffs).

In the absence of better measurements, exposure to lead from cigarette smoking can be estimated by making some relatively arbitrary assumptions. If it is assumed that an average cigarette contains 10 μg of lead and that 5 percent of that lead is transferred to the mainstream smoke when a cigarette is smoked, each cigarette could contribute 0.5 μg of inhaled lead to the total exposure of an adult who smokes. Smoking 30 cigarettes per day therefore could result in the inhalation of 15 μg of lead. This amount is the same as was calculated above for the "average" adult in an urban area, who inhales an assumed 20 m^3 of air containing a national mean value of 0.75 μg/m^3 of lead. It appears, therefore, that heavy smoking could double the typical exposure to inhaled lead of an average urban adult, but improved information is needed to support or modify this highly tentative conclusion. Also, since the particle size and chemical form of lead in cigarette smoke are largely unknown, lead from this source might differ from lead in ambient air in its availability for absorption.

Integrated Assessment of Exposures

Exposure to lead for the general adult population can be summarized as follows.

Diet: Average ingestion, about 200 to 300 μg/day; estimated range, less than 100 to more than 2,000 μg/day. Knowledge of the range of exposure is very uncertain.

Water: Average ingestion, about 20 μg/day; estimated range, less than 1 to more than 500 μg/day. Neither the average nor the upper limit of the estimated range is well established.

Air: Average inhalation, about 15 μg/day in urban areas; estimated range, less than 1 μg/day in some rural areas to more than 100 μg/day at some urban sites. Both average exposures and the estimated range are based on extensive monitoring data, but local variation in exposures within urban regions is not well documented.

Tobacco: Estimated inhalation, about 10 μg of lead per pack of cigarettes smoked. Insufficient information is available to determine the accuracy of this estimate, or the likely range of variation.

Dust, Soil, and Paint: Ingestion is assumed to be negligible for most adults. A tentative upper limit of 10 μg/day ingested accidentally with foods is proposed in this report.

These estimates make it clear that the average person is exposed to lead chiefly through the diet; however, the relative importance of different environmental pathways of exposure cannot be determined without considering the extent to which inhaled or ingested lead is absorbed (see Step 4). The summary here also makes it clear that there may be subsets of the general population whose total exposure to lead is well above average. Excessive exposures usually are the result of personal habits of food or water intake or tobacco use, combined with exposure to levels of lead in the environment that are in the higher regions of typical ranges. The identity of such subpopulations, the fraction of the total population that falls into such categories, and the extent to which their exposure to lead exceeds that of the average person have not been extensively documented.

Step 4: ESTABLISH THE ASSOCIATION BETWEEN EXPOSURE AND LEAD IN THE BODY FOR THE SPECIFIC POPULATION

The present state of knowledge about relationships between exposure to lead and levels of lead in the bodies of humans was discussed in some detail in the previous example on urban children. The discussion here emphasizes aspects of the absorption and distribution of lead that apply to the general adult population. As in the case of urban children, most of the available information about body burdens of lead in adults involves measurements of lead in blood.

Absorption of Lead

The literature on absorption of lead is reviewed in detail by the EPA (1977a), the WHO (1977), Drill et al. (1979), Ewing et al. (1979), and Jaworski (1979). Holtzman (1978) summarized available data derived from studies with radioisotopes of lead. Although they are not based on knowledge of absorption rates, some empirical regressions have been calculated for relationships between concentrations of lead in the blood of adults and lead in the air (U.S. EPA 1977a), workplace atmospheres (U.S. OSHA 1978), and water supplies (U.S. EPA 1979), but such relationships have not been defined for the contributions of food or tobacco to typical blood lead levels.

Absorption from Air   The EPA (1977a) and the WHO (1977) reviewed available studies of respiratory absorption of lead by adults and concluded that about 30 ± 10 percent of inhaled lead particles are deposited in the lung under general ambient conditions of exposure. The deposition rate depends on the size distribution of the particles and the frequency of respiration. Most of the available summary documents agree that there is insufficient knowledge of the rate of absorption of lead from deposited particles to determine the fate of lead deposited on lung surfaces. The EPA (1977a, 1979) therefore emphasized empirical evidence that relates air lead levels to blood lead levels, and did not attempt to estimate the fraction of inhaled lead that is absorbed. On the other hand, Drill et al. (1979) reviewed the available literature and concluded that 40 percent is a reasonable value for absorption of lead into blood from ambient air in the average adult. If this estimate is considered along with the estimated fraction of inhaled lead particles that is deposited, it appears to assume essentially complete absorption of deposited lead.

The EPA (1977a) reviewed in detail the published literature on relationships between levels of lead measured in ambient air and levels of lead in the blood of adults. Relationships of this sort are of uncertain meaning, since the relative importance of inhalation and of ingestion of deposited lead particles cannot be separated; there are also serious uncertainties about the appropriateness of existing air monitoring data for estimating exposures of the individuals whose blood was sampled. However, a few studies involving inhalation of lead by volunteers under controlled conditions have produced results generally in agreement with population surveys. The EPA concluded, as did the WHO (1977), that at typical ambient concentrations of lead in air the concentration of lead in blood is elevated by approximately 1 to 2 $\mu g/100$ ml for each 1 $\mu g/m^3$ of lead in air. The (blood lead)/(air lead) ratio varies according to age, sex, geographic location, and other characteristics of populations, and the exact functional relationship is still unknown (U.S. EPA 1977a).

Absorption from Water   Little of the available information on absorption of lead from the human gastrointestinal tract pertains specifically to lead ingested in water; most data refer to absorption from mixtures of food and beverages (see discussion of absorption from foods, below). According to the EPA (1979), recent studies indicate that the fraction of ingested lead that is absorbed is up to 8-fold higher when lead is ingested between periods of fasting than it is when lead is taken with meals. This difference suggests that lead in water and other beverages ingested between meals may have a greater proportional impact on total absorption of lead than the lead ingested with food. Additional information on absorption of lead from water per se is an important need, especially for establishing drinking water standards.

The EPA (1979) reviewed three available studies that show relationships between concentrations of lead in tap water and concentrations of lead in the blood of populations using the water supplies. Although the available data are insufficient to establish conclusively either the exact form of the relationship or the magnitude of the effect of lead in water on lead in blood, the three studies agree that the relationship is nonlinear. The contribution of lead in drinking water to blood lead appears to be proportionally smaller for large doses of ingested lead than for small doses of lead. For instance, by averaging the results of the three studies, the EPA estimates that blood lead would be elevated by 4.07 $\mu g/100$ ml at a concentration of 5 $\mu g/l$ in water, and by 8.57 $\mu g/100$ ml at a level of 50 $\mu g/l$ in the water supply. This empirically derived relationship suggests that a change in the concentration of lead in drinking water from 50 to 25 $\mu g/l$ would lower the average blood lead level in adults by about 1.7 $\mu g/100$ ml (U.S. EPA 1979).

However, information on mean population responses is insufficient to judge the importance of variations in the responses of individuals. In Step 3, above, it was noted that the amount of water ingested varies significantly from person to person. It is important to know the relationship between lead in blood and the total dose of lead ingested from water supplies containing different concentrations of lead. An individual who consumes 10 l of water containing 10 $\mu g/l$ of lead and one who drinks 2 l containing 50 $\mu g/l$ would both ingest 100 μg of lead in water, but the data summarized by the EPA (1979) suggest that the amount of lead absorbed and its effect on blood lead concentration might be significantly different in the two cases. An approach that is based on average population responses may fail to consider differences that are critical for determining the degree of protection required. A relationship between absorption of lead from water and the dose of lead ingested could perhaps be estimated from the data in the three studies summarized by EPA, or might require gathering additional data. In either case, an effort to shed light on this question seems justified.

Absorption from Food   Results of numerous studies that used either balance methods or radiolead tracers are in rather close agreement that adults absorb, on the average, 8 to 10 percent of the lead ingested in the diet (WHO 1977; U.S. EPA 1977a, 1979; Jaworski 1979; Holtzman 1978; Drill et al. 1979). However, Barltrop (1978) and Moore et al. (1979)

have reported on balance studies in adults that suggest that some individuals absorb up to 40 percent of ingested lead; it seems likely that there is wide individual variation in this regard. Most of the studies have not separated gastrointestinal absorption of lead in foods from absorption of lead in beverages. In addition, gastrointestinal absorption of lead is known to be affected by the kinds of foods ingested, the amounts of fat, protein, calcium, zinc, and phosphorus present, the chemical and physical forms of the lead compounds, and certain characteristics of individuals' health, physiology, and perhaps genetic makeup. The influence of any of these variables (or combinations of them) on the absorption of lead can be estimated only qualitatively with present knowledge (see Case I, Step 4).

A quantitative relationship between lead in foods and lead in blood has not been determined, chiefly because insufficient information is available on amounts of lead ingested by individuals for whom blood lead data have been obtained. The WHO (1977) and the EPA (1979) summarized available estimates and suggested that each 100 μg/day of oral intake of lead may be associated with increases in blood lead levels of from 4.4 to 18.3 μg/100 ml. Improving the precision of such estimates will require further research, as will estimates of the range of normal human variation in this relationship, and determination of whether the relationship is a linear function.

Absorption from Tobacco Smoke   Virtually no information is available on the absorption of lead from inhaled tobacco smoke. In the absence of better data on the particle size, chemical form, and concentration of lead inhaled by smokers, Patterson (1965) assumed that the efficiency of absorption of lead from cigarette smoke by the lung is equivalent to the efficiency of absorption of lead from ambient air. This assumption is still unsupported by data, but is probably the most reasonable one under the circumstances.

Epidemiological data generally have shown that smokers have somewhat higher blood lead levels than nonsmokers, although some studies have shown no significant differences between the two groups (WHO 1977). The magnitude of differences reported is typified by results of a study by Johnson et al. (1978), who found blood lead levels of 11.2 μg/100 ml in female smokers, 8.7 μg/100 ml in female nonsmokers, 12.9 μg/100 ml in male smokers, and 11.5 μg/ml in male nonsmokers, all residents of suburbs of Dallas, Texas. These results are consistent with the hypothesis advanced above (in Step 3) that heavy smokers may inhale as much lead from cigarette smoking as they do from the ambient air in many urban and suburban areas. It is also possible, however, that smoking impairs mechanisms that clear particles from the lung, and that the higher blood lead levels of smokers could be due at least in part to increased retention of lead from ambient air.

Absorption from Soil and Dust   No reliable estimates are available on the efficiency of gastrointestinal absorption of lead from soil and dust in adults. The particle size and chemical form of lead in soil and dust are probably quite different from those characteristics of lead in the diet, but the effects of any differences of this sort on absorption are matters for speculation. In the absence of other information, it may be assumed that the absorbed fraction of lead ingested in dust and soil is comparable to the fraction absorbed from other materials in the gastrointestinal tract, i.e., about 8 to 10 percent in typical adults. Relationships between blood lead levels and concentrations of lead in soil and dust have been demonstrated for children (see Case I, Step 4), but not for adults. Given the estimated differences in exposure of adults and children to this source of lead, a significant effect of lead in soil and dust on the lead in blood of average adults is not expected.

Integrated Assessment of Absorption   As in Case I, the question of the relative contributions of different sources to lead in the bodies of typical adults is a crucial element of the assessment of exposures. The question can be approached in two ways; each approach has both advantages and disadvantages.

The first method is to estimate exposures and absorption rates for each environmental pathway and to add up the fractional contributions. This approach requires assuming values for exposures and absorption factors that are often highly uncertain; however, such a model is flexible enough to test a large number of different assumptions (see Drill et al. 1979).

The second approach is to apply empirically derived general relationships between levels of lead in the environment and lead in blood to specific cases of interest, and to estimate the relative fraction of blood lead derived from each source of exposure. The empirical approach is limited by significant gaps in information, and by uncertainties about the appropriateness of applying existing data to the populations being considered. This approach does not require making assumptions about poorly understood variables, such as the efficiency of absorption of lead from the lung. At the same time, it fails to account for the fact that the concentration of lead in blood is the result of a complex and dynamic process of absorption, excretion, and interchanges among various compartments of the body, rather than a simple function of exposure.

Estimates of the relative contributions of various sources of general exposure to the lead absorbed by typical adults, derived by the modeling approach, are shown in Table 2.6 and Figure 2.8. Two cases are presented:

an urban resident who smokes, and a nonsmoking rural resident. As in the examples for urban children (Table 2.2), these are hypothetical cases, and the apparent significance of any particular source of exposure can be changed substantially by making different assumptions. For example, if the concentration of lead in urban air is assumed to be 3 $\mu g/m^3$ (which might be typical for areas adjacent to heavily traveled highways) and other assumptions are unchanged, the contribution of atmospheric lead to total absorption would be 38.1 percent, not 13.3 percent. Many other cases involving quite different assumptions about typical exposures can be calculated in the same manner.

Distribution of Lead in the Body

Current knowledge about the distribution, storage, mobilization, and excretion of lead in the human body was summarized in Case I. Figure 2.5, presented in Step 4 of that example, is based on measurements obtained in adult males. As the figure shows, in adults about 94 percent of the body burden of lead is stored in the skeleton, about 4 percent is in the blood, and 2 percent is in soft tissues.

The concentration of lead in bone increases throughout most of the average person's lifetime, and in adulthood the total amount of lead in the body may be between 100 and 200 mg in average residents of industrially advanced nations (Barry 1978). Males generally accumulate more lead than females, presumably because men have greater exposures and larger bones. Barry (1978) has reviewed the extensive literature on the accumulation and distribution of lead in human tissues. Studies published over the last 20 years show no marked trends of either increasing or decreasing average lead body burdens in typical adults.

Some significant gaps remain in knowledge of the distribution of lead in the body. It is not known, for instance, what factors regulate the mobilization of skeletally stored lead, or how pregnancy or other physiological stresses affect the equilibrium balance of lead among various tissues of the body. Since lead crosses the placenta, and concern exists over potential toxic effects on the fetus (see Step 5), the lack of knowledge about possible changes in the distribution of lead during pregnancy is an important information gap.

As was noted in the discussion of the body burden of lead in children earlier in this chapter, the total amount of lead in the body is probably less significant in terms of possible physiological effects than the amount in blood and soft tissues. The most common method of measuring the lead in these pools in adults is to measure the concentration of lead in blood, as in children.

TABLE 2.6 Two Hypothetical Examples of Estimates of Contributions of Specific Sources of Exposure to Total Absorption of Lead for Subsets of the General Adult Population[a]

Route of Exposure	Concentration of Lead in Environment	Amount Inhaled or Ingested Per Day	Absorption Factor	Amount of Lead Absorbed (μg/day)	Percent of Total Lead Absorbed
Case I: Urban Residents Who Smoke Cigarettes					
Air	$0.75 \, \mu g/m^3$	$20 \, m^3$	0.4	6	13.3
Water	$10 \, \mu g/1$	2 1	0.1	2	4.4
Food	$0.15 \, \mu g/g$	2,000 g	0.1	30	66.7
Soil/dust	$500 \, \mu g/g$	0.02 g	0.1	1	2.2
Tobacco	$0.5 \, \mu g/cig$	30 cigs	0.4	6	13.3
TOTAL				45	100
Case II: Rural Residents Who Do Not Smoke					
Air	$0.083 \, \mu g/m^3$	$20 \, m^3$	0.4	0.7	2
Water	$10 \, \mu g/1$	2 1	0.1	2	6
Food	$0.15 \, \mu g/g$	2,000 g	0.1	30	91.7
Soil/dust	$50 \, \mu g/g$	0.02 g	0.1	0.1	0.3
TOTAL				32.8	100

[a] Based on the method developed by Drill et al. (1979). The basis of assumed values for exposure and absorption factors is discussed in the text.

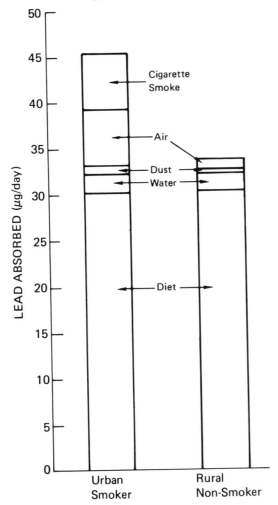

FIGURE 2.8 Estimated contributions of different sources of exposure to the total lead absorbed by two different subsets of the general population.

Epidemiological Data on Blood Lead Levels in Adults

To assess the potential for biological effects of lead in the general adult population, information is needed about the range of levels of lead in adults who have no occupational or other unusual exposures. It is important to know not only the average level of lead in the body for the population or for particular subsets of it, but also the statistical distribution of individual blood lead values about the mean.

The EPA (1977a) and the WHO (1977) have reviewed published data on the blood lead levels of adult populations. Sufficient data are available to suggest in at least a qualitative way the influences of several variables other than exposure on the average blood lead levels of specific subsets of the general population. Age does not appear to affect blood lead levels in adults, but females commonly have slightly lower blood lead values than males. Smokers of both sexes have somewhat higher blood lead levels than nonsmokers. Limited data suggest that blacks have higher blood lead levels than whites; this difference has also been documented in children (see Figure 2.6 in Case I). Proximity to sources appears to be highly significant; urban populations consistently exhibit higher blood lead levels than suburban populations, and both groups usually have more lead in their blood than rural or remote populations do. However, the size of the difference between urban and suburban or rural groups has varied in different studies, and other geographic variables, such as climate, deserve to be examined, along with source density, in seeking explanations for the variation. (See U.S. EPA [1977a] for a detailed discussion.)

Typical blood lead levels in different populations of adult males have been summarized by the WHO (1977). Residents of a rural California county had an average blood lead level of 12 μg/100 ml. Suburban populations had average values of from 11 to 15 μg/100 ml, while groups who lived or worked in downtown areas of several major cities had average blood lead levels that ranged from 19 to 26 μg/100 ml. Groups with higher-than-average exposure to sources of airborne lead, such as traffic policemen, tunnel or parking garage attendants, and garage mechanics, had average blood lead values of from 28 to 38 μg/100 ml. Within a population of military recruits from urban areas, average blood lead levels were 31 μg/100 ml for whites, and 38 μg/100 ml for blacks (Creason et al. 1976). In addition to the racial difference, these last data suggest that young adult males, who on the average eat more food per capita than any other subset of the general population, have higher-than-average blood lead levels. This is in keeping with the estimated contribution that the diet makes to exposure to lead.

While it has been estimated by many authors that the average blood lead level of adults in urban areas of the United States is between 20 and 25 μg/100 ml, that estimate is relatively uncertain. Preliminary analysis of data from the HANES II survey, described in Case I, showed mean blood lead levels of 17.7 μg/100 ml in males and 12.8 μg/100 ml in females in a sample of 2,646 juveniles and adults (aged 16 to 75). Within that sample, the fractions exhibiting blood lead levels above 30, 40, and 50 μg/100 ml were 3.5, 0.76, and 0.32 percent, respectively (Mahaffey et al. 1979).

The reported differences among populations that have been studied can be attributed in part to differences in exposures, in part to differences in the characteristics of the populations themselves, and in part to differences in the methods and reliability of sampling and analytical techniques employed in the various studies (U.S. EPA 1977a). It is difficult, however, to assign appropriate weights to each of these sets of variables in order to explain differences in average blood lead levels, and it is still more difficult to define a "typical" blood lead level for the general adult population. It seems likely that typical average values for different, relatively homogeneous subpopulations may range from less than 10 to more than 30 μg/100 ml.

In addition, the available data base is insufficient to determine trends over time in blood lead levels in the adult population. Some data on urban children suggest that average blood lead levels have decreased in recent years (see Figure 2.6). Information is needed on trends in blood lead levels in adults. Such data could suggest the effects that reductions in emissions of lead from motor vehicles and other contributions to general exposures may have had on the total exposure to lead of both adults and urban children.

Most analyses of the statistical distribution of individual blood lead levels in populations have shown an approximately log-normal distribution (U.S. EPA 1977a). In such cases, the best measure of the median value of a set of data is its geometric mean, and the proper measure of variation is the geometric standard deviation. However, most available data sets have not been analyzed to yield these parameters, and the average values given in the literature (including many of those discussed above) generally are arithmetic means. It is also apparent that measurement variance, rather than real differences, could explain a significant part of the variation in reported blood lead levels (U.S. EPA 1977a). These problems make estimates of the statistical distribution of adult blood lead values among the general population difficult and tenuous today. Studies on populations of children have reported geometric standard deviations in blood lead levels that fall between 1.3 and 1.5 (U.S. EPA 1977a); however, these limits are not firmly established, and there is scant basis to choose a specific value from within that range. A precise estimate of the geometric standard deviation of blood lead values is essential for setting environmental standards, since it is required in order to predict the fraction of a population whose blood lead will exceed any particular level if the geometric mean blood lead value of the population is known.

Step 5: ESTABLISH THE ASSOCIATION BETWEEN LEAD IN THE BODY AND BIOLOGICAL CHANGE IN THE SPECIFIC POPULATION

It has generally been assumed by most regulatory and public health agencies that the levels of lead in the bodies of typical adults are unlikely to result in significant adverse effects on health. This attitude is based on a lack, at least until recently, of substantial evidence that demonstrates adverse effects on normal physiological functions associated with typical blood lead levels (i.e., about 10 to 40 $\mu g/100$ ml). In fact, the magnitude of hazards to groups that are singled out as being at higher risk (such as children, adults with occupational exposures, or others with unusually high exposures to lead) has usually been estimated by comparing the population "at risk" with a "normal control" population whose blood lead levels fall in the range just given.

The possibility exists, however, that adverse effects on human biochemical and physiological functions might occur in adults at typical levels of lead in the body, and that they are so widespread or common in the population that they are not distinguishable as "abnormal." The hypothesis that typical levels of lead in modern adults cause undetected and perhaps undetectable toxic effects is provocative, but by its nature is beyond proof with current knowledge. On the other hand, the contrary hypothesis, that no such effects exist, is fundamentally unprovable. However, additional insight on this question can be gained by examining evidence related to the natural occurrence of lead in humans. If natural background levels of lead in adults are much lower than typical present-day levels, it might be inferred that the possibility of toxicity is significant (Patterson 1965). This topic is the subject of Case III, later in this chapter.

For purposes of making public policy, several pertinent questions can be identified: first, are there any cases in which typical levels of lead in the bodies of adults are known to be associated with biological changes? If so, what effects are observed, and how large is the fraction of the general population in which they are likely to occur? And, regarding effects that are known to occur at higher levels of exposure to lead but have not been demonstrated at typical levels, how wide is the margin between the levels of lead found in typical adults and the levels at which the effects have been observed?

The dose–effect and dose–response data needed to answer most of the questions listed above are incomplete for most effects. However, a great deal of research has been done on the effects of lead on adults with substantially higher-than-average exposures, including workers in lead industries and populations exposed to environmental pollution or lead-laden drinking water. The evidence provides extensive qualitative information about effects of lead on human health, and some quantitative knowledge of levels of lead in the body (as indicated by blood lead levels) associated with the effects.

Target Organs and Systems

Step 5 of Case I emphasized effects of lead on heme synthesis and on behavioral and intellectual functions, because those effects are believed to be the most sensitive signs of lead' toxicity in children. The same effects are central concerns in regard to the adult population as well, but many other possible effects of lead in adults also need to be examined. In particular, the likely sensitivity of the developing fetus to toxic effects of lead makes the exposure of women of childbearing age to typical levels of lead a matter for special attention. A more general need, however, is an assessment of whether lifelong exposure to commonplace levels of lead in the environment and diet can produce effects in some members of the general adult population similar to effects observed in groups whose exposures to lead are much greater.

As noted in Case I, lead may have chronic toxic effects on many organs and systems of the body. In addition to the hematopoietic system and the central nervous system, the target systems include the kidneys, the skeleton, and the gastrointestinal, cardiovascular, endocrine, immune, reproductive, and peripheral neuromuscular systems. In addition, the effects of lead on cellular functions need to be examined in terms of possible relationships between lead in the body and the aging process, chromosomal abnormalities and mutations, and cancer.

Extensive reviews of current knowledge of effects of lead on various physiological systems in adults have been published recently by the WHO (1977), the EPA (1977a, 1979), NIOSH (1978), OSHA (1978), and the National Research Council of Canada (Jaworski 1979). The discussion here is therefore concise and emphasizes gaps in knowledge.

Effects on Heme Synthesis

The nature of the effects of lead on heme synthesis was described in the case on urban children. The same effects occur in adults, in association with about the same concentrations of lead in blood (see Figure 2.7, in Case I). The evidence indicates that significant (> 40 percent) inhibition of ALAD occurs in some individuals at blood lead levels above about 15 μg/100 ml. Although Figure 2.7 suggests that women are more sensitive than men to inhibition of heme synthesis, as indicated by the elevation of

FEP levels, other factors, including iron deficiency and endogenous steroid metabolism, also affect FEP responses. The possibility of sex differences in sensitivity therefore is unresolved, and merits further study.

As is true for children, the significance to health of the inhibition of heme synthesis is unknown. Clinically detectable anemia (lower-than-normal hemoglobin level) has recently been associated with blood lead levels of 40 to 80 μg/100 ml in lead workers (U.S. OSHA 1978), but is not believed to occur at blood lead levels typical of most adults. However, as noted in Case I, heme is a precursor for the biological synthesis of respiratory pigments (cytochromes) that are essential to cellular respiration, and inhibition of heme synthesis might be associated with as-yet-unmeasured interference with cellular functions (see U.S. OSHA [1978] for discussion).

A general toxic effect on such a fundamental cellular process could underlie effects of lead on many different tissues and organs. However, further investigation will be required to determine whether cellular respiration in various tissues is significantly affected by typical levels of lead in the body.

Effects on the Nervous System and Behavior

Adults presumably have passed the developmental stages that make children especially vulnerable to effects of lead on the nervous system (see Case I), but the central and peripheral nervous systems are nevertheless sensitive to lead toxicity. Peripheral neuropathy (as indicated by slowed reflexes and muscular weakness) and altered sensitivity to pain have been observed in workers whose blood lead levels exceed 50 μg/100 ml, but clinical encephalopathy has not been reported in adults with blood lead values below about 100 μg/100 ml (Repko and Corum 1979).

Evidence from studies on animals, discussed in Case I, has shown that very small amounts of lead in nerve cells can alter the functions of the cells. However, it is currently unknown whether such effects occur in humans at typical levels of lead in the body, or if they do, what impact they might have on health or intellectual capacity.

Behavioral tests have been widely used recently to evaluate biological effects of lead, and blood lead levels between 40 and 80 μg/100 ml have been correlated with various effects on sensory, psychomotor, and psychological functions in adults (WHO 1977, U.S. OSHA 1978, Repko and Corum 1979). Some effects were detected only by specific functional tests in workers who by other indications were asymptomatic.

The term behavioral effects is also frequently applied to a large class of subjective complaints that have been attributed to lead. The effects include fatigue, insomnia, headaches, loss of appetite, loss of libido, and assorted personality changes, such as irritability, anxiety, depression, hostility, and moodiness (Repko and Corum 1979). Such effects vary widely among individuals, and may be outward signs of toxic effects on any of several systems of the body, not merely the nervous system. Because subjective effects of this sort usually must be described by the patient, they have been frequently reported in adults with occupational exposures, but are less documented in children.

Subjective complaints of the kinds just described have often been among the symptoms noted in cases of clinical lead poisoning, but few dose–response data for such effects are available (Repko and Corum 1979). One recent study, however, found subjective and psychological changes in 55 percent of a group of workers whose mean blood lead level was 60 µg/100 ml (Lilis et al. 1977). At present it is not possible to specify a blood lead level below which such symptoms do not occur. Additional epidemiological data, collected by screening populations with different degrees of exposure to lead using carefully standardized questionnaires, would provide a better definition of the dose–response curve (Zielhuis 1975b).

There have been no surveys of the general population that would shed light on a possible relationship between typical blood lead levels and subjective complaints of the sort attributed to occupational exposures. Schroeder (1974) made the provocative suggestion that, "That tired, run-down feeling, nervousness, depression, apathy, lack of ambition, frequent colds and other infections, and mild psychoneuroses" may be results of exposure to lead. However, the effects listed by Schroeder are extremely common, nonspecific responses to many forms of stress, including numerous environmental toxins in addition to lead, many medications, certain diseases, and other conditions of modern urban life. Only extensive and meticulously collected epidemiological evidence could indicate the extent to which any single factor such as exposure to lead is associated with effects on the mental health of the general adult population; and even a statistical association could not establish a causal relationship.

Effects on the Developing Fetus

The possibility that lead is teratogenic (produces congenital malformations in infants exposed during gestation) is considered here because pregnant women, the vehicles of exposure of fetuses, are part of the general adult population.

There is conclusive evidence in both humans and animals that lead crosses the placenta and accumulates in fetal tissues, at least after the twelfth week of pregnancy in humans (NIOSH 1978, Jaworski 1979). Fetal blood lead levels correspond closely to maternal blood lead levels, and the distribution of lead among fetal tissues is similar to its distribution after birth; however, a proportionally much greater fraction of the total body burden is concentrated in the brain of the fetus (NIOSH 1978, Drill et al. 1979).

There is little evidence that lead causes overt congenital malformations. A few animal experiments have produced deformations in offspring of pregnant rats and hamsters given very large doses of lead (e.g., 25 to 70 mg/kg), and injection of lead into chicken eggs caused developmental abnormalities (Jaworski 1979). There is virtually no epidemiological evidence of such effects in humans. One case has been reported of retarded development and neurological damage in an infant born to a mother who habitually drank lead-contaminated illicit whiskey (U.S. EPA 1977a), but the effect of alcohol must also be considered in this case. Women employed in lead industries and some women who ingested lead in attempts to induce abortions have not been found to bear abnormal children (U.S. OSHA 1978). On the other hand, a great deal of evidence suggests that lead is associated with an increased hazard of miscarriage or stillbirth (see next section).

The most critical concern in regard to effects of lead on the developing fetus is the possibility of subtle toxic effects, especially on mental functions, which would not be evident at birth. Animal experiments have produced convincing evidence of behavioral and learning deficiencies following intrauterine exposure to lead, and exposure of pregnant rats to lead is known to delay the development of the brain in newborn pups (U.S. EPA 1977a, NIOSH 1978, Bull et al. 1979). The effects have been induced at maternal blood lead levels of 34 $\mu g/100$ ml in sheep and 32 $\mu g/100$ ml in rats (Jaworski 1979, Bull et al. 1979).

There is too little evidence of effects on mental functions in humans to permit an assessment of the hazards of prenatal, as opposed to pre- plus postnatal, exposures to lead. An association between mental retardation and high concentrations (more than 800 $\mu g/l$) of lead in drinking water used during pregnancy and in the first year after birth has been reported by Beattie et al. (1975); subsequent analysis of blood obtained from the retarded infants 2 weeks after birth showed a mean blood lead level of 25.5 $\pm$ 8.9 $\mu g/100$ ml (U.S. EPA 1977a).

The dearth of data on effects of lead on human fetal development led the EPA (1977a) and the WHO (1977) to conclude that no dose–effect relationships could be described. However, the EPA's water quality criteria document (U.S. EPA 1979) concluded, in the absence of convincing dose–effect data on either, that embryotoxic effects (discussed in the next section) probably occur at lower levels of lead in the body than the levels that produce teratogenic effects.

Effects on Reproduction

Extensive evidence on occupationally exposed populations, supported in many cases by data from animal experiments, demonstrates that heavy exposure to lead has serious adverse effects on the mammalian reproductive system. Effects include disruption of the ovarian cycle in women and of spermatogenesis in men, reduced fertility in both sexes, reduced libido and impaired potency in men, and an increased likelihood of abnormal pregnancy, spontaneous abortion, miscarriage, or stillbirth. The evidence has been reviewed in detail by the EPA (1977a), the OSHA (1978), and Jaworski (1979).

Most of the evidence of effects of lead on human reproduction is drawn from early reports involving occupational exposures in which levels of lead in the body were unmeasured but were assumed to be very high. Only a few recent studies have examined populations with relatively low blood levels for such effects. OSHA (1978) and Jaworski (1979) cited evidence from four recent epidemiological studies that showed significant effects on male and female reproductive functions in association with blood lead levels in the range of 25 to 40 $\mu g/100$ ml. OSHA noted, however, that there has been "appallingly little research on this problem."

On the basis of the very limited evidence that human reproduction is adversely affected by lead at blood lead levels of 25 to 40 $\mu g/100$ ml, it seems possible that some segments of the general adult population (and most adults with occupational exposures) could experience some reduction in fertility at typical current levels of exposure. The need for research to better define this dose–response relationship is clear.

Genetic Effects

Several studies of lead workers have reported an elevated frequency of chromosomal abnormalities in lymphocytes (white blood cells) relative to that found in populations with lower exposures to lead. The effects observed include gaps in the chromosomal strands, which are generally held to be defects that can be repaired by cellular processes, and complete breaks in the chromosomes, which are regarded as irreparable. Jaworski (1979), OSHA (1978), and EPA (1977a) have reviewed the literature on chromosome damage associated with lead; the evidence is somewhat contradictory and inconclusive.

No clear dose–response relationship has been defined for the effects of lead on chromosomes. Four studies reviewed by Jaworski (1979) found increased frequency of abnormal chromosomes in groups of workers with mean blood lead levels that ranged from 19.3 to 91 $\mu g/100$ ml. OSHA

(1978) cites a study that found no excess of chromosomal abnormalities in workers whose blood lead ranged from 50 to 100 μg/100 ml, but suggests that the study lacked a suitably unexposed control group. In one recent study, smelter workers were divided into three groups according to blood lead levels: high (mean of 65 μg/100 ml), medium (39 μg/100 ml), and low (22 μg/100 ml). The incidence of chromosomal abnormalities in the workers was compared with that in a control group with a mean blood lead level of 13.6 μg/100 ml. Both the high- and the medium-exposure group had significantly more chromosomal breaks and gaps than the control group; workers in the low-exposure group had more chromosomal gaps, but no more breaks, than controls did (Beckman 1978). The author concluded that the risk of chromosome damage is increased in adults whose blood lead levels exceed 25 μg/100 ml.

Interpretation of this evidence is difficult. The studies cited above examined cells grown in laboratory cultures, and the occurrence of chromosomal aberrations in cultured lymphocytes does not guarantee that the same effects occur in the human body. In addition, most of the worker populations studied were probably exposed to arsenic, cadmium, and other potential mutagens as well as to lead. Jaworski (1979) concludes that lead probably is a weak environmental mutagen at current levels of environmental contamination.

The biological significance of chromosome damage in white blood cells is unknown. OSHA (1978) and EPA (1979) state that no known effects on health are linked to chromosome breaks in lymphocytes, but raise the possibility that chromosome damage may occur in other cells as well, including eggs and sperm. Noting that spontaneously aborted fetuses and stillborn infants exhibit a high frequency of chromosomal abnormalities, the two agencies suggest that effects of lead on reproduction (discussed in the previous section) may be caused at least in part by effects on the genetic material. This hypothesis is being explored through further research (see Appendix B).

An additional concern is that substances that are carcinogenic frequently are also mutagenic. The effects of lead on human chromosomes therefore add some weight to the hypothesis that lead may cause or promote human cancer (see next section).

Carcinogenic Effects

There is convincing evidence that lead can produce cancer in laboratory animals. Six studies have reported that inorganic lead salts cause renal tumors in rats, and one study each has associated lead with renal cancer in mice, lung tumors in hamsters, and brain tumors in rats. The EPA

(1979) reviewed the animal studies in detail and analyzed the available dose–effect data. All of the experiments involved very high doses of lead; on a mg/kg basis, the doses were more than 1,000 times greater than typical human exposures. While the EPA concluded that there is little doubt that lead is a carcinogen or at least a cocarcinogen for some species, the available data are inadequate to determine a dose–response relationship that could be extrapolated to estimate the possible incidence of cancer at much lower levels of exposure.

Epidemiological evidence on the incidence of cancer in human populations with exposure to lead is equivocal at best. The few available retrospective surveys of causes of death among people with occupational exposure to lead have generally shown no excess of cancer deaths above expected rates. One recent study, reviewed by the EPA (1979), showed statistically significant elevations in cancer mortality among battery workers, the majority of whom had recorded blood lead levels of from 40 to 70 μg/100 ml during the period of employment. However, there was no evidence of increased incidence of the specific forms of cancer suggested by animal studies, and no consistent association could be shown between cancer mortality and either length of employment or estimated exposure to lead.

A study of the relationships between cancer mortality and trace elements in water supplies of the United States showed statistically significant (p < 0.01) correlations between lead and cancer of the stomach, large intestine, and small intestine (NRC 1978a). However, such a result must be interpreted with great caution. Exposures to lead were estimated from average concentrations of the element in surface waters of different river basins, rather than levels in tap water. A correlation by itself is no proof that a causal relationship exists, and lead might in fact be a surrogate for another variable with a similar distribution. Correlation studies serve primarily to generate useful hypotheses; subsequent research in which differences in the exposure of populations to the element in question can be measured is required to establish and quantify a causal relationship. Since studies on populations with occupational exposures have not yet confirmed an increase in gastrointestinal cancer among lead workers, the hypothesis remains highly tentative.

It seems likely that if lead is a human carcinogen, it is a relatively weak one. The existing data base is too small to confirm or refute the possibility that lead plays some role in the incidence of human cancer. Further research is needed, and should examine both additional groups with high exposures to lead and subsets of the general population for which exposure data are available. On the basis of animal studies and geochemical correlations, the most likely sites of effects would appear to be the kidney and the gastrointestinal tract.

Effects on the Kidneys

It was noted in the summary of effects of lead on children in Case I that lead is known to produce both an acute form of renal tubular damage and a chronic reduction in the ability of the kidneys to remove substances from the bloodstream. The U.S. OSHA (1978) has thoroughly reviewed current knowledge of effects of chronic exposure to lead on the kidneys of adults. OSHA concluded that possible renal effects have been inadequately investigated, but are potentially of equal significance to effects on the hematopoietic, nervous, or reproductive systems.

The prevalence of kidney disease among lead workers is poorly known; about 4 percent of the general population has some form of kidney impairment, and demonstration of a causal relationship with exposure to lead is difficult, even in individuals with lengthy occupational exposure. Standard diagnostic procedures cannot detect the early stages of renal disease, and an individual may lose up to two-thirds of the functional capacity of the kidneys and remain asymptomatic (U.S. OSHA 1978). OSHA therefore believes that the occurrence of kidney disease in lead workers has been underestimated in the past. Several recent studies, including one that used more sensitive, more elaborate diagnostic procedures, suggest that as many as 10 percent of people with occupational exposures to lead may have reduced kidney function (U.S. OSHA 1978, Lilis et al. 1979). A number of cases have shown improvement in response to prolonged chelation therapy, indicating that the effects may be reversible if the disease is detected at an early stage (U.S. OSHA 1978, Wedeen et al. 1979).

The relationship between the amount of lead in the body and loss of kidney function is currently unclear. The blood lead levels of most workers with reduced renal clearance were below 80 μg/100 ml, and many of them were below 60 μg/100 ml (U.S. OSHA 1978). The EPA (1979) suggested that 50 μg/100 ml may be the lower limit for effects of lead on kidney function. However, blood lead levels indicate primarily recent exposure, and blood lead values obtained at the time of diagnosis are unreliable markers of levels of lead in the body that might be associated with the chronic development of progressive renal disease.

It is not possible to say whether or not the amounts of lead in the bodies of typical adults could produce some loss of kidney function. Since the body has a large reserve capacity in this regard (individuals can live normally with one kidney), mild reductions in renal clearance are unlikely to have immediate impacts on health. However, such effects are probably additive with those due to other factors, such as advancing age, that also are associated with loss of kidney function. Low-level lead stress on the kidneys therefore might conceivably contribute to a shortening of the functional lifetime of the organ.

In addition, lead workers with impaired kidney function showed reduced urinary excretion of lead (U.S. OSHA 1978). It is not known whether lead clearance is affected by the early, mild stages of reduced kidney function; however, it is possible that even slight impairment of this excretory mechanism could increase the retention of lead, and thus elevate the body burden and the potential for other physiological effects.

It was noted above that about 4 percent of the adult population of the United States has identifiable kidney disease; an unknown additional fraction may have mild, undetectable early stages of reduced renal function. While it would be important to know the role played by lead (and other environmental toxins) in causing kidney disease, the large number of factors that affect the kidney and the difficulty of diagnosis of early stages of the disease make it unlikely that research on the general population could be fruitful. However, additional studies on populations with occupational exposures probably would improve understanding of the relationship between low-level exposure to lead and loss of kidney function.

Effects on Other Organs and Systems

Lead has been associated with effects on several additional organs or systems in adults. The evidence of effects on the liver, gastrointestinal tract, endocrine system, and immune responses was discussed in Case I (see U.S. EPA [1977a] and Jaworski [1979] for details). In addition, there is some evidence that lead is associated with cardiovascular disease, and largely unexplored possibilities have been raised of effects on skeletal metabolism and the process of cellular aging.

Cardiovascular Effects   Jaworski (1979) reviewed evidence that the heart and vascular system are targets of lead toxicity, at least at high doses. Studies in several animal species demonstrated effects ranging from vasoconstriction to abnormal heartbeats, structural damage to heart tissues, and arteriosclerosis (hardening of the arteries) following exposure to lead. Evidence of abnormal heart function has been associated with other symptoms of clinical lead poisoning in both adults and children, but the evidence of effects at lower exposures is conflicting (U.S. EPA 1977a, 1979; WHO 1977). Some epidemiological studies have shown both an elevated prevalence of hypertension and an excess mortality rate from cerebrovascular diseases among lead workers, but other studies have shown no effects of this sort in similar populations.

Assessment of the possible role of lead in causing hypertension must consider that kidney disease is a known cause of high blood pressure, and the reverse may also be true (U.S. EPA 1979, U.S. OSHA 1978). If lead is a factor in hypertension, therefore, it might be either through direct action on the cardiovascular system or as an indirect consequence of renal effects.

Reliable dose–effect and dose–response data for effects of lead on cardiovascular functions in humans are not available, and it is unknown whether such effects could occur in the general population at typical levels of exposure. The hypothesis that lead may be one factor in the observed differences in the incidence of cardiovascular disease that are associated with hard and soft water supplies is currently being tested by the EPA, through experimental and epidemiological studies (see Appendix B).

Effects on the Skeleton   Since approximately 95 percent of the body burden of lead is stored in the skeleton (see Step 4), the possibility of toxic effects on bone metabolism as a result of long-term accumulation of lead must be considered. Only a small amount of research has been done on this topic. The results clearly suggest that accumulation of lead affects the functions of the bone cells responsible for deposition and resorption of bone mineral, but dose-effect relationships in humans are rather poorly understood. Jaworski (1979) reviewed studies that show that the "lead lines" visible in X-rays of the bones of children with lead poisoning are caused by perturbation of bone formation, and are not deposits of lead; these visible changes in bone density have been associated with blood lead levels above 50 μg/100 ml (Betts et al. 1973). Possible less marked effects of lower but longer-term elevations of blood lead have not been documented in humans. Anderson and Danylchuk (1977) found that bone formation was adversely affected in beagles fed low doses of lead. The blood lead levels of the lead-fed dogs ranged from 55 to 82 μg/100 ml over the 6-month experimental period, compared to 12 to 20 μg/100 ml in control dogs. The experimental group exhibited no anemia or other symptoms of lead intoxication except disturbed bone formation.

The scanty evidence available suggests that chronic exposure to low levels of lead may affect skeletal metabolism in humans, and that further research is needed. Osteopenia, a decrease in bone production and resorption, is a common condition in people over the age of 40; and osteoporosis, a more serious condition of loss of mineral mass and fragility of the bones, is an increasingly widespread disease of the elderly. The causes of osteopenia and osteoporosis are not well understood. The hypothesis that cumulative toxins such as lead may play some role in causing these conditions is worthy of exploration.

Effects on Cellular Function Most if not all toxic effects of lead may have at their base changes in the biochemical functions of cells. In addition to concern over the disease processes already discussed, the possibility exists that toxic trace elements may play some role in causing or accelerating the natural process of aging (Patterson 1965, Schroeder 1974). However, research has only begun to explore cellular aging, and there is little substantive evidence as yet to support a specific role for lead.

Nevertheless, a toxic substance that affects many routine cellular processes would be a good candidate for the postulated role, and lead meets that criterion well. Lead is known to affect the activity of many enzymes and to disturb cellular respiration, carbohydrate metabolism, protein synthesis, metabolism of DNA and RNA, and cellular replication. Jaworski (1979) and the EPA (1977a) have compiled extensive recent reviews on subcellular effects of lead.

Most evidence of effects of lead on cellular processes has been gathered from *in vitro* studies, and many of the studies used relatively high concentrations of lead. Some effects have been reported at concentrations of lead lower than those found in human blood; however, since it is not known whether blood lead levels accurately represent levels at subcellular sites of effects, no inferences can be drawn about effects in living humans.

Better understanding of the toxic effects of lead at the subcellular and molecular levels is an important key to improved understanding of lead's role in human diseases, but the assessment of relationships between changes in fundamental cellular processes and effects at the organism and population levels is a formidable task. In addition, in order to determine whether typical levels of lead in the environment affect cellular functions, it is necessary to measure those functions in cells that are essentially free from any contamination by lead. Because of the pervasive distribution of lead in the modern environment, effectively "clean" controls are frequently difficult to achieve. The implications of this problem for biological research on the effects of low levels of lead are examined in Case III.

Interactions among Effects

The attempt to determine dose–effect and dose–response relationships for any one effect of lead in humans is complicated by the fact that more than one kind of effect can occur at once, and the different effects are not independent. For instance, it has been noted that reduced kidney function may be associated with hypertension and with increased skeletal accumulation of lead, and that inhibition of heme synthesis may affect cellular respiration or the biochemistry of the nervous system.

Although some interrelationships among toxic effects of lead are known and others may be postulated, the full health implications of such interactions are unknown. Because of the complexity of human responses to lead, the concept of a "critical" effect (i.e., a single effect observed at the lowest level of lead in the body known to produce biological changes) can be usefully applied to adult populations as well as to children. In adults, as in children, inhibition of heme synthesis appears to be the most sensitive effect that can presently be measured at typical levels of exposure. Further research may reveal additional biochemical indicators that can serve as markers for biological changes induced by lead at typical blood lead levels.

Factors that Affect Toxicity

Jaworski (1979) and the WHO (1977) have reviewed what is known of the effects of various dietary, environmental, and human physiological variables on the toxicity of lead in adults; some of the variables were discussed in Step 2, above. As in the case of children, only crude qualitative conclusions about the likely direction of influence of specific factors can be drawn from available knowledge.

If the goal of standards set by government is to provide a reasonable margin of protection against adverse effects of lead for the most sensitive subsets of the general population, it is important to know the identity of the groups at greatest risk, and to have specific dose–response data for those subpopulations. This knowledge does not exist at present. Neither the variation in typical exposures nor the variation in human susceptibility to toxic effects of lead have been well measured. It is currently impossible, therefore, to determine how many people may be at significantly greater-than-average risk, or to what extent the hazard to such people exceeds the hazard to the average adult.

In considering this question it is important to remember that the general adult population includes substantial subsets who are aged, infirm, or physiologically handicapped. Most of the available dose–response data have been obtained from populations of industrial workers, who on the whole are healthy adult males. It therefore seems likely that some sectors of the general population are susceptible to toxic effects at lower levels of lead in the body than those indicated by data on occupational groups. Carefully controlled epidemiological studies of adults with typical exposures would be necessary to determine whether significant differences in sensitivity exist; however, there have been very few studies in which members of the general public were treated as anything but control populations.

TABLE 2.7   Summary of Lowest Blood Lead Levels Associated with Specific Biological Changes in Adults

Blood Lead Level (μg Pb/100 ml)	Effect	Reference
10	Inhibition of ALAD	U.S. EPA (1979)
15	Elevation of FEP	U.S. EPA (1979)
20-25	Chromosomal abnormalities	Jaworski (1979) Beckman (1978)
30	Toxicity to fetus	U.S. OSHA (1978)
30-40	Reduced fertility (women)	U.S. OSHA (1978)
30-40	Altered spermatogenesis (men)	U.S. OSHA (1978)
40-50	Anemia	U.S. OSHA (1978)
40-60	Psychological, sensory, and behavioral changes	U.S. OSHA (1978)
50	Impaired kidney functon	U.S. EPA (1979)
50-60	Peripheral neuropathy	U.S. EPA (1979)
100-120	Encephalopathy	U.S. EPA (1979)

Summary of Biological Effects

At the outset of Step 5, three questions were identified as crucial for policy making: Do typical body burdens of lead produce biological changes in adults? If so, what fraction of the general population is likely to experience such effects at typical levels of exposure? For effects known to occur only at higher levels of exposure, what is the margin between the lowest level of lead in the body that produces the effect and typical levels in the bodies of adults?

Table 2.7 summarizes available estimates of the lowest levels of lead in blood that have been associated with a variety of toxic effects of lead in adults. The effects on the hematopoietic and nervous systems have been relatively well documented at the indicated levels of lead in blood, but the estimates for effects on chromosomes, toxicity to the fetus, interference with reproduction, altered behavior, and reduced kidney function are based on much less conclusive evidence. The majority of the estimates are drawn from a small number of recent studies on populations with occupational exposures to lead, and need to be confirmed and better defined by additional research. For several other possible effects of lead, such as cancer, cardiovascular effects, or interference with bone formation, not even approximate dose–effect estimates are available.

It was estimated in Step 4 that typical blood lead values in the adult population fall between 10 and 40 μg/100 ml, with a mean of about 15 to

20 μg/100 ml, and that about 3.5 percent of the population may have blood lead levels above 30 μg/100 ml. Table 2.7 therefore suggests that inhibition of heme synthesis, chromosomal damage, toxicity to the fetus, and reproductive effects could occur in apparently asymptomatic members of the general population. The table also shows that the margin between the upper range of typical blood lead levels and the lower levels of lead in the body associated with subjective and behavioral effects, anemia, marginal changes in kidney function, and peripheral neuropathy is quite small. About 0.3 percent of typical adults may have blood lead levels above 50 μg/100 ml, based on the data from the HANES II survey, discussed in Step 4. In a population of 150 million adults, 450,000 might fall into this relatively high-risk subset of the general population. On the basis of the same (HANES II) survey, 3.5 percent, or about 5 million adults, may have blood lead levels above 30 μg/100 ml.

The available dose–response data do not permit a precise estimate of the incidence of any effects of lead in the general population, except for inhibition of heme synthesis. At an average blood lead level of 15 to 20 μg/100 ml, about 10 percent of adults might have depressed ALAD activity and elevated FEP levels (see Figure 2.7), but even on this thoroughly studied topic dose–response data in this range are very uncertain. An important information gap is the lack of dose–response data for any effect in subsets of the larger population who may be hypersensitive to toxic effects of lead.

In cases that involve the progressive development over a period of years of a chronic disease condition (such as neurological damage or kidney disease), blood lead levels at the time of diagnosis are unreliable indicators of the actual level of exposure associated with the onset of toxic effects. In the absence of careful prospective epidemiological studies, blood lead data may be the best index of exposure available, but reliance on this marker adds substantially more uncertainty to estimates of dose–effect relationships.

The evidence summarized here makes it clear that few if any members of the general public are likely to become obviously ill as a result of daily exposure to lead in foods, water, air, or tobacco. However, it seems highly likely that some fraction of the adult population (perhaps 3 to 4 percent) could experience biochemical and physiological effects of lead that are not presently associated with overt symptoms of dysfunction. Some evidence suggests that subtle effects on reproductive processes and on the health of unborn children also might occur in some "average" adults. In addition, current evidence suggests that a small fraction of the population (<1 percent) might experience behavioral effects or subjective complaints, and implies that a few individuals might exhibit mild anemia, slight loss of kidney function, or minimal neuromuscular effects. These are obvious areas on which additional research should concentrate.

Epidemiological research on possible effects of lead in the general population faces substantial obstacles. First, many of the effects in question are difficult to measure, and may have many causes. Second, it is unlikely that specific comparable subsets of the U.S. population can be identified that will have mean blood lead levels that differ by more than a factor of 3 or 4. In order to demonstrate significant differences in health over this range of exposure, large populations would need to be surveyed.

Because the "baseline" level of lead in blood in the U.S. population is apparently about 10 to 15 μg/100 ml, it is likely to be virtually impossible to demonstrate effects of lead at lower blood lead levels. Nevertheless, in theory some dose–effect curves might extend nearly to zero, and the physiological states now defined as "normal" might actually be "abnormal" conditions associated with typical levels of lead in the body. The hypothesis that people would be healthier in subtle ways if the average blood lead level were 1 to 2 μg/100 ml (or less) deserves sober consideration, and is examined again in Case III.

Step 6: ESTIMATE THE LIMIT OF NON-DETRIMENTAL BIOLOGICAL CHANGE DUE TO LEAD AND THE ASSOCIATED LEVEL OF LEAD IN THE BODY

As noted in Step 6 of Case I, the scientific basis for judging precisely how much biological change is detrimental is scanty, and the definition of a toxic effect requires considerable subjective judgment. The nature of some of the judgments involved was discussed in the example on urban children. In considering the adult population, some additional problems arise. It is possible that effects that are detrimental in children might not be harmful in adults, for a variety of reasons. However, the number of effects that may occur in adults is greater (compare Tables 2.4 and 2.7), and the likelihood of simultaneous effects on different systems of the body makes it more difficult to define harmful degrees of change.

There is no clear consensus about whether several of the effects discussed in Step 5 are detrimental. It is uncertain whether adverse effects on health are associated with moderate inhibition of heme synthesis or with chromosomal abnormalities in white blood cells. The argument that these effects should be considered detrimental rests on largely subjective judgments, such as that the effects may be considered initial stages of a progressive disease process, or that they are indicative of potential (but as yet unobserved) effects of the same sort in other cells or systems. Other effects, including reduction of kidney function, interference with reproduction, toxicity to the developing fetus, and subjective and psychological disorders, would probably be regarded as detrimental by most people;

however, dose–effect relationships are too poorly defined to specify levels of lead in the body at which detrimental degrees of change in these functions occur. For a third set of effects, including cancer, high blood pressure, and disturbances of bone metabolism, there is undoubtedly a consensus that the effects are harmful, but there is only weak and generally nonquantitative evidence that they may be caused by lead.

In short, although there is considerable knowledge about detrimental effects of lead at higher levels in the body, the dividing line between "detrimental" and "non-detrimental" degrees of biological change associated with the typical range of blood lead levels is subject to great uncertainty and controversy. It can be stated with some confidence, however, that the margin between levels of lead in the body associated with acknowledged detrimental effects and the mean level of lead in typical adults is narrow, perhaps no more than a factor of 2 or 3.

Once an agency had confronted the uncertainties and made its estimate of a detrimental level of lead in the body, it would need to examine available dose–response data in order to estimate the fraction of the population at risk of harm, given the current distribution of blood lead values in the adult population. This information is required in order to choose an acceptable level of exposure of lead (in Step 8, below). However, as Step 5 explained, reliable dose–response data are not available for any effects except inhibition of heme synthesis. Although an agency might establish a definition of a detrimental degree of biological change for effects on other organs or systems, it would be unable to estimate reliably the number of people expected to exhibit that degree of effect at current or projected levels of exposure to lead.

Step 7: IDENTIFY AND DESCRIBE ALTERNATIVE CONTROL STRATEGIES

The information gathered and evaluated in Steps 5 and 6 supports the conclusion that there is at least a possibility that adverse health effects are associated with current levels of exposure of adults to lead. In fact, two agencies concerned with protecting the general population—EPA and FDA—have already reached this conclusion (see Chapter 3 and Appendix C). Because biological evidence supports such a view, it is essential to assess opportunities that exist for reducing exposures, and to determine the effectiveness, costs, and benefits of different control strategies involving different combinations of measures and different schedules for implementing them.

Reduction of exposures for the general adult population is at least in theory less complicated than controlling lead exposures of urban children, because the important modes of exposure are fewer for adults. Also, strategies for general reductions in exposure for the entire population do not depend on some approaches to control, such as population screening.

It was shown in Step 3 that the diet, air, water, and (for heavy smokers) tobacco products are the important known sources of exposure to lead for the average adult. Soil, dust, and lead-based paint are generally insignificant contributors to lead in adults' bodies. Of the known sources, current knowledge suggests that food provides by far the greatest fraction of the lead absorbed into the blood of adults.

Opportunities for Control

Because general exposures via food, air, and water are fundamental parts of the baseline of exposure of urban children to lead, techniques for reducing exposures by these three routes were discussed in some detail in Case I. Although many methods are available and some measures have already been implemented, there are few quantitative estimates of the effectiveness of different measures in reducing total exposures, especially for adult populations. Uncertainties are particularly great regarding the control of ingestion of lead in foods. (For detailed discussion, see Step 7 of Case I.)

Exposure to lead through smoking tobacco could be controlled by establishing limitations on the permissible lead content of tobacco products, in the same manner that limits could be set on the levels of lead in other agricultural products. It is not clear, however, whether any agency of the government currently has authority to set such limits on tobacco products.

Alternative Control Strategies

Several alternative combinations of current and contemplated control measures could be proposed in order to reduce the total exposure to lead of the average adult. The multimedia nature of exposures makes a coordinated interagency assessment of control strategies a practical necessity.

The current program of phased removal of lead from gasoline, if carried out to the full extent anticipated by EPA's regulations, should reduce total emissions of lead to the atmosphere by 60 to 65 percent (see Appendix C). Although the exact relationship between emissions and exposure to lead is uncertain, some roughly proportional reduction in the contribution of inhaled lead to body burdens would be expected. In addition, reduction in emissions of lead will decrease the deposition of aerosol lead onto crops and soils, and as a result will lower the amount of lead in the diet. However, the magnitude of this effect is highly uncertain at present (see Case III).

On the other hand, since the air at most sites and about 98 percent of water supplies currently comply with the EPA's standards for lead in air and drinking water, those measures are not expected to have great impacts on the average person's exposure to the element. One component of an assessment of potential strategies to reduce general exposures would be to determine whether more stringent limits on lead in the air and water or different kinds of limits (such as restrictions on the lead content of tap water) would significantly lower typical levels of exposure.

Since the diet is the greatest contributing source of lead for the average adult and the only major route of exposure not yet subject to significant regulations, reduction of the amounts of lead in foods is a natural focus for possible new control efforts (Ewing et al. 1979). Very little is known currently of the extent to which lead can be eliminated from different foods, either by reduction of aerosol deposition noted above or by elimination of contamination during food processing and canning. As noted in Step 7 of Case I, substantial information needs exist regarding the effectiveness and feasibility of different approaches to reducing dietary intake of lead.

One of the fundamental approaches discussed in Case I, the elimination of lead products or uses of lead that contribute significantly to environmental exposures, may be especially important in terms of reducing exposure for adults. Because adults in the general population are not exposed to extraordinary sources of lead, the key to significant reduction of levels of lead in people may depend primarily on the phasing-out of "ordinary" sources. The gradual removal of lead from gasoline is an important example of this approach. Research needs to explore further opportunities, such as phasing-out the use of lead solders in food containers, were discussed in Case I.

Costs and Benefits

The current state of knowledge of the economic costs and benefits of some specific control measures that would reduce general exposure to lead was discussed in Step 7 of Case I. Until recently, government agencies have emphasized the more urgent need to protect workers and children at risk of greatly excessive exposure; there has been little impetus to examine approaches for or to estimate the costs of reducing the exposure of the general adult population. Likewise, the economics of replacing major uses of lead with other materials has not been the subject of serious research.

It is unlikely that a definitive analysis of the costs and benefits of controlling current general environmental pollution by lead could be achieved now; better information on the hazards lead poses to health and on how those hazards can be reduced is needed first. However, even a crude attempt at economic assessment could be valuable. Since the questions posed by economic analysis are central to the policy-making process, research to estimate costs and benefits of control would be one important method for better definition of information needs.

Step 8: APPLY RISK-BENEFIT, COST-BENEFIT, AND OTHER CONSIDERATIONS, COMPARE ALTERNATIVES, AND MAKE A DECISION

This step in the decision process requires, first, a summary of the factual information and judgments about the hazards associated with lead in the environment and the feasibility of reducing general exposures, and second, the assignment of subjective weights to the various risks, costs, and benefits that have been identified. Ideally, policy makers would complete this step for several alternative control strategies, and choose one that was most desirable by their criteria.

Current knowledge is insufficient to provide definitive answers to most of the questions an agency would need to address in completing this step. The summary that follows therefore stresses tentative conclusions and major unknowns.

Risk Considerations

Step 5 showed that a number of biological changes are associated with blood lead levels that probably occur in some fraction of the general population, and that other effects may occur in some individuals whose blood lead levels are only slightly higher than the typical range. There is no consensus at present about whether inhibition of heme synthesis or the presence of chromosomal abnormalities in somatic cells are detrimental to the health of adults (Step 6). Reproductive and fetotoxic effects, as well as others that currently have been demonstrated primarily in occupationally exposed populations, are more generally regarded as adverse effects. However, there is still considerable uncertainty about the possible occurrence of these effects in the general population.

Step 5 indicated that dose–response data are unavailable for almost all of the suspected toxic effects of lead on adults. It is therefore not possible to determine the exact fraction of the population that might be subject to specific effects at a given average blood lead level. However, some data now suggest that effects can occur in association with blood lead levels in the range of 20 to 40 μg/100 ml. The limited available surveys indicate that blood lead levels in American adults typically fall between 10 and 20 $\mu g/100$ ml, and about 3 percent of the population—roughly 5 million adults—may have blood lead levels above 30 $\mu g/100$ ml. These data suggest that, at best, the margin between typical body burdens and those associated with detectable biological changes is extremely narrow, and that the number of adults who may experience biochemical changes of uncertain but potentially toxic significance is large.

The relationships between major routes of exposure to lead (air, water, tobacco, and food) and the levels of lead in the bodies of average adults are still somewhat uncertain, and gaps exist in understanding of individual differences in both rates of absorption of lead from the lung and gut and the magnitude of exposures (Steps 2, 3, and 4). However, the diet appears to be the greatest source of exposure for the general population; air also may contribute significantly in some urban centers.

Control Considerations

Neither the effects on average exposure to lead of control measures now in effect nor the extent to which additional control measures could further reduce exposures can be reliably determined with available information. In order to know the degree of health protection conferred by a particular combination of control measures, it would be desirable to know the reduction in exposure to lead that could be achieved, the effect of reduced exposure on the mean blood lead level of the population, and the effect of a reduced mean blood lead level on the fraction of the population exposed to a risk of detrimental biological changes. Insufficient information on these questions is available for the adult population, because of the unknowns and uncertainties described above. In addition, little or no information has been developed on the costs of different degrees of reduction in exposure to lead, either through further limitations on environmental exposure or through elimination of additional uses of lead. The uncertainties noted in available information have thus far prevented definitive estimates of the costs and benefits of reducing general exposure to lead.

The Decision-Making Step

Because of the limited information on most topics, judgments about whether or not the potential risks to the health of the general population associated with current levels of lead in the environment are acceptable contain large subjective elements. Since neither defensible probabilities of harmful effects nor credible estimates of the cost of reducing risks are available, regulatory agencies probably could make only qualitative judgments at this point. On the whole, the decisions reached by most agencies in the past have been that hazards to adults are too small or too poorly documented to require specific controls. It has been recognized that actions taken to reduce exposure of children to lead (e.g., removal of lead from gasoline) also are beneficial in that they reduce general exposure; but no agency has yet offered a scientific assessment of risks associated with lead in the general adult population as the primary basis for measures to reduce exposures. Some further perspectives on this question and the implications of the current state of ignorance are examined in Case III.

Step 9:   EVALUATE THE PROCESS AND THE DECISION

Each of the preceding steps has commented on the appropriateness, accuracy, and adequacy of available data about general exposures to lead. It is clear that knowledge is very incomplete and that improvements in the quality of data are needed on almost every topic.

Since the protection of the general adult population from exposure to lead has not been the primary objective of regulatory measures implemented to date, little information has been generated that would permit an assessment of the effectiveness of the actions in terms of protecting the adult population as a whole. Better information is needed to determine how effective current air, water, and emission standards have been in that regard. In addition, it is critical that proper procedures to permit future evaluations of the effectiveness of programs be an integral part of future regulatory actions, including the pending establishment of limitations on lead in foods.

CASE III: THE NATURAL OCCURRENCE OF LEAD AND THE MAGNITUDE OF NATURAL CONTRIBUTIONS TO HUMAN EXPOSURES

This section examines the natural geochemical cycle of lead and what is known about the likely range of natural exposures to lead. "Natural" conditions with respect to lead are defined here as those that prevailed before humans began to extract the element from the Earth's crust. Lead ores have been mined and smelted for more than 4,000 years, and during that period myriad uses of the metal have contaminated the human environment. Contamination by lead-containing aerosols has been particularly extensive, especially since the introduction of lead alkyl fuel additives in the 1920s.

To what extent has the baseline of human exposure to lead been elevated above its natural range because of human activities? An answer to this question requires close examination of the geochemistry of lead and the responses of ecosystems to added anthropogenic (originating with human activity) input of the element. The subject has direct bearing on present and future policy decisions, especially those regarding exposures through the diet, since naturally occurring levels of lead probably represent the lowest achievable limits.

If present-day exposures to lead greatly exceed natural levels, it is possible that current exposures might pose a general hazard to health. That proposition has been highly controversial within the scientific community, and was much debated within this committee. On the one hand, scientific judgment has progressively lowered the level of lead in the body considered a likely hazard to health during the past 20 years, and future biological research probably will support further reductions of the definition of an acceptable level of exposure. On the other hand, present regulatory programs have not yet eliminated higher-than-typical exposures to lead, which pose an acknowledged present hazard to the health of some members of the population. Information on natural exposures can help put immediate problems in perspective, and may suggest future regulatory concerns. A return to a pretechnological state with respect to lead is probably impossible (and possibly undesirable), but typical current (American) exposures to the element could be reduced substantially over the long term if society were willing to bear the costs. Results of research on the potential biological significance of exposures above the natural range may suggest whether or not those costs are worth bearing.

To facilitate comparisons, the assessment of knowledge in this section is presented in the same step-by-step, decision-oriented format used in previous sections. However, there are substantial differences between this and the two earlier cases. This discussion proceeds only as far as Step 5 of the decision process. An examination of the natural occurrence of lead is of interest primarily to gain insight into the implications of present-day typical exposures; and the issues that would be raised in subsequent steps would apply to the present situation, addressed in Case II.

Current scientific knowledge about the natural occurrence of lead is much less complete than the information base on most other topics addressed in this report. Few recent review documents have compiled and weighed specific evidence on the behavior of lead in unperturbed ecosystems. Gaps in knowledge are wide, and the uncertainties associated with estimated ranges are therefore especially great. Research needs on questions raised in this section may be fundamental or "basic," in contrast to the often more focused research needs identified in the two previous cases. Although fundamental research can be critical for identifying and attaining long-term health and environmental goals, research in this subject area has seldom received high priority, especially in the context of assessments that weight information needs in favor of immediate utility for decision making.

Step 1: IDENTIFY SOURCES OF LEAD AND PATHWAYS OF ENVIRONMENTAL TRANSFER

Natural Ecological Pathways

Under natural conditions, biogeochemical transfers of lead would result in some human exposures through inhalation of airborne lead or ingestion of lead in water, food, nonfood items, or soil particles.

The natural biogeochemical cycle of lead can be described rather simply in qualitative terms. Most (> 90 percent) of the lead in terrestrial ecosystems is in the soil reservoir (Nriagu 1978b). Native lead in soils originates primarily from natural weathering of parent rocks, and is distributed chiefly via the hydrological and sedimentary cycles. Wind dispersion of soil particles and translocation in biomass play smaller roles in the movement of lead in soils on a global scale (Nriagu 1978b). The primary natural sources of lead in air include wind-blown soil particles, volcanic emissions, gaseous emissions from rocks, sea salt spray, smoke from combustion of vegetation, and organic emissions from plants (Nriagu 1978a). Natural transfers of lead into waters include leaching from soils or rock strata, transport of sediment particles in surface runoff, and deposition of aerosols onto water surfaces.

Although vast amounts of data are available on the lead content of various plants and animals, few systematic studies have been made on the transfer of lead within natural food chains. In qualitative terms, it is known that terrestrial and aquatic plants absorb some lead from the soil or the aquatic habitat. Unlike some other metals and organic compounds, lead generally does not accumulate to progressively higher concentrations in wildlife food chains. Instead, the opposite often occurs: lead exhibits progressive decreases in concentrations in organisms at higher trophic levels (Elias et al. 1975, Rolfe et al. 1977, Wong et al. 1978).

In most organisms, lead, barium, and strontium are closely associated with physiological reservoirs of calcium in tissues, and some investigators have examined Pb/Ca ratios (as well as Ba/Ca and Sr/Ca ratios), rather than absolute concentrations of lead, in ecological studies (Elias et al.

1975, Settle and Patterson 1979). As discussed later, Pb/Ca, Ba/Ca, and Sr/Ca ratios also exhibit progressive decreases with transfers to higher trophic levels in vertebrate food chains. This phenomenon has been attributed to inefficient absorption of the trace elements from the intestine of animals, relative to uptake of calcium. Although the concept of successive biochemical diminutions of Pb/Ca ratios appears to be a useful qualitative model for food-chain transfers of lead, exceptions to the general principle are known to exist (e.g., in invertebrate food chains), and quantitative applications of the concept are still fraught with uncertainty.

Nature of Human Perturbations

Solid and liquid wastes that contain lead can affect the geochemical cycle of the element on a local scale or throughout a watershed, and lead in aerosols may have local to global impacts. Some fertilizers, sludges, and soil conditioners can transfer lead into agricultural soils. Such additions of lead also can elevate concentrations of the element in soil, surface runoff, soil solution, plants, dust on plant surfaces, and animals.

Effects of this sort have been demonstrated conclusively at heavily contaminated sites, such as near ore smelters or adjacent to highways. The critical questions in an assessment of the natural occurrence of lead, however, involve the quantitative applications of this knowledge to more typical rural and remote locations. It is important to determine whether or not natural background conditions corresponding to the pretechnological lead cycle currently exist anywhere on earth; if not, reported "natural" background levels of lead in air, soil, water, and biota at most sites may be higher than pretechnological levels at the same sites, and the magnitude of changes resulting from human activities could be underestimated. Knowledge of the quantitative aspects of the cycling of lead in the environment is discussed in Step 3, below.

Step 2: IDENTIFY SPECIFIC HUMAN POPULATIONS WITH EXPOSURES TO LEAD

Levels of exposure to lead under natural conditions were undoubtedly somewhat variable, because natural levels of lead in the environment differed from place to place and specific human populations had significantly different dietary habits. Current knowledge about the natural occurrence of lead permits estimation of a range of possible values for most parameters of exposure (see Step 3). However, the specific combinations of factors that might influence the exposure to lead of specific populations under natural, unperturbed conditions are too poorly known to permit estimation of the range of variation in total exposure experienced by different pretechnological populations. Instead, a crude, order-of-magnitude calculation of the "average" natural level of exposure for a typical adult will be developed and compared with typical current exposures of adult Americans (see Step 4, below).

Step 3: ESTIMATE QUANTITATIVELY THE LEVEL OF EXPOSURE TO LEAD BY EACH PATHWAY THAT AFFECTS THE TARGET POPULATION

The estimates in this step are based on the same assumptions about respiratory volumes and amounts of food, water, and soil ingested by typical adults that were used to estimate exposures for the general adult population in the previous section. It is assumed that the significant

TABLE 2.8   Natural and Anthropogenic Sources of Emissions of Lead to the Atmosphere

	Estimated Global Emissions	
Source	10^9 g/yr	Range
Natural		
Windblown dusts	16	0.19-35
Volcanogenic particles	6.4	4.2-96
Vegetation	1.6	1.6-21
Forest fires	0.5	0.04-2.8
Sea salt spray	0.02	0.01-0.05
Rock degassing	?	?
TOTAL	24.5	6.0-155
Anthropogenic[a]		
Mining	8.2	
Primary lead production	31	
Other primary nonferrous metal production	45.5	
Secondary smelting	0.8	
Iron and steel production	50	
Industrial uses of lead	7.4	
Coal combustion	14	
Gasoline combustion	273	
Waste incineration	8.9	
Miscellaneous	10.4	
TOTAL	449	
TOTAL EMISSIONS	474	

[a] Anthropogenic emission estimates are for 1975.

SOURCE: Adapted from Nriagu (1979).

differences between natural exposures and those of present-day Americans depend only on the concentrations of lead in the media of exposure; unknown effects of possible physiological differences between populations cannot be estimated.

Lead in the Atmosphere

Sources Estimated present-day annual emissions of lead from natural and anthropogenic sources are shown in Table 2.8 (from Nriagu 1979). Settle and Patterson (1979) have estimated a somewhat lower total for pretechnological natural emissions (5×10^9 g/yr). The disparity suggests that a substantial fraction of present-day "natural" emissions in fact has an anthropogenic origin. As the range of values given in Table 2.8 suggests, there is still considerable uncertainty about the exact magnitude of some of the natural geochemical fluxes. However, the preponderance of evidence suggests that the correct values are most likely to be in the lower portions of the ranges indicated by the table.

The best available estimates therefore suggest that natural emissions of lead can account for no more than 5, and perhaps as little as 1 percent, of the present-day flux of the metal into the atmosphere (Nriagu 1978a, 1979; Settle and Patterson 1979). As noted above, some emissions listed as "natural" have partially anthropogenic origins; for example, the lead released by forest fires is in large part anthropogenic lead deposited on vegetation surfaces.

About 90 percent of present-day emissions of lead occur in the Northern Hemisphere (Robinson and Robbins 1971). Atmospheric transport across the Equator is very slight; it may therefore be appropriate to consider the Northern and Southern Hemispheres separately in assessing the atmospheric cycle of lead aerosols (Nriagu 1978a).

Current Levels in Air Using estimates of emission rates and certain other parameters, current global "background" levels of lead in the air can be estimated by mass-balance methods. Then, if comparison with actual measured background levels of lead validates the model, the same mass-balance approach can be used to estimate natural, pretechnological background concentrations of lead in the air.

Parameters of the mass-balance model include *emission rates* from natural and anthropogenic sources; the *particle-size distribution* of emissions, which determines the extent to which lead aerosols may remain suspended and be transported long distances; the atmospheric *volume* in which the emissions are mixed; and the atmospheric *residence time* of the lead-containing particles. Residence time, the average interval between emission and removal of particles, depends in turn on the rates of removal processes, primarily scavenging by precipitation (wet deposition) and gravitational settling (dry deposition). In the model used here, the two mechanisms are considered as a single flux, which may be described in terms of a net *deposition velocity*.

In order to calculate a background concentration of lead in the air, values must be selected for each of the parameters. In addition, it is assumed that different sources (natural as well as anthropogenic) are essentially similar in terms of the behavior of particles from the various sources in the atmosphere. This, like assumptions about other variables, is an oversimplification, but for making a rough estimate of the sort sought here, it is satisfactory.

The following values are assumed for variables in the mass-balance calculation:

Emissions: 4.3×10^{11} g/yr, or 90 percent of the total shown in Table 2.8. This represents emissions in the Northern Hemisphere.

Particle-size distribution: It is assumed that 50 percent of the mass of emitted lead (2.2×10^{11} g/yr) is in fine particles that enter into long-term transport.

Atmospheric volume: The volume of air to a depth of 10 km in the Northern Hemisphere is 2.5×10^{18} m^3.

Residence time: 10 days. This value corresponds to a net deposition velocity of 0.6 cm/sec. Estimates for the residence time of lead in the atmosphere range from about 1 to 40 days; estimates based on lead-210 average about 7 days (Turekian et al. 1977), but other workers have used values of 10 to 20 days (Lantzy and Mackenzie 1979). Deposition velocities for dry fallout have been well measured; an average value is about 0.3 cm/sec (Davidson 1979). Deposition in precipitation is more rapid, though less frequent. The relative importance of the two mechanisms has been determined only at a few sites and for relatively short periods, and it is difficult to support general conclusions; however, estimates for the contribution of dry fallout at typical rural locations range from about 30 to 60 percent of total deposition. It is therefore assumed here that 0.6 cm/sec represents a reasonable average deposition velocity for wet-plus-dry removal processes.

Using the values just given, the average present-day background concentration of lead in the air of the Northern Hemisphere is calculated to be about 2.4 ng/m^3. It would be reasonable to expect that background levels over land and near sources would be somewhat higher than the average, and that levels over the oceans and at very remote points would be lower than the average. Since emissions in the Southern Hemisphere are only a fraction of those in the Northern Hemisphere, lead levels in the air from points below the equator should be lower than the levels at comparable sites in the Northern Hemisphere.

The validity of the model can be checked by comparing the estimate with measured lead levels in the air at various remote or "background" sites. In fact, this calculation fits rather well with levels of lead in air that have been measured at various points on the Earth's surface. Table 2.9 displays recorded atmospheric lead levels at a number of representative rural and remote sites. Published data have been reviewed in more detail by the EPA (1977a), Nriagu (1978a), and Lindberg (1979). The table shows that concentrations of lead in the air at remote sites in the Northern Hemisphere are of the same order of magnitude expected from mass-balance assumptions, and values in the Southern Hemisphere are generally lower than those from comparable sites in the Northern Hemisphere.

Natural Levels in Air   Several methods have been used to estimate the natural range of concentrations of airborne lead. The same model used to calculate present-day background levels can be applied to the inventory of natural emissions. If global emissions of lead from natural sources are about 25×10^9 g/yr (Table 2.8), if the mean residence time for 100 percent of naturally emitted particles is 10 days, and if natural sources are of equivalent importance in both hemispheres, the estimated average global natural background level of lead in the air to a depth of 10 km is roughly 0.1 ng/m^3. Because of the uncertainty in estimates of natural emissions, the range of reasonable estimates of the global average natural background level of airborne lead might be at least 0.02 to 0.5 ng/m^3. As in the case of present-day concentrations, considerable site-to-site variation would be expected.

A second approach for estimating natural levels is to calculate the atmospheric lead burden attributable to wind-entrained soil particles, the principal natural source. The National Research Council (1979) estimates that natural levels of airborne particles in regions with average precipitation and vegetative cover are probably about 5 to 10 μg/m^3; much higher values may be observed in regions with sparse vegetation, and much lower levels occur over oceans, polar ice caps, and other sites remote from soil sources. If typical soils contain 5 to 25 μg Pb/g (see below) and the natural background level of particulate matter in air is 5 to 40 μg/m^3, airborne lead concentrations from this source would be about 0.025 to 1.0 ng/m^3. However, this estimate may be high, since surface soils at many sites contain deposited anthropogenic lead as well as native lead.

Conclusions The two methods suggest that a reasonable range for the natural concentration of lead in the atmosphere is about 0.01 to 1.0 ng/m^3, with the lower end of the range reflecting expected values at remote and oceanic sites, and the upper portion of the range typical of land areas likely to be inhabited by humans. This estimated natural range for comparable sites is exceeded by about 1 to 2 orders of magnitude by present-day levels at remote points on the Earth's surface, and by 2 to 4 orders of magnitude in areas inhabited by human populations.

Two additional lines of evidence support these estimates of natural levels. Chemical compositions of aerosols collected at remote sites commonly show an enrichment of more than 100-fold in the abundance of lead relative to its occurrence in natural source materials such as soils and sea salt spray (NRC 1978b, Lantzy and Mackenzie 1979). This enrichment indicates a possible anthropogenic origin for the lead-enriched particles. Mass-balance considerations suggest that volcanogenic particles, which may also be enriched in lead, could not account for the present-day background levels of lead aerosols observed globally; and although it is possible that some natural process could emit particles with enriched trace metal contents (Duce et al. 1975), the weight of other evidence suggests that this is not the case for lead. In particular, Murozumi et al. (1969) showed that lead deposited in polar ice layers increased 200-fold since about 3,000 years ago; that observed increase closely matches historical use of lead (Settle and Patterson 1979). This observation adds convincing support to the conclusion reached from mass-balance estimates that present-day background levels of lead in the air are largely if not almost entirely anthropogenic in origin.

Deposition of Atmospheric Lead

The primary transfer of atmospherically transported lead to terrestrial and aquatic ecosystems can be expressed as a deposition flux, i.e., the mass of lead deposited per unit of area per unit of time. Examination of deposition fluxes suggests the potential magnitude of effects that the atmospheric burden of anthropogenic lead could have on levels in soils, surface waters, and organisms.

Natural Fluxes   If natural levels of lead in air are 0.01 to 1.0 ng/m^3 and the mean deposition velocity (averaging wet and dry deposition) of particles containing lead is 0.6 cm/sec, the range of natural deposition fluxes for lead is approximately 2 to 200 μg/m^2/year (0.002 to 0.2 mg/m^2/year).

Current Fluxes   Measured deposition fluxes for atmospheric lead at a variety of sites are shown in Table 2.10. Values representative of heavily contaminated sites, typical inhabited and agricultural regions, and remote areas have been selected from a much larger number of values in the literature, reviewed in more detail by Nriagu (1978a) and Lindberg (1979).

Some caution is required in comparing and interpreting the measurements listed in Table 2.10. Annual deposition fluxes are difficult to measure accurately, because of variations over time and limitations on extrapolation from short-term samples (Turekian et al. 1977). Different reported fluxes are based on different sampling methods, which can produce substantially different results, depending on the collecting devices used, the analytical methods, and whether samples consisted of bulk precipitation, only wet precipitation, or only dry precipitation. Some of the data in the table suggest that dry deposition alone can account for about half of total rates; calculated fluxes that are based on rainfall or dryfall alone therefore are probably underestimates. Despite these uncertainties, the values in the table for rural and remote sites correspond rather closely to reported levels of atmospheric lead at comparable sites (Table 2.9).

Additional estimates of deposition fluxes at other locations can be calculated from measured atmospheric levels of lead. If it is again assumed that lead-containing aerosols have a mean deposition velocity of 0.6 cm/sec, the deposition fluxes implied by data in Table 2.9 range from 0.02 mg/m^2/year at the South Indian Ocean site to roughly 5 to 50 mg/m^2/year for representative rural locations. These estimates also are consistent with measured values.

The recent report by Boutron (1979) provides an interesting contrast between the Northern and Southern Hemispheres (Table 2.10). The deposition flux he measured in Antarctica (0.01 mg/m^2/year) is the lowest yet recorded, and is about 2 orders of magnitude lower than the flux he measured using the same techniques in Greenland.

Conclusions   The data in Table 2.10 suggest that observed rates of transfer of lead from the atmosphere to the Earth's surface at sites representing present-day background conditions are consistently 1 to 2

TABLE 2.9   Measured Concentrations of Lead in Air at a Variety of Rural and Remote Sites[a]

Site	Lead in Air (ng Pb/m^3)
Rural	
Chadron, Nebraska, 1973-1974	45 (9-90)
Walker Branch Watershed, Tennessee, 1976-1977	107 (63-172)[b]
Rural background, Belgium, 1972	230
Oceanic, New York Bight, 1974	130 (20-300)
Chacaltaya, Bolivia, 1974	37 (18-76)
Puerto Montt, Chile, 1975	12 (9-15)
Remote	
Novaya Zemlya, USSR, 1968-1969	0.23
Jungfraujoch, Switzerland, 1973-1974	8.7 (0.13-25)
Northern Norway, 1971-1972	4.0 (0.6-20)[c]
White Mountains, California, 1969-1970	8.0 (1.2-29)
Bermuda, 1971-1972	3.0 (0.1-20)[c]
Hawaii, 1969-1970	2.0 (0.3-13)[c]
Thule, Greenland, 1965	0.5
Antarctica, 1971	0.4
South Pole, 1974	
North Atlantic, 1971-1972	0.049
North Atlantic, 1971-1972	1.6
South Atlantic, 1971-1972	0.18
North-Central Pacific, 1967	1.0 (0.3-1.5)
South Indian Ocean, 1971-1972	0.13
South China Sea, 1971-1972	0.32

[a] Except as noted, data are representative examples taken from a much larger compilation in Nriagu (1978a).
[b] Lindberg (1979).
[c] NRC (1978b).

orders of magnitude higher than estimated natural fluxes for comparable sites. Inhabited rural and agricultural regions generally exhibit deposition rates that are an order of magnitude higher than remote, uninhabited areas. Fluxes in urban locations and near specific sources of emissions are 1 to 3 orders of magnitude higher than rural background values, and up to 5 orders of magnitude higher than estimated typical natural rates.

To determine whether a change of this magnitude in a geochemical flux of lead is significant in terms of potential human exposure to the element, it is necessary to examine the reservoirs and transfers of lead in the ecosystems that receive the atmospheric deposition.

TABLE 2.10   Measured Atmospheric Deposition of
Lead at Selected Contaminated, Rural, and Remote Sites[a]

Site	Deposition flux ($mg\ Pb/m^2/yr$)
Near Sources	
Toronto, near secondary smelter	>6,000[b]
Missouri, 800 m from smelter	1,265[b]
Cincinnati, <10 m from highway	304[b]
Toronto, near expressway	600[b]
Urban	
New York City	350
New York City	547[b]
Central Los Angeles	365-8,000[b]
Los Angeles Basin (Pasadena, California)	102-296[b]
Los Angeles Suburbs	17-120[b]
San Diego, California	350[b]
London, England	54
Madison, Wisconsin	>25
Rural	
France (11 locations)	14.6[c]
Northwest England	<19.6
Walker Branch Watershed, Tennessee	15.0
Delaware River watersheds	6.2[c]
Mt. Moosilauke, New Hampshire	19.6
Upper Great Lakes Basin	12.0
Lake Michigan	15.0
Off Southern California Coast	34.1
Remote	
Scandinavian glaciers	4.2
Sierra Nevada Mountains, California	4.0[d]
French Congo	0.2[b]
North-Central Pacific Ocean	0.6[e]
Eastern Pacific Ocean	0.09
North Atlantic Ocean	1.4[f]
Northern Greenland	0.04
Greenland	0.08[g]
Antarctica	0.01[g]

[a] Representative data have been selected from larger compilations of
reported values in Nriagu (1978a) and Lindberg (1979), unless otherwise noted. Deposition fluxes are bulk precipitation (rain, snow, and
dustfall) unless otherwise noted.
[b] Dry deposition only.
[c] Wet deposition (rainfall) only.
[d] Shirahata et al. (1979).
[e] Schaule and Patterson (1979).
[f] NRC (1978b).
[g] Boutron (1979).

Lead in Soils

Sources and Distribution   The source of most native lead in soils is weathering of parent rocks. Nriagu (1978b) cites an estimated average global lead concentration of 12 to 20 $\mu g/g$ in the Earth's crust, and 17 to 20 $\mu g/g$ in soils. Under natural conditions lead is transferred only very slowly from sites of high concentrations, because of the limited solubility of the element in water. Wind dispersal of soil particles and transport of sediment particles in surface runoff are significant in redistribution of soil lead; the former process operates on a local scale, and the latter on a global one.

Anthropogenic activities add lead to nonurban soils via atmospheric deposition, by disposal of lead-containing liquids or solid wastes on land sites, and through a variety of agricultural practices. Nriagu (1978b) noted that some fertilizers, limes, composts, manures, sludges, fly ash, and other soil conditioners may contain substantial amounts of lead, and he calculated that the lead content of the surface 10 cm of soil could be doubled over a few years if such materials were added in substantial amounts on a regular basis. Lead pesticide residues may be responsible for concentrations of several hundred μg Pb/g in some surface soils (Cannon 1976). In general, agricultural practices and waste disposal have localized impacts on lead in soils. Atmospheric deposition, on the other hand, has the potential to affect measured background soil lead concentrations on a much broader scale.

Concentration gradients have been observed in the lead content of soils at many rural and remote sites; surface layers to a depth of 1 to 5 cm generally are enriched with lead in comparison to layers from depths of 10 cm or more (Nriagu 1978b). A natural mechanism has been invoked to explain this phenomenon: lead may be absorbed by roots at depth, translocated to aboveground portions of plants, and returned to surface soils in decaying plant or animal tissues (Nriagu 1978b). In addition to this natural process, however, the possible effects of atmospheric deposition of anthropogenic lead on surface soil lead concentrations must be examined.

Soil Chemistry of Lead   Lead in soils is relatively insoluble and immobile, although it may be leached by acid waters and removed in complexes with soluble organic compounds. Lead is transferred within soils by combinations of oxidation and reduction reactions, adsorption of cations on soil components, chelation by organic matter and other metal oxides, and cycling within the biota. Site-specific factors such as mineral composition, organic content, and acidity of the soil influence each of these processes (Tidball 1976, Rickard and Nriagu 1978). Soil conditions vary greatly from one location to another, but in general the primary factor governing the availability of lead for leaching or uptake is its very low solubility.

Current Levels in Soils   Nriagu (1978b) summarized the extensive literature on the occurrence of lead in soils. Reported concentrations span 5 orders of magnitude, from < 1 μg/g in some remote sites to > 100,000 μg/g near ore outcroppings. Soils at relatively uncontaminated sites in the United States contain < 10 to 700 μg Pb/g, with a geometric mean of about 16, and only 6 percent of samples contain more than 30 μg/g (Tidball 1976). Estimates of the average global lead content of soil range from 15 to 20 μg/g, and the WHO (1977) estimates that a range of 5 to 25 μg/g encompasses the great majority of reported present-day background levels.

Effects of Atmospheric Deposition   The potential effects of deposition of lead on concentrations of the element in soils can be readily calculated. Assuming an initial lead concentration of 15 μg/g and a soil density of 2 g/cm^3, a surface soil layer 1 m square and 1 cm deep contains 300 mg of lead. If all deposited lead remains in the top 1 cm of soil, the relative increase due to deposition is simply the deposition flux times the duration of the flux, divided by 300 mg.

Under the assumptions just given, the estimated natural atmospheric deposition flux (0.002 to 0.2 mg/m^2/year) represents an annual increase of about 0.0007 to 0.07 percent of the lead content of surface soils. Also, since most of the natural flux is in wind-entrained soil particles, it may be assumed that there would be little net change in soil lead content on a global basis as a result of this natural transfer.

The effects of the present-day deposition rates shown in Table 2.10 clearly are substantial in urban areas and near sources. At an annual deposition rate of 300 mg/m^2/year, typical of many urban sites, the input to soil each year would equal the estimated average initial native lead content. Nriagu (1978b) tabulates numerous published reports of lead concentrations in soils at such locations; elevations of 1 to 4 orders of magnitude above the typical background range have commonly been observed.

In rural areas, typical fluxes of 6 to 30 mg/m^2/year represent annual increases of 2 to 10 percent of the estimated native lead in the upper 1 cm of soil. Nriagu (1979) estimates that total anthropogenic emissions of lead since the beginning of technological civilization amount to approximately 2×10^{13} g, or roughly 44 times recent annual emissions. If current deposition rates were continued for 44 years, the lead content of surface layers of many rural soils could be elevated 2 to 5 times above its original natural level. Although there are reasons to expect that this calculation overestimates possible effects on soil lead (see below), it is plausible that surface soils at many sites taken to represent natural background conditions may be contaminated significantly by anthropogenic lead deposited from the atmosphere. Such errors in estimates of natural lead concentrations would be especially likely for samples taken from only the top few centimeters of soil.

Several considerations, however, could reduce the calculated effect of atmospheric deposition on soil lead concentrations. It was assumed that all lead deposited on soil remains in the uppermost layer (1 cm); however, if leaching occurs, even at a very slow rate (e.g., 1 cm/year), the added lead could be dispersed through a sufficient volume of soil to make the net impact of typical rural and remote deposition fluxes virtually negligible. In addition, many agricultural soils are effectively mixed to a depth of 10 to 20 cm by plowing; this mixing could dilute the impact of atmospheric inputs to a small fraction of its surface effect at most cultivated sites.

Geochemical studies using lead-210 provide evidence that most of the lead deposited from the atmosphere remains in the soil. Servant and Delapart (1979) measured low lead levels (12 μg/l) in rivers in southern France, and concluded that almost none of the lead deposited on nearby urban and suburban soils was transferred to the streams. Turner et al. (1977) measured an export flux of 0.2 mg/m^2/year in streamflow from a Tennessee watershed receiving atmospheric inputs of 15 mg/m^2/year of lead, and Siccama and Smith (1978) found an atmospheric input/stream output ratio of 31.7/1.1 in the Hubbard Brook watershed in New Hampshire. Rolfe et al. (1977) measured atmospheric lead inputs of 130 mg/m^2/year and stream lead outputs of 3.64 mg/m^2/year in a cultivated watershed in Illinois.

Benninger et al. (1975) estimated that less than 2 percent of the annual atmospheric input of lead-210 was leached to groundwater in a deciduous forest in Maryland. They determined that 0.8 percent of the annual atmospheric flux, or less than 0.02 percent of the total amount of lead-210 present in the soil, was removed in streamborne particles each year. These mass-balance studies indicate that the residence time for lead-210 in soils, relative to erosion, is 2,000 to 5,000 years (Lewis 1977, Benninger et al. 1975, Siccama and Smith 1978).

The same studies have demonstrated that most of the lead in soils is associated with soil organic matter. While the majority of the results cited apply to soils in deciduous forests, sandy soils and some agricultural soils may be lower in organic matter, and may have lower capacities to retain lead. In soils where that sorptive capacity is initially low or is already saturated by accumulated lead, the fraction of lead retained may be lower, and significant removals of atmospheric lead from soil via erosion may be more likely (Rolfe et al. 1977).

In addition, it seems evident from Tables 2.9 and 2.10 that there may be some places on the earth's surface where atmospheric deposition fluxes of lead are small, and where significant impacts on the lead content of even the surface layer of soils are unlikely. Fluxes of less than 1 $mg/m^2/year$ would increase the lead content of most soils by less than 0.3 percent/year. Atmospheric deposition rates of 0.01 to 1 $mg/m^2/year$ have been measured at some locations, especially in remote regions of the Southern Hemisphere. Although present deposition fluxes at such sites may be an order of magnitude or more greater than they are believed to have been in pretechnological times, the amount of lead in the soil reservoir at some sites is sufficiently large relative to this rate of annual deposition that significant changes in the soil pool seem unlikely.

Conclusions   It seems will established that lead deposited from the atmosphere is largely retained in soils, and it is therefore probable that the average present-day lead content of surface soils is somewhat higher than the average natural level. However, it seems likely that the increase that has occurred at many remote and rural sites is small. Mass-balance considerations show that even if the atmospheric deposition flux is 2 orders of magnitude greater than the natural flux, it still represents a relatively small input compared to the reservoir of native lead in most soils. In some truly remote sites on the Earth's surface, soils in approximately natural conditions with respect to lead probably can still be observed. In soils of regions inhabited by human populations, the increased lead content is generally in the upper few centimeters of the soil layer.

Several important questions about lead in soils will benefit from further research. Pertinent problems include the effect of an increase of lead levels above natural levels on the geochemical cycling of lead within soils, the extent to which the lead content of the soil organic matter pool has been increased, and the importance of such an increase in terms of the biological availability of lead in soil. Better understanding also is needed of the differences in long-term retention of lead and of variation in losses of lead by erosion from soils of different types.

Lead in Surface Waters and Sediments

Sources   Lead enters streams, lakes, and oceans as soluble ions leached from rocks and soil, in insoluble sediment particles, by wet or dry deposition from the atmosphere on water surfaces, and by direct discharge of sewage, industrial wastes, and urban runoff. Contributions by direct discharge of wastes and atmospheric deposition are almost entirely anthropogenic fluxes, whereas the soluble and insoluble lead transferred from soils to surface waters is of both anthropogenic and natural origins. As noted in the previous section, exogenous lead deposited on soil is believed to remain there; however, human activities—such as irrigation, logging, or cultivation—that increase the rate of soil erosion also increase the flux of soil lead to surface waters.

No complete national or global inventory of inputs of lead to aquatic ecosystems has been compiled, but the relative importance of specific contributions has been determined from mass-balance studies at a number of sites. Patterson and Kodukula (1978) estimated that stream inputs accounted for 63 and 60 percent of the lead entering Lakes Superior and Huron, respectively; atmospheric deposition made up 37 and 39 percent of total inputs. Municipal and industrial wastes were 0.4 percent of the total input to Lake Huron and 0.2 percent of that to Lake Superior. Lantzy and Mackenzie (1979) estimated a global mass transfer of lead in stream flow of 4.7×10^{11} g/yr. Since global atmospheric emissions are also estimated at about 4.7×10^{11} g/yr (Table 2.8), atmospheric inputs and continental runoff may contribute roughly comparable amounts of lead to the oceans. Duce et al. (1976) determined that atmospheric deposition could account for 13 percent of total lead inputs to surface ocean waters in the New York Bight, a site where impacts of stream deliveries would be expected to be great. Schaule and Patterson (1979) estimated that in the central North Pacific, more than 1,000 km from shore, atmospheric deposition exceeds input from fluvial sources by more than an order of magnitude. The magnitude of the atmospheric input and its recent origin were confirmed by analysis of the isotopic composition and mass deposition rates of lead in aerosols and sediments.

In contrast to the general transfer processes that move lead into large surface water bodies, discharges from erosion, urban runoff, and other specific anthropogenic sources may predominate in rivers, streams, and coastal waters that drain heavily industrialized areas, agricultural and urban regions, or mining sites.

TABLE 2.11   Mean Deposition Fluxes of Lead Into Recent Sediments of Lakes and Coastal Waters[a]

Site	Deposition Fluxes (mg Pb/m^2/yr)	
	Recent	Preindustrial
Urban and Near-Urban		
Lake Erie	110	7
Lake Ontario	70	10
Lake Mendota (Madison, Wisconsin)	60-100	
Lake Monona (Madison, Wisconsin)	200-300	
Rural and Remote		
Lake Michigan	13	1.6
Lake Huron	22	7
Trout Lake (N. Wisconsin)	20	
Minocqua Lake (N. Wisconsin)	15	
Devil's Lake (N. Wisconsin)	5-23	
Near-Shore Oceanic		
Pacific, near Santa Monica	9	2.4
Pacific, near San Piedro	17	2.6
Pacific, near Santa Barbara	21	10
Pacific, near San Clemente	0.4	

[a] Adapted from Nriagu (1978b).

Changes in Sources with Time   Sediments offer a readily accessible record of the total amount of lead entering a quiescent body of water over long periods. The sedimentation process is subject to various perturbations that prevent metal concentrations in sediments from being a precise chronological record of concentrations in the overlying water (NRC 1978b). Nevertheless, sediments record gross changes in the amount of lead in the aquatic environment.

Lead concentrations in sediments of numerous freshwater lakes, estuaries, and coastal marine waters commonly show increases that range from 2-fold to 100-fold over the last century or more (Nriagu 1978b). Natural (pretechnological) levels of lead in sediments vary, usually approximately matching those of bedrocks in the drainage basin. Sediment records may reflect local impacts of intense sources of lead, but even sediments at remote sites exhibit significant increases in lead with time. Shirahata et al. (1979) measured a 4-fold increase in the rate of deposition of lead in sediments of the last 100 years from a pond in a remote canyon in the Sierra Nevada Mountains.

Table 2.11 summarizes estimates of mass deposition rates of lead to recent and preindustrial sediments of several North American lakes and near-shore ocean waters. A comparison with estimates of atmospheric deposition rates suggests that natural atmospheric fluxes of lead (estimated earlier to be 0.002 to 0.2 mg/m^2/year) could account for only a small fraction of the estimated natural transfer of lead to sediments, and that stream inputs are the chief source of lead in preindustrial sediments. However, recent deposition rates of atmospheric lead in urban and rural areas (Table 2.10) are of about the same order of magnitude as deposition fluxes to sediments of lakes in comparable locations. This comparison suggests that deposition of atmospheric lead could account for most of the observed historical increase in lead in sediments at many sites. This inference has been supported by more complete mass-balance studies of several lakes, and confirmed by isotopic analysis in a few cases (Robbins 1978, Shirahata et al. 1979).

Fate of Lead in Aquatic Systems   Although mass-balance data and sediment records provide convincing evidence that inputs of lead to surface waters have been greatly increased by human activities, changes in lead concentrations, and subsequent changes in human exposure through drinking water, depend on removal processes as well as on inputs. A great deal of qualitative knowledge of the dynamics of lead in aquatic systems is available. As noted previously, lead is only slightly soluble in water, although exceptions exist (e.g., in complexes with organic ligands). The extent to which soluble lead is present in the aquatic environment is influenced by particle size and chemical forms of the lead compounds and the pH, hardness, alkalinity, sediment load, organic content, temperature, biological activity, and other characteristics of the receiving waters. Complex interactions among many of these variables are likely, and the fate of added lead may be very different in different bodies of water (Hem 1976, Wershaw 1976, Rickard and Nriagu 1978).

Much of what is presently known quantitatively about the behavior of lead in waters has been learned by investigations of lead-210; Robbins (1978) has prepared a comprehensive review of that body of evidence. Available data suggest that, in many lakes and rivers, soluble lead is rapidly scavenged by particulate matter. Lewis (1977) found that lead in the Susquehanna River remained in solution for extended times in a section of the stream with pH less than 4.5 (caused by mining activities in the watershed), but where the pH was 6.5 to 7.0, lead was quickly adsorbed on particles composed of iron and manganese oxides and organic complexes. The estimated residence time in that portion of the river was less than 1 day. Studies on several rivers in the western United States produced estimated residence times of a few days to a few weeks (Robbins 1978).

In estuaries, much of the particle-bound lead becomes soluble at first mixing, but rapidly becomes associated with particles again (Benninger 1978). Mass-balance studies show that deposition fluxes of lead-210 to estuarine sediments account for essentially all inputs of the isotope, suggesting that little lead is transported through estuaries and into the open oceans (Benninger 1978, Turekian 1977). In the oceans, scavenging by particles is much more efficient near shore; Turekian (1977) estimated that the residence time of lead-210 in coastal mixing basins is one day or less, and that in near-shore waters the residence time is tens of days.

Chow (1978) cited several estimates of the residence time of lead in the oceans that ranged from 600 to 2,000 years. However, more recent data based on lead-210 measurements suggest that residence times for lead may be much shorter. Nozaki et al. (1976) estimated that the residence time for lead is 0.6 year in coastal waters, 1.7 years in mid-ocean surface waters, and 50 to 100 years in deep ocean waters.

Current knowledge, therefore, suggests that the residence times of soluble lead in many bodies of fresh water are short. Great site-to-site variation, related especially to the efficiency of scavenging by particles, has been observed, and adds uncertainty to quantitative comparisons based on sediment records in different lakes. It is also noteworthy that most lead in fresh waters appears to be associated with particles, rather than in soluble ionic form. Since modern water treatment essentially removes all particulate matter from drinking water, the lead added to bodies of water by human activities may not reach consumers. It is possible that exposures to lead in drinking water under natural conditions may have been higher than many typical exposures today, because of particles ingested in the water.

Current Concentrations Fishman and Hem (1976) and Chow (1978) reviewed surveys of lead in natural waters. Rivers, streams, and lakes in the United States have been reported to contain from no detectable lead to 890 $\mu g/l$, with an average of about 4 $\mu g/l$. Many similar surveys in this and other countries report average concentrations of 1 to 10 $\mu g/l$. Ground and spring waters may contain from < 1 to > 100 μg Pb/l, with concentrations as high as 5,000 $\mu g/l$ reported in a few springs near ore deposits. Concentrations of 100 $\mu g/l$ or more have been observed in surface waters near sources of sewage, urban runoff, or industrial wastes. Some streams and lakes in remote, pristine areas have lead concentrations as low as 0.006 to 0.05 $\mu g/l$ (Settle and Patterson 1979). The number of reliable measurements at the low end of the range is small, because of analytical insensitivity and contamination of samples (see Appendix D). If high values attributable to localized natural or anthropogenic contamination are excluded, the range of typical current concentrations still spans 3 orders of magnitude, i.e., <0.01 to 10 μg/l.

Chow (1978) reviewed available estimates of the lead content of sea water. The data show progressively lower values as the sensitivity and reliability of analytical procedures has improved. Chow estimated the current lead content of surface sea waters to be about 0.07 to 0.2 μg/l, and that of deep ocean waters to be 0.03 to 0.05 μg/l; but he noted that analysis by isotopic dilution in a clean laboratory had measured lead concentrations as low as 0.002 μg/l in deep waters. He concluded that more accurate measurements were needed to improve the tentative current information. More recently, Schaule and Patterson (1979) conducted analyses in an ultra-clean laboratory, and reported lower concentrations of lead in ocean waters than any previously published. They measured 0.005 to 0.015 μg/l in surface samples and about 0.001 μg/l in deep waters (>3,500 m). Concentrations in waters near the California coast (50 to 120 km offshore) were similar to those 1,000 to 2,000 km offshore, suggesting that natural removal mechanisms offset the expected greater inputs to coastal waters.

Effects of Human Activities   It seems unlikely that typical natural levels of lead in fresh waters fall much outside the range that is observed today (<0.01 to 10 μg/l). However, it is possible that the average natural concentration may be lower than the present-day average. The conditions that affect concentrations of lead in fresh waters are so heterogeneous that there is at present no basis for a quantitative estimate that could apply to freshwater environments in general. However, several mass-balance approaches offer some qualitative insights. For instance, the mass of lead emitted to the atmosphere each year in the United States would be sufficient to raise the lead concentration of all stream runoff from the 48 contiguous states by about 150 μg/l (Fishman and Hem 1976). Obviously, most of the emitted lead never reaches surface waters; the greatest part is deposited on soils, where it is largely retained (see earlier section on lead in soils). Nevertheless, the atmospheric flux is so large that the fractions of the total that are deposited directly on water bodies or carried to them by surface runoff or erosion can have significant effects on the cycle of lead in aquatic ecosystems, as confirmed by sediment records.

Chow and Patterson (1962) estimated that natural, pretechnological levels of lead in fresh waters were about an order of magnitude lower than present-day levels. Their estimate was based on the average rate of deposition of lead in oceanic sediments over several hundred thousand years (1.7 $\times$ 10^{10} g/yr), and the estimated volume of fluvial inputs to the seas (3.7 $\times$ 10^{16} l/year); these figures suggest an average lead concentration of 0.5 μg/l in ancient stream waters. However, more recent knowledge indicates that removal processes in estuaries prevent most streamborne lead from entering the oceans (discussed above). The average lead content of ancient continental runoff therefore may have been considerably less than an order of magnitude different from current mean levels.

A crude mass-balance calculation suggests the approximate magnitude of possible effects of atmospheric deposition on soluble lead concentrations in freshwater bodies. Assuming an average present-day atmospheric deposition flux over water surfaces of 20 mg/m^2/year (see Table 2.10), an average water depth of 10 m, 20 percent solubility for deposited lead, and a mean residence time of 0.1 year, atmospheric fallout of lead could increase the average concentration of the element in surface waters by about 0.04 μg/l, or about 1 percent of the present-day average reported value for North American rivers. The values chosen for this calculation were selected arbitrarily from a range of possibilities; most of the variables are highly uncertain. For example, the residence time might be an order of magnitude or more shorter than the value selected, and deposition fluxes at some sites are an order of magnitude higher than the value chosen here. If the full range of plausible values for each variable is considered, the estimated effects range from undetectable to more than present concentrations of lead in waters. Better information on the most appropriate values of the parameters, and especially the residence times for soluble lead in various surface waters, will be required to reduce the current uncertainty in this approach.

The calculation above applies to fresh waters, where atmospheric deposition is only one of several possible anthropogenic sources of lead. Schaule and Patterson (1979) made a similar calculation for remote ocean sites, where they measured an atmospheric deposition flux of 0.6 mg/m^2/year. They estimated that lead from continental runoff reaching the site was a much smaller flux (0.05 mg/m^2/year). Using an estimated residence time of 2 years for lead in the upper 100 m of the seas, they calculated that the average concentration of lead in the ocean surface layer should be 0.01 μg/l. They estimated that the atmospheric deposition rate in prehistoric times was <0.005 mg/m^2/year, and that ancient fluvial inputs, estimated at 0.03 mg/m^2/year, produced an average natural concentration of lead of 0.0006 μg/l in surface ocean waters. Their measured values for surface waters (0.005 to 0.015 μg/l) corresponded to the present-day concentration predicted by their model; and they concluded that the concentrations in deep ocean waters (0.001 μg/l) represent approximate natural background levels.

Conclusions The assumptions used in the various mass-balance calculations described here are based on relatively few reliable data. As more and better measurements become available, estimates of natural lead concentrations in waters and of the impacts of human activities on those concentrations will be subject to much refinement.

The estimate by Schaule and Patterson (1979) that lead in ocean surface waters has been increased by about an order of magnitude by atmospheric fallout is based on what appear to be the most reliable measurements of lead in sea water yet published. The mass-balance model they employed is probably the best starting point for continued assessments of the impacts of atmospheric lead on the oceans.

Fewer conclusions can be supported regarding effects of human activities on levels of lead in fresh waters and on human exposure through drinking water. It seems plausible that in certain remote, clear lakes and streams, atmospheric deposition of lead might have increased concentrations in water above the natural levels; in such cases, both the original and the augmented concentrations would be very low. In general, however, the great inherent variability of present-day background lead concentrations in surface waters effectively masks any differences that might be attributed to anthropogenic inputs, other than obvious problems associated with proximate sources. The mass-balance and isotope studies examined here suggest that increases due to atmospheric deposition of lead would probably be small, and that the total lead removed from the land surfaces of the earth in streamflow has increased by less than an order of magnitude since prehistoric times. As in the case of soils, it seems likely that some surface waters in remote reaches of the Southern Hemisphere may be very slightly perturbed (if at all) from their natural condition with respect to lead.

Even if the average lead content of drinking water currently were severalfold greater than the average natural concentration, drinking water contributes only a very small portion of present-day exposure to lead for most populations. The demonstrable increases in fluxes of anthropogenic lead into aquatic ecosystems therefore may be of concern chiefly in terms of the potential they create for lead to enter aquatic food chains (see next section).

Lead in Aquatic Food Chains

Wong et al. (1978) have compiled an extensive review of published data on the occurrence of lead in aquatic organisms. Table 2.12 presents a summary of representative data on typical organisms from different trophic levels.

TABLE 2.12 Reported Lead Content of Representative Organisms of Different Trophic Levels in Aquatic Ecosystems[a]

Organism and Tissue Sampled	Lead Content (µg/kg, dry wt.)	Measured Level of Lead in Water (µg/l)	Reference
Vegetation			
Phytoplankton, various sp.	2,000-53,000	0.43	Wong et al. (1978)
Marine algae, various sp.	90-1,940	—	Wong et al. (1978)
Seaweeds, various sp.	3,000-35,000	0.2-27.4	Wong et al. (1978)
Freshwater macrophytes	14,900-347,000	7.1	Wong et al. (1978)
Freshwater macrophytes	1,450-20,000	15-20	Wong et al. (1978)
Invertebrates			
Freshwater zooplankton	3,990-18,300	15-20	Wong et al. (1978)
Marine zooplankton	2,100-7,900	0.43	Wong et al. (1978)
Marine copepods	13,000-170,000	—	Wong et al. (1978)
Marine mollusks (muscle)	18-23,000	—	Wong et al. (1978)
Freshwater mollusks (soft parts)	900-5,100	1-18	Wong et al. (1978)
Marine crustaceans (whole body)	<1,000-42,000	5.9	Wong et al. (1978)
Freshwater crustaceans (whole body)	4,700	—	Wong et al. (1978)
Freshwater worms (whole body)	6,000-143,900	1-18	Wong et al. (1978)
Freshwater insects (whole body)	50-120	(low)	Wong et al. (1978)
Freshwater insects (whole body)	854,000-1,117,000	(near mine)	Wong et al. (1978)
Freshwater bottom-dwellers	12,600-367,000	—	Rolfe et al. (1977)
Freshwater swimming varieties	4,700-11,000	—	Rolfe et al. (1977)

Fish			
Freshwater, 75 sp.	<100-4,900	—	U.S. FWS (unpublished data)
Marine, 204 sp.	300-700 (mean)	—	Hall et al. (1978)
Freshwater, various sp.	90-2,130	2	Wong et al. (1978)
Freshwater, various sp.	11,500-34,000	13	Wong et al. (1978)
Marine, various sp. (muscle)	254-14,000	1.6-13	Wong et al. (1978)
Marine, various sp. (gill)	4,000-50,000	1.6-13	Wong et al. (1978)
Codfish muscle, fresh	320	(market)	Ewing et al. (1979)
Shellfish, edible parts	280-550	(market)	Ewing et al. (1979)
Canned fish	340-720	(market)	Ewing et al. (1979)
Birds and Mammals			
Cormorants and darters (whole)	280-2,400	4-12	Greichus et al. (1977)
Birds' diets (fish) (composite)	<100-1,000	4-12	Greichus et al. (1977)
Seals (muscle, liver, kidney)	30-740[b]	—	Harms et al. (1977/1978)
Dolphins, porpoises, and whales	30-430[b]	—	Harms et al. (1977/1978)
Mammals' diets (fish)	10-800[b]	—	Harms et al. (1977/1978)

[a] Reported lead contents are ranges of data reported in more detail and for individual species in Wong et al. (1978). Comparable values for organisms of similar kinds are combined in this table.

[b] Data on marine mammals expressed as $\mu g/kg$ fresh weight.

Aquatic Plants Reports cited by Wong et al. (1978) indicate that lead is taken up from water and sediments quite efficiently by some aquatic plants, over a wide range of environmental lead concentrations (Table 2.12). Many algal species secrete an extracellular polysaccharide sheath that has a high affinity for lead; the metal may be removed quite rapidly from solution and either bound on algal surfaces or absorbed into cells. Aquatic macrophytes can absorb lead both from water (into leaves) and from sediments (into roots); such plants commonly show higher lead content in the roots. Algal species from the sediment zone generally contain more lead than those from surface samples, reflecting the typical distribution of lead in the aquatic environment (Gale et al. 1972).

Data summarized by Wong et al. indicate that some aquatic macrophytes can accumulate lead to concentrations 100 to 4,600 times higher than that of the surrounding water, over a range of lead levels in water of 10 to 270 $\mu g/l$. Comparable average concentration factors for algae are not available. Not all species have been shown to accumulate significant lead; those that do, however, appear frequently to concentrate the element to levels 2 to 4 orders of magnitude greater than those of the surrounding water.

It seems clear that aquatic vegetation can effectively scavenge lead from water; in fact, some aquatic plants are commonly used to cleanse industrial effluents of toxic metals. The evidence suggests that aquatic plants may play a significant role in maintaining equilibrium concentrations of lead in water, and that some fraction of added (anthropogenic) lead rapidly enters aquatic food chains, increasing the likelihood of exposure of organisms at higher trophic levels to elevated amounts of the metal in their food.

Aquatic Animals In addition to ingesting lead through the food chain, aquatic animals may absorb some lead directly from water; and soluble or particulate lead can be adsorbed on external surfaces (mucous membranes, gills, fur, skin).

Levels of lead in freshwater and marine invertebrates exhibit close relationships with lead content of water, dietary habits (e.g., herbivore, detritivore, or filter-feeder), habitat (e.g., planktonic versus bottom-dwelling), and the size (age) of the specimens (Wong et al. 1978). Typical ranges of lead content (dry weight) for various invertebrates are shown in Table 2.12. Values for some human food organisms were expressed as whole-body averages; levels in edible tissues may be an order of magnitude lower than those in shells, except for certain organs such as kidneys. The data suggest that invertebrate tissues may contain lead concentrations at least 2 to 4 orders of magnitude higher than those of the surrounding water, or roughly the same relative elevation observed in aquatic vegetation.

Lead concentrations in most varieties of marine and freshwater fishes are generally lower than those in plants and invertebrates, suggesting that the lead content of organisms diminishes, rather than increases, at higher (vertebrate) trophic levels in aquatic food chains. One recent study (Burnett 1979) has examined lead transfers in a multistep marine food chain; the lead content of organisms at successive levels (given as Pb/Ca ratios) exhibited sequential decrements, amounting to a decline of about 2 orders of magnitude through four trophic levels (algae, zooplankton, anchovy, tuna).

Very few reports are available on lead levels in organisms above the level of fish in aquatic food chains. Harms et al. (1977/1978) reported notable accumulation of mercury and organochlorine compounds, but not of lead, in seals, porpoises, and whales. However, Greichus et al. (1977) found lead concentrations in fish-eating birds that were 2-fold to 10-fold greater than those in fish.

Most published data on levels of lead in fish and other biological samples have been criticized as being based on faulty analytical procedures (Patterson and Settle 1976, Settle and Patterson 1979). Using stringent "clean-room" techniques, Settle and Patterson (1979) measured lead levels of 0.0003 μg/g in tuna muscle, and 0.006 μg/g in abalone, values 2 to 3 orders of magnitude lower than those previously reported. More thorough evaluation of the accuracy of existing data is urgently needed, since the work of Patterson and his colleagues clearly suggests that estimates of human dietary exposure to lead may be substantially in error (see Appendix D).

Natural Lead Content   Settle and Patterson (1979) argue that the approximate 10-fold enrichment of lead in surface ocean waters (discussed above) results in comparably elevated lead burdens at all trophic levels of aquatic food chains, i.e., that the observed process of successive diminution operates independently of initial environmental or dietary concentrations of lead. They conclude, therefore, that the average present-day levels of lead in all marine organisms are about an order of magnitude higher than natural levels. Unfortunately, other evidence is too sparse to confirm or modify this tentative estimate.

Available evidence strongly supports a qualitative conclusion that lead added to aquatic systems has entered food chains in significant amounts; however, the general magnitude of effects on the lead content of seafoods and other unprocessed human dietary items must be regarded as unknown. Accurate measurements of lead levels in aquatic biota from relatively uncontaminated sites (such as lakes in remote regions of the Southern Hemisphere) could shed light on this question, but apparently have not yet been attempted.

Lead in Terrestrial Food Chains

Terrestrial plants and animals comprise the bulk of the human diet; since food is the primary source of typical present-day exposure to lead (see Case II), information about the fraction of lead in foods that is of natural origin has direct and critical bearing on matters of health and environmental policy. Aspects of this issue, particularly estimates of the extent to which atmospheric lead contributes to lead in plants, have been the subject of extensive scientific debate. Recent comprehensive reviews by Cannon (1976), Peterson (1978), and Forbes and Sanderson (1978) have examined most of the available data.

Terrestrial Plants   Cannon (1976) and Peterson (1978) summarized the extensive available data on levels of lead in vegetation, and Ewing et al. (1979) compiled information from recent surveys of the lead content of edible grains, fruits, and vegetables. Most unprocessed food items derived from plants typically have been reported to contain lead levels of 0.1 to 0.2 $\mu g/g$ (fresh weight), but levels in specific samples exhibit variation of more than an order of magnitude on either side of the mean. Lead concentrations in natural vegetation from rural and remote sites show means and ranges similar to those observed in crops (Table 2.13). Lead content varies with species, tissue sampled, season of year, and site-specific conditions, especially soil characteristics and levels of lead in the air. Cannon (1976) notes that the lower end of the range of published data in most reports reflects the limit of the analytical method employed. With more widespread use of the most reliable and sensitive techniques for detecting lead, mean values probably would be lower than those now accepted, especially for samples from remote areas (see Appendix D).

Lead in plant tissues may have two principal origins: absorption from soil (presumed to be a largely natural source) and deposition from the atmosphere (assumed to be largely an anthropogenic flux). Lead added to soils by agricultural practices and by atmospheric deposition onto soils also might increase the amount of the element absorbed through roots, and wind-blown or rain-splashed soil particles could contribute additional topical lead, especially on low-growing plants.

Numerous reports have shown that the lead content of vegetation is affected markedly both by soils that contain anomalously high levels of the metal (e.g., near ore deposits) and by heavy atmospheric fallout (e.g., near highways, around smelters) (Cannon 1976). Effects at heavily contaminated sites, however, are of little relevance to typical human dietary exposures to lead, which are attributable chiefly to the ordinary occurrence of the metal in the rural environment where most crops and forages are grown.

Data presented earlier indicated that the present-day atmospheric deposition fluxes at typical rural sites appear to be about 2 orders of magnitude greater than estimated natural fluxes. Soil lead content, on the other hand, appears to have been increased above its natural level only modestly, if at all, in soils at root depth at most rural sites. This comparison suggests that if plants accumulate lead from both air and soil under natural conditions, present levels of airborne lead could potentially elevate levels of the element in plant tissues substantially.

Most plants appear to absorb relatively little lead from soils, and experimental data suggest that absorbed lead is translocated to only a small degree. Peterson (1978) reviewed estimates that a 10-fold increase in soil lead was followed by about a 2-fold increase in root uptake. Zimdahl and Arvik (1973) measured approximately an order-of-magnitude difference between the lead content of roots and that of stems and leaves of several varieties of crops grown in nutrient solutions with added lead; and other evidence suggests that there may be an additional order-of-magnitude reduction in lead content from stems and leaves to flowers and fruit (Peterson 1978). However, these observations do not exclude the possibility that lead levels of 0.1 to 0.2 $\mu g/g$ in edible plant tissues, especially root crops, could be derived primarily from soils. Furthermore, both uptake and translocation of lead in plants are influenced by soil conditions, the availability of nutrients, climatic factors, and other variables. Under some conditions, elevated accumulation of lead from soil in edible parts of plants might occur; but the combinations of factors that could cause this to happen are not currently well understood.

Many investigators have reported that the lead content of aboveground portions of some plants, especially leafy vegetables, is higher than that of roots of the same specimens (Peterson 1978); because this pattern reverses the gradient observed in experimental studies, this evidence also suggests an atmospheric origin for the lead. Such findings, however, are insufficient proof of either a causal relationship or of a quantitative contribution of lead in air to the total lead in plants.

Several lines of evidence suggest that atmospheric deposition of lead makes a substantial contribution to the measured lead content of plants, but the amount of that contribution is still controversial. Cannon (1976) reviewed her own work and that of others on relationships between lead in vegetation and proximity to sources of lead emissions, particularly highways. She concluded that the preponderance of evidence supports

TABLE 2.13 Reported Lead Content of Representative Organisms of Different Trophic Levels in Terrestrial Ecosystems

Organism and Tissue Sampled	Site Sampled	Lead Content (μg/g, dry weight)	Reference
Vegetation			
Composite sample	Urban	67	Rolfe et al. (1977)
Composite sample	Rural, near highway	34	Rolfe et al. (1977)
Composite sample	Rural, away from roads	4.1-8.6	Rolfe et al. (1977)
Garden vegetables (lettuce)	Urban	5.3-64.6	Rolfe et al. (1977)
Lichens (entire)	Remote	12.3-150	Cannon (1976)
Mosses (entire)	Various, remote-urban	<0.8-500	Cannon (1976)
Mosses, collected ca. 1860	Rural	25	Ruhling and Tyler (1968)
Mosses, collected 1968	Rural	100	Ruhling and Tyler (1968)
Ferns (fronds)	Various	<0.8-50	Cannon (1976)
Grasses (stalks and leaves)	Wilderness	<0.8-5.6	Cannon (1976)
Herbs (stalks and leaves)	Wilderness	<1.2-3.0	Cannon (1976)
Shrubs (leaves)	Wilderness	0.6-8.2	Cannon (1976)
Deciduous trees (leaves)	Wilderness	<0.6-9.1	Cannon (1976)
Coniferous trees (branch tips)	Wilderness	1.0-10	Cannon (1976)
Tree rings, 1910-1920	Rural	1.9	Rolfe et al. (1977)
Tree rings, 1963-1973	Rural	7.9	Rolfe et al. (1977)
Vegetables (edible parts)	Market-basket samples	0.1-7.0	Ewing et al. (1979)
Fruits (edible parts)	Market-basket samples	0.1-3.0	Ewing et al. (1979)
Grains	Market-basket samples	0.16-2.6	Ewing et al. (1979)
Leafy vegetables	Market-basket samples	1-159	Ewing et al. (1979)
Potatoes	Market-basket samples	0.3-14	Ewing et al. (1979)
Invertebrates			
Earthworms	Within 3 m of road	331	Gish and Christensen (1973)
Earthworms	More than 50 m from road	38.5	Gish and Christensen (1973)

Woodlice and millipedes	0-30 m from road	50-700	Forbes and Sanderson (1978)
Sucking insects (composite)	Rural, away from road	5.4-7.8	Rolfe et al. (1977)
Sucking insects (composite)	Near traffic	15-29.5	Rolfe et al. (1977)
Chewing insects (composite)	Rural, away from road	4.8	Rolfe et al. (1977)
Chewing insects (composite)	Near traffic	57.5-77.4	Rolfe et al. (1977)
Predatory insects (composite)	Rural, away from road	5.5-10.4	Rolfe et al. (1977)
Predatory insects (composite)	Near traffic	39.6-99.1	Rolfe et al. (1977)
Vertebrates			
Frogs and toads	Rural and urban	2.7-3.5	Rolfe et al. (1977)
Songbirds, 5 sp. (bones)	Rural	6.9-41.3	Rolfe et al. (1977)
Songbirds, 5 sp. (bones)	Urban	9.1-213	Rolfe et al. (1977)
Small mammals, 8 sp. (whole)	Rural, away from road	2.7-7.4	Rolfe et al. (1977)
Small mammals, 8 sp. (whole)	Urban and near road	11.2-31.7	Rolfe et al. (1977)
Birds, 28 sp. (bone)	Rural background	4-26	Forbes and Sanderson (1978)
Doves (bone)	Rural	13	Forbes and Sanderson (1978)
Doves (bone)	Urban	84	Forbes and Sanderson (1978)
Rats (bone)	Rural	10.3	Forbes and Sanderson (1978)
Rats (bone)	Urban	200	Forbes and Sanderson (1978)
Small mammals (kidney)	Near road	7.0	Forbes and Sanderson (1978)
Small mammals (kidney)	Far from road	4.2	Forbes and Sanderson (1978)
Bats (whole body)	Near highway	49-145	Clark (1979)
Shrews (whole body)	Near highway	22-76	Clark (1979)
Mice and voles (whole body)	Near highway	6-22	Clark (1979)
Caribou (whole body)	Remote tundra	1.8-2.6	Forbes and Sanderson (1978)
Caribou diet (lichens)	Remote tundra	1.5-7.7	Forbes and Sanderson (1978)
Hamburger	Market-basket samples	0.25	Ewing et al. (1979)
Pork	Market-basket samples	0.5-1.3	Ewing et al. (1979)
Poultry and eggs	Market-basket samples	0.1-0.2	Ewing et al. (1979)
Turkey	Market-basket samples	2.9-3.4	Ewing et al. (1979)

the view that atmospheric lead is a significant source of the element in plants. Ter Haar (1970) measured lead in crops grown near highways and in greenhouses, and found no accumulation of atmospheric lead in 8 of 10 varieties. He measured some increase in lead levels in two species grown near highways, but concluded that even if all crops were grown at such sites the lead deposited on crops from the air could account for only 0.5 to 1.5 percent of the lead in the human diet. In contrast, most other investigations have shown more substantial contamination of crops by airborne lead. Lagerwerff (1971) grew radishes 200 m from a highway and estimated that 40 percent of the lead in the tops of the plants (but not in the edible roots) came from the air. Cannon and Bowles (1962) compared lead levels in vegetation at a rural site in Maryland and a remote site in New Mexico, and found a 5-fold greater amount of lead in the crops from the inhabited region. The same investigators showed a 10-fold increase in the lead content of grass in an urbanizing region of Denver, Colorado, associated with increasing automotive traffic, over a 10-year period (Cannon and Anderson 1971).

As investigative techniques have improved and the ability to reliably measure small differences in amounts of lead has increased, research has begun to suggest the magnitude of atmospheric contributions to the lead in plants with more clarity. Rabinowitz (1972) used isotopic tracers to distinguish soil lead from atmospheric lead contributions to the lead in oats and lettuce. His results suggested that more than 90 percent of the lead in lettuce grown in rural California was from the atmosphere. Elias et al. (1975) determined elemental ratios in organisms in a remote mountain ecosystem, and demonstrated a 10-fold increase of lead above natural background levels, attributed to an annual deposition flux of about 4 mg/m^2. Tjell et al. (1979) used lead-210 as a marker for soil uptake, and grew rye grass in a rural area of Denmark with a background level of lead deposition (about 12 mg/m^2/year). Results showed that only 0.2 to 10 percent of the lead in the grass at the end of the growing season came from soil.

These independently confirming results suggest that, even at rural and remote sites where atmospheric deposition of lead is at "background" levels, 90 to 99 percent of the lead in some varieties of plants may be atmospheric, and therefore anthropogenic, in origin. Research to date has involved too few reports to provide a general estimate of the origins of lead in crops, and in plant-derived human foods. The extent to which plants accumulate lead from the air depends on many species-specific factors, such as leaf size, configuration, and surface characteristics (Chamberlain 1966, 1974; Wedding et al. 1975). The degree to which lead deposited on leaves enters the human diet depends on the portions of plants consumed, and on whether lead is translocated within the plant. However, lead deposited on leaves and grasses also can affect human exposure indirectly, through the food chain.

Additional insights may be gained by studies of specific rates and mechanisms of transfer of atmospheric lead to plant surfaces of different types. Some research has attempted to measure the deposition of lead onto vegetation surfaces. Davidson and Friedlander (1978) reviewed the literature and conducted experiments on mechanisms and rates of atmospheric deposition of metals onto plants, using wild oat grass as a model; they concluded that plants are capable of significant scavenging of atmospheric lead. Lindberg (1979) measured mass transfers of several heavy metals in a deciduous forest watershed. He determined that 99 percent of the lead flux to the forest floor was deposited from the atmosphere, at an average rate of 15 mg/m^2/year. Dry deposition accounted for about 52 percent of the total flux, and vegetation (the forest canopy) initially captured almost all (88 percent) of the dry deposition flux. However, rainfall washed slightly more than half of the scavenged lead off the leaves; the net retention by the forest canopy was 22 percent of total annual deposition. Lindberg also measured deposition to individual leaf surfaces, and determined that the film remaining on leaves after a single dry/wet period of 7 days contained an amount of lead equivalent to approximately 70 percent of the total present in the leaf. Dry deposition over the growing season was found to deliver 1 to 2 orders of magnitude more lead to the leaf surface than was initially present in the entire leaf (Lindberg 1979).

Lead deposited from the atmosphere must be retained by the plant if the concentration of the element in vegetation is to increase. Cannon (1976) and Peterson (1978) reviewed reports in the literature that lead is not readily washed from the surfaces of plant samples. Peterson concludes that the fraction of the total lead in plants that can be removed by washing is about 50 percent on the average, with a range from 8 to 80 percent. Lindberg's data suggest that about half of the dustfall onto leaves is removed by rainfall; however, he also measured directly the degree to which deposited lead could be washed from leaves. Comparison of leaves and inert surfaces of sampling devices showed that an order of magnitude less lead could be washed from the leaves. Other substances studied (cadmium, zinc, manganese, and sulfate) exhibited no significant differences in leaching from the two surfaces. The results suggest that some vegetation surfaces may have a particular affinity for lead (Lindberg 1979).

There has been considerable scientific debate about the fate of lead that cannot be washed from plant surfaces. Most available evidence suggests that lead is not absorbed through the leaf cuticle (Cannon 1976, Peterson

1978), but several reports of apparent absorption of atmospheric lead by leaves have been published (Krause and Kaiser 1977, Zimdahl 1976). Particles also might be bound tightly to the external surface of the leaf. There is little information available on the extent to which lead deposited on leaves might be translocated to other portions of plants; in general, significant transfers of this sort appear unlikely (Zimdahl 1976).

In summary, a growing number of reliable recent reports appear to indicate that most of the lead content of typical vegetation, perhaps as much as 90 to 99 percent of the total lead in plants, originates with recent atmospheric pollution. This estimate cannot be applied yet to crops in general, and it specifically cannot be applied to edible portions of many crops. Nevertheless, it seems clear in a qualitative way that the present-day lead content of plant biomass, and therefore of most food chains, is substantially higher than natural levels.

A limited amount of historical evidence supports this qualitative conclusion. Samples of mosses from the 1860s in herbarium collections contained only 20 to 25 percent of the lead measured in recent specimens (Ruhling and Tyler 1968). Lee and Tallis (1973) measured 40- to 50-fold increases in the lead content of peat layers deposited from 3,000 years ago to the present, but the site was subject to contamination above background levels by nearby mining and industrial activities. Chronological increases of up to an order of magnitude have been observed in the lead content of tree rings, but the quantitative accuracy of the tree-ring record has been questioned because of possible translocation of lead within the xylem (Cannon 1976).

The reports by Elias et al. (1975) and Tjell et al. (1979), cited above, suggest that atmospheric deposition fluxes of lead of 4 to 12 mg/m^2/year can increase the lead content of vegetation by an order of magnitude or more. It was concluded previously (see section on Atmospheric Deposition, above) that deposition fluxes at some remote sites in the Southern Hemisphere may be an order of magnitude lower than those present in the recent studies. It seems possible, therefore, that plants growing at such remote locations may have lead levels much closer to (perhaps no more than double) the natural levels. The collection of more extensive data on the occurrence of lead in vegetation from unperturbed sites therefore seems essential, to indicate the extent to which typical levels of lead in plants in inhabited areas exceed natural levels.

Terrestrial Animals　The extensive literature on the lead content of wild and domestic animal species has recently been reviewed by Forbes and Sanderson (1978). Excessive accumulation of lead and associated toxic effects have been reported in livestock grazing near smelters, small mammals near roadways and mining sites, animals in urban zoos, waterfowl that have ingested lead shot, and other animals exposed to heavily contaminated forage, soil, air, water, paint, or lead wastes. The differences in body burdens of lead that occur in urban and rural populations of dogs, rats, pigeons, and songbirds exhibit striking parallels with those that occur in humans.

Typical, "normal" levels of lead in animals today are the result of general exposures to the metal via diet, air, and water which, as for humans, have been elevated above natural levels by human activities. As in the human case, an assessment of the magnitude and origin of the increase above natural body burdens is difficult, and most research on lead in animals has been concerned only with unusually high exposures.

Table 2.13 presents reported data on lead levels in organisms representing several trophic levels in terrestrial ecosystems. Relatively few data are available on the accumulation of lead by invertebrates. Earthworms and woodlice collected near roadways contained enough lead to pose a toxic hazard to predators (Forbes and Sanderson 1978). Levels in some specimens were elevated even at distances from the road at which soil lead was at background levels, suggesting that deposition on vegetation or sorption on soil organic matter may have contributed to the lead in the organisms' diets. Rolfe et al. (1977) reported decreasing lead levels in insects with distance from traffic sources. Predatory species had higher body burdens than herbivorous varieties, a difference that suggests some biomagnification in the food chain.

Extensive reports are available on the accumulation of lead in wild birds. Waterfowl and other game birds frequently have high levels of the metal in their tissues (often because of ingestion of lead shot), but most predatory birds have relatively low body burdens (Forbes and Sanderson 1978). Marked urban/rural differences in lead levels were noted in populations of five varieties of songbirds, but no differences could be attributed to dietary habits (Rolfe et al. 1977).

Most information on lead in wild mammals has been collected in reference to a particular source, usually a highway. Proximity to sources correlates strongly with lead levels in animals, as it does for levels in air, soil, and vegetation (Forbes and Sanderson 1978). Differences in feeding habits appear to be significant in mammals; insectivores (shrews and bats) accumulated higher levels of lead than herbivores (voles) or granivores (mice, ground squirrels) (Rolfe et al. 1977, Clark 1979). In each of the studies, lead residues in animals were generally lower than concentrations in their foods, which suggests that, as in aquatic ecosystems, lead levels in vertebrate food chains tend to decrease, rather than increase, at higher trophic levels. (As noted, however, invertebrate food chains may exhibit some biomagnification.)

Very few studies have been conducted on the occurrence of lead in animals in remote, uninhabited areas. Forbes and Sanderson (1978) cite two reports of elevated lead absorption in caribou and reindeer, attributed to accumulation of atmospheric lead by lichens and other forage plants. Elias et al. (1975) studied ecological transfers of lead in an alpine ecosystem in Yosemite National Park. They observed step-by-step diminutions of lead burdens (measured as Pb/Ca ratios) in a four-stage food chain; the total relative decrease in lead burden was about 30-fold between soil-forming rocks and a carnivorous mammal (Table 2.14).

Elias et al. (1975) also attempted to ascertain the effects of anthropogenic lead (atmospheric deposition, measured at 4 $mg/m^2/year$) on the flow of lead through the food chain, and to estimate natural lead burdens in wildlife. They concluded that anthropogenic lead increased natural exposures of animals by deposition onto vegetation, deposition onto soil followed by plant uptake, and deposition onto fur followed by ingestion through grooming or predation. Elias et al. estimated that exogenous lead had elevated body burdens in animals (Pb/Ca ratios) about 30-fold higher than natural burdens: i.e., that 97 percent of the lead in animals was anthropogenic in origin. They concluded that under natural ecological conditions the lead burdens (Pb/Ca ratios) in terrestrial animals should be about 3 orders of magnitude lower than those in the earth's crust (i.e., the observed 30-fold differences, multiplied by the 30-fold effect of exogenous lead).

Although present-day levels of lead in animals probably are greater than natural levels, the implications for human exposure remain unclear. As in humans, the lead burden in most vertebrates is primarily in the skeleton, and the effect of a general increase of lead in the food chain on levels of the metal in edible tissues is uncertain. There is little basis at present, therefore, for an estimate of the precise increase in the contribution of animal products to total human dietary intake of lead. However, Settle and Patterson (1979) addressed this problem and, by making certain assumptions, estimated that present levels are about 100-fold higher than natural levels of lead in the animal portions of the human diet. This highly tentative estimate is discussed further in the section on Lead in Human Diets, below.

Potential Hazards to Wildlife If evidence reviewed here is inconclusive on the matter of natural human dietary exposure, the available data suggest with some clarity that potential toxic effects of lead on animals

TABLE 2.14 Transfers of Lead and Barium in a Food Chain in a Small Subalpine Ecosystem in the Sierra Nevada Mountains

Food	Organism	Ba/Ca[a]	Pb/Ca[a]	Pb/Ca[a] Corrected for Contamination	Material Analyzed
	rock	30	0.35	0.35	Wall rocks
Plant food		10	0.23	0.12	Soil moisture
	sedge	2	0.045	0.0048	Sedge leaves
Herbivore food	herbivore	3	0.1 to 1.5	0.01 to <0.8	{ Pine cones, sedge leaves, feces
		0.09	0.0077	0.00029	{ Chipmunk, squirrels, voles
Carnivore food	carnivore	0.10	0.039	(?)	Feces, herbivores
		0.02	0.012	~-0.00039	Martens

[a] Atomic elemental ratios, ×1,000.

SOURCE: Elias et al. (1975).

themselves may be a more serious possibility than has heretofore been recognized. Under natural conditions, the observed diminution of lead burdens in terrestrial vertebrate food chains probably would limit accumulation of lead to very low levels in animals. But exogenous lead deposited on food bypasses part of the diminution process, as does inhaled or otherwise nondietary lead. The results reported by Elias et al. suggest that even in the absence of evident biomagnification, levels of lead in some animals may be 1 to 2 orders of magnitude higher than they are believed to be under natural conditions of exposure. This estimate is at present a rough approximation, and its general applicability has not been established. Improved information on this topic clearly is needed.

Current understanding of potential biological effects of lead in most domestic animals and wildlife species is considerably less definitive than comparable knowledge for humans. "Clinical lead poisoning" is well known in many species, although its incidence is difficult to verify (Forbes and Sanderson 1978). Potential subtle effects on behavior, reproduction, or other critical functions have been investigated only sparsely, and chiefly in laboratory animals and economically important livestock species. It was concluded in Case II that the margin between typical human exposures to lead and those that are potentially toxic is uncomfortably narrow. The same concern probably should be extended to myriad animal species, whose environments also are contaminated by lead, and whose sensitivity to the toxic effects of the element might equal or exceed our own.

Lead in Human Diets

In order to determine the extent to which present-day dietary exposure to lead is anthropogenic in origin, it is essential to establish a valid baseline. The needed information includes accurate measurements of present background levels of lead in foods, to assess the impacts of specific activities, such as canning. It also includes reliable estimates of natural background levels of lead in foods, to assess the impact of general environmental contamination by lead on human dietary exposure to the element.

Efforts to establish such baselines face several methodological obstacles. Although massive amounts of data exist on lead levels in various organisms (see reviews cited in Tables 2.12 and 2.13), the analytical accuracy of many of the data may be questioned (see Appendix D). It is therefore difficult to determine whether present-day background levels in foods have been accurately determined; if errors exist, they are most likely to involve overestimation of background levels. Regardless of the accuracy of the measurements, conventional data-gathering studies offer little insight into possible differences between modern background levels and natural levels of lead in plants and animals.

Viewed against the bulk of conventional data, the research by Patterson and his associates, discussed at several points in the sections above, is almost a unique body of evidence. For example, conventional data show wide measurement variations for specific food items and great differences among lead levels in various foods; estimates of current "typical" dietary intakes of lead, discussed in Cases I and II, therefore are only crude averages. Data reviewed in the section on lead in terrestrial food chains suggest that atmospheric deposition is a signficant source of lead in foods, but cannot provide a quantitative estimate. Conventional measurements also support the conclusion that lead levels in canned foods are generally about 2 or 3 times higher than levels in similar fresh foods (see Case I). While it is known qualitatively that cooking and processing also may add lead to foods, no general quantitative estimates of these additions are available.

In contrast, the work of Patterson and his associates suggests some different and much more specific conclusions. By assiduously controlling for contamination during sampling and analysis, Patterson's group has shown that organisms from remote areas contain substantially lower levels of lead than previously reported. This finding suggests that differences between "background" levels and typical levels of lead in domestic crops and animals probably have been underestimated. Using novel techniques to measure small geochemical transfers of lead in food chains from remote terrestrial and marine areas, Elias et al. (1975) and Burnett (1979) have developed estimates of natural levels of lead in a few organisms. The results indicate that most organisms, even at remote sites, contain 5 to 30 times more lead than they would under natural conditions, and that the source of this added lead is primarily deposition of anthropogenic lead aerosols. Settle and Patterson (1979) have inferred from this data base that human food chains in less remote, more heavily contaminated areas are subject to even greater elevations of lead levels above the natural range. Finally, they showed that if the lead concentration in fresh tuna fish is accurately measured, the increase due to canning and processing is not 2-fold, but 4,000-fold.

Taken as a whole, these results are consistent with the hypothesis that there has been a large increase above the natural level of lead in the diet. Settle and Patterson (1979) estimate that the general increase is about 2 orders of magnitude. However, this estimate is still extremely tentative. Although Patterson and his colleagues have avoided the problem of analytical inaccuracy and have developed an effective approach for discriminating between natural and anthropogenic transfers of lead in ecosystems, other methodological limitations still impose major uncertainties on current knowledge. The number and nature of the food chains examined to date are too small to support general estimates with confidence. It has not yet been determined whether the same quantitative geochemical relationships observed in a remote alpine food chain also occur in domesticated food chains (e.g., soil/air—corn—beef—humans). Patterson and his associates have emphasized the importance of examining elemental ratios (e.g., Pb/Ca) as geochemically more meaningful measures of the occurrence of lead than absolute concentrations of the metal, whereas other researchers have generally reported only lead levels. This fact, and differences in analytical reliability, make it difficult to determine by reference to other work whether the results published by Patterson's group are consistent with or contradictory to other evidence.

Conclusions Conventional research approaches have thus far largely failed to shed light on the important question of the magnitude to which human dietary exposure to lead may have been increased by the dispersal of lead in the environment. The approach developed by Patterson and colleagues seems better suited to address that problem, and has already produced some provocative results. The answers generated thus far cannot be regarded as more than tentative, but this research has certainly set the stage for future attacks on the problem.

While it is supported by very few data, Settle and Patterson's estimate that the human diet now contains about 2 orders of magnitude more lead than it did under natural conditions is probably the best available estimate and deserves to be treated as a serious working hypothesis. That hypothesis is consistent with evidence presented in earlier sections that the level of lead in the air in inhabited regions is 2 to 4 orders of magnitude higher than natural levels, and that lead deposited from the air may enter food chains in significant amounts. Furthermore, evidence to be discussed in Step 4, below, suggests that the level of lead in the body of a typical present-day American is 2 to 3 orders of magnitude higher than levels in pretechnological, prehistoric humans. None of these estimates is presently more than an order-of-magnitude approximation; taken together, however, they form a consistent picture that suggests that the general increase in environmental lead levels is reflected in the human diet.

Because the question of human impacts on dietary exposure to lead is central to pending policy actions (see Appendix C), research to improve the basis for quantitative estimates is an important need. It is essential that other investigators apply the methods and models developed by Patterson and his associates to other ecosystems, and obtain data that can corroborate, modify, and refine the results so far available. It is clear that careful attention to contamination controls in sampling and analysis should be a fundamental part of such research. Further insights into the rigor of the methods and better estimates of baseline levels of lead in foods can be gained by additional studies of ecological transfers of lead both in remote, relatively unperturbed ecosystems and in the more heavily contaminated ecosystems that produce the staples of the human diet. Because of differences between estimated dietary exposures of Americans and those of Scandinavians (discussed in Case II), it would be valuable to replicate such studies in at least those two different industrialized regions.

Summary of Natural Exposures

Table 2.15 summarizes current estimates of natural levels of lead in the environment, and compares those estimates with typical present-day levels, discussed in Case II. The ranges of values in the table reflect both the heterogeneity of the natural world and the uncertainties associated with a small number of data points. The estimated differences between the typical natural level and typical present-day levels of lead in various media are meant only as tentative, order-of-magnitude approximations, and will be subject to revision as knowledge improves. However, the table makes it clear that the greatest increases in exposure above natural levels have occurred in air and diet, the two media that contribute most to typical urban residents' present-day exposures (see Table 2.6). Levels of lead in soils and fresh water have increased only slightly, if at all; but these two environmental pools contribute much less to direct human exposure, at least in typical adults.

Despite the quantitative uncertainties, a general qualitative conclusion is depicted in Figure 2.9. In the strictest terms, no place on the Earth's surface has been completely unaffected by atmospheric dispersal of lead aerosols. Nevertheless, evidence reviewed here suggests that there are probably some sites at which the natural cycle of lead in terrestrial ecosystems has been perturbed only slightly in comparison to sites that have been studied. Relatively pristine conditions are most likely to be found in the Southern Hemisphere, especially in areas remote ($>1,000$ km) from urban centers or industrial sources of lead emissions. Populations residing in such regions may experience very low exposures to lead, especially if they are at a premetallurgical stage of technological development, subsist on native diets, and have little cultural exchange with the outside world. Conditions in such present-day primitive cultures might not be totally representative of typical, prehistoric exposures to lead. However, as Figure 2.9 shows, the hypothetical natural range and the range of present-day remote, relatively undisturbed exposures probably overlap to a significant degree.

It seems highly probable, therefore, that knowledge about approximate

TABLE 2.15 Comparison of Estimated Natural Levels of Lead in the Environment with Typical Present-Day Levels

Medium	Estimated Natural Lead Concentrations	Typical Present-Day Lead Concentrations[a]	Approximate Ratio, Present-Day/Natural
Air			
Rural/remote	0.01-0.1 ng/m^3	0.1-100 ng/m^3	10-1,000
Inhabited	0.1-1.0 ng/m^3	0.1-10 µg/m^3	100-10,000
Soil			
Rural/remote	5-25 µg/g	5-50 µg/g	1-2
Inhabited	5-25 µg/g	10-5,000 µg/g	2-200
Water			
Fresh	0.005-10 µg/l	0.005-10 µg/l	1
Ocean	0.001 µg/l	0.005-0.015 µg/l	10
Foods	0.0001-0.1 µg/g	0.01-10 µg/g	100

[a] See Cases I and II for basis for estimates of typical present-day levels.

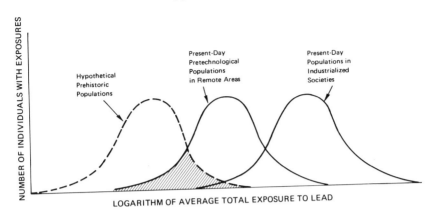

FIGURE 2.9 A qualitative comparison of exposures to lead encountered by pretechnological human populations exposed only to natural sources in prehistoric times, present-day pretechnological populations, and present-day populations of industrialized nations. The shaded zone suggests populations that, if studied, might provide additional insights into natural conditions of exposure to lead. Present data are inadequate to determine the exact degree of overlap between the three curves, or the precise form of the curves (see text for discussion).

natural exposures to lead and other topics examined here could be improved substantially if such sites could be identified, and levels and critical transfers of lead there could be accurately measured.

Step 4: ESTABLISH THE ASSOCIATION BETWEEN EXPOSURE AND LEAD IN THE BODY FOR THE SPECIFIC POPULATION

Four approaches can be used to estimate natural levels of lead in the human body. The first is to use a simple exposure/absorption model to calculate daily uptake of lead. A second approach relies on attempts to locate populations with extremely low exposures to lead, and to measure levels of lead in their bodies. It is also possible to measure the lead content of human tissues that have been preserved from ancient, premetallurgical cultures. Finally, the theoretical natural burden of lead in humans might be predicted from studies of the natural geochemistry of the element.

Exposure/Absorption Estimate

Table 2.16 presents a hypothetical set of assumed conditions of exposure to and absorption of lead under natural conditions. The same approach was used in Cases I and II earlier in this chapter (see Tables 2.2 and 2.6);

TABLE 2.16 Estimated Exposures to and Absorption of Lead for a Typical Adult under Arbitrarily Defined Natural Conditions[a]

Route of Exposure	Concentration of Lead in Environment	Amount Inhaled or Ingested Per Day	Absorption Factor	Amount of Lead Absorbed (μg/day)	Percent of Total Lead Absorbed
Air	$0.0001\ \mu g/m^3$	$20\ m^3$	0.4	0.0008	0.03
Water	$1\ \mu g/l$	2 l	0.1	0.2	8.5
Diet	$0.01\ \mu g/g$	2,000 g	0.1	2.0	85.1
Soil	$15\ \mu g/g$	0.1 g	0.1	0.15	6.4
TOTAL				2.35	100.0

[a] The values selected for the exposure variables are, arbitrarily, the approximate midpoints of wide ranges (see Table 2.15). The value and limitations of making such assumptions are discussed in the text.

the usefulness and limitations of the methodology were discussed in those earlier sections. However, additional caution is needed when this approach is applied to the natural background case. Because of the uncertainties associated with estimates of natural levels of lead (discussed in previous sections), the choice of specific values for those variables in this case is relatively arbitrary. The estimated level of lead in air shown in Table 2.16 represents the approximate midpoint of the natural range. Values shown for lead in soil and water are only slightly lower than typical present concentrations in these media; there is no persuasive scientific basis to support the selection of other values. The estimated natural levels of lead in foods are based on data reviewed by Settle and Patterson (1979); this is acknowledged to be a very limited data base for such a general estimate. Plausible outcomes of this modeling approach could include both higher and lower estimates of total absorption than the one in Table 2.16. Despite currently irreducible uncertainties, the procedure followed is believed to be valuable, because even a crude, order-of-magnitude estimate of human absorption of lead under natural conditions offers some useful insights.

It is assumed here that the fractional absorption of lead from the human gastrointestinal tract and lung was comparable in ancient humans to that observed today, and that proportional uptake is unchanged over a 100-fold range of absolute exposures. However, the fractions of lead absorbed at very low levels of exposure are in fact unknown, and the possibility cannot be excluded that they might be significantly different from fractions absorbed at typical present-day levels of exposure.

The natural daily uptake of lead estimated in Table 2.16 is about 5 percent of the estimated amount absorbed by a typical present-day urban resident (Table 2.6). The distribution of lead in the body at very low levels of absorption is unknown, but it might reasonably be expected that most of the absorbed lead would be stored in the skeleton, and that the fraction of total body burden in blood and soft tissues would be small. Empirical relationships between blood lead levels and present-day exposures are nonlinear; that is, proportionally greater increases of blood lead levels are observed at low dose levels than at higher dose levels (see earlier sections). The physiological basis for this differential response is not well understood, and an extrapolation to predict "natural" blood lead levels is not feasible.

Present-Day Body Burdens in Populations with Low Exposure

A few measurements of blood lead levels in groups of individuals from several largely pretechnological cultures have been reported in the literature. The EPA (1977a) summarized reports of blood lead levels in Brazilian Indians, African Bushmen, New Guinea tribesmen, and other remote populations; mean lead levels reported were 12 to 23 μg/100 ml. However, it seems likely that spuriously high values may have been obtained; blood lead analysis is difficult and prone to positive error under even the best laboratory conditions (see Appendix D). Furthermore, no extensive assessment was conducted of environmental and dietary lead levels, and it could not be demonstrated that the populations examined had no significant exposure to lead of anthropogenic origin.

Three more recent studies have reported much lower blood lead levels in remote populations. Hecker et al. (1974) measured heavy metal body burdens in 90 Orinoco Indians of the Amazon River Basin, and observed a mean blood lead level of 0.83 μg/100 ml. Piomelli (1979) measured mean blood lead levels of 3.5 μg/100 ml in children and 3.4 μg/100 ml in adult residents of Nepal. Poole et al. (1979) sampled blood from children in a remote rural area of Papua, New Guinea, and reported an average blood lead level of 5.2 $\pm$ 2.5 μg/100 ml. These recent data suggest that if careful attention is paid to proper controls for contamination, lower, more accurate estimates of blood lead levels in remote populations than those previously published can be obtained.

Unfortunately, the limited data on blood lead levels of populations in remote regions have very rarely been supported by analyses of air, water, soils, or diets for lead content. Piomelli (1979) reported a mean air lead level of 0.022 μg/m^3 in the Nepalese village where blood lead measurements were obtained, but information on other possible sources of exposure is not available. No well-designed, systematic study of exposure and body burdens of lead in populations with very low blood lead levels has been carried out to date. Such research is the only presently practical way to obtain data on low levels of lead in living humans, and such studies should be encouraged before remaining modern-day primitive cultures become exposed to additional technological sources of lead.

Lead in Ancient Human Tissues

Barry (1978) reviewed reported lead levels in tissues, chiefly bones, from several hundred specimens of human remains preserved by mummification or burial. The use of such remains to estimate natural levels of lead in humans is subject to significant sources of possible error. First, some ancient cultures made extensive use of lead. Gilfillan (1965) suggested on the basis of lead burdens in Roman bones that lead poisoning was endemic in Roman times and may have contributed to the fall of the Roman Empire. Lead levels in bones from medieval and more recent cultures correspond well to archaeological evidence of use of lead artifacts, and can be useful for inferring historical human exposures to anthropogenic lead (Grandjean 1978).

An additional confounding factor is the possibility that lead levels in skeletal remains may have been altered after burial, either through exchange of lead with the soil moisture or through contamination with lead of anthropogenic origin. Unless it is reasonably certain that such changes have not occurred, measured levels may not represent natural levels, even in specimens from cultures that made no known use of lead. Such errors, and contamination during sample preparation and analysis, would tend to result in overestimation of natural levels, and underestimation of the degree to which present-day body burdens exceed natural levels.

Because of these limitations, relatively few studies of ancient bones meet criteria that permit inferences about natural levels of lead in humans. Grandjean and Holma (1973) measured lead in 136 skeletons from five cultural periods in Denmark; median lead values increased from less than 0.2 $\mu g/g$ (dry weight) in specimens more than 3,000 years old to 6.8 $\mu g/g$ in 250-year-old bones. Grandjean et al. (1979) reported an average lead content of 0.6 $\mu g/g$ in temporal bone and 0.9 $\mu g/g$ in dentine of 9 ancient Nubians who lived between 4,800 and 5,300 years ago in an arid, desert environment. Matched control samples from present-day Denmark contained about 10 times more lead in bones and 30 times more lead in teeth, and comparable analyses of teeth from Philadelphia contained 200 times more lead than the Nubian samples. In a similar study, Ericson et al. (1979) measured an average lead content of 1 $\mu g/g$ in bones and 0.11 $\mu g/g$ in tooth enamel of 6 partial skeletons of Peruvian Indians from a desert archaeological site dating back 1,400 to 2,000 years. Specimens from 4 individuals were excluded because of evidence of more recent contamination; the lead content of the remaining 2 skeletons, normalized to a mean age of 45 years, was 0.08 $\mu g/g$.

Considering the possible sources of error, the available data are relatively consistent. Typical levels of lead in present-day human bones are about 5 to 30 $\mu g/g$, and in teeth, 5 to 200 $\mu g/g$ (Barry 1978). The reported values from ancient bones (0.08 to 0.6 $\mu g/g$), dentine (0.9 $\mu g/g$), and tooth enamel (0.1 $\mu g/g$) are therefore roughly 1 to 3 orders of magnitude lower than typical present levels. Some uncertainty remains as to whether the available measurements actually represent unaltered, natural skeletal burdens of lead; and the sites from which suitable remains have been obtained are too few to represent the full range of variation of natural human environments. Nevertheless, the available data suggest that present-day lead burdens in Scandinavian adults are 1 to 2 orders of magnitude higher than natural levels, and skeletal burdens in Americans may be 2 to 3 orders of magnitude higher than natural levels. The difference observed between Scandinavians and Americans may be related to a difference in dietary exposures, suggested by the recent report by Schutz (1979), discussed in Case II.

Although the evidence supports a conclusion that natural levels of lead in bones are 0.001 to 0.1 times current typical levels, it does not necessarily follow that natural concentrations of lead in blood and soft tissue are the same degree lower than typical present-day levels. A qualitative inference of this sort may be justified, but the dynamics of low levels of lead in the body are too poorly known to permit quantitative estimates.

Prediction from Ecosystem Studies

Knowledge of natural ecological transfers of lead (Table 2.14) has been used to predict the expected occurrence of lead in an organism in an ecological niche analogous to that of humans, i.e., an omnivore at a high level in the food chain. Ericson et al. (1979) used this approach to estimate Pb/Ca and Ba/Ca ratios in human bones under natural conditions, then compared predicted values with measured values in modern bones and in the ancient Peruvian skeletons described above. The results, summarized in Table 2.17, show that the predicted abundance of barium is close to the observed ratio in all cases, and that the lead content of ancient Peruvian bones is also close to the expected level. However, the Pb/Ca ratios in bones of British and American adults are between 350 and 600 times higher than those of the ancient Peruvian bones. This result is consistent with the range of natural lead levels in bones inferred from lead content alone in the previous section, and appears to confirm the approximate magnitude of the historical increase.

Step 5: ESTABLISH THE ASSOCIATION BETWEEN LEAD IN THE BODY AND BIOLOGICAL CHANGE IN THE SPECIFIC POPULATION

No research has been conducted to determine the health status of populations exposed to natural levels of lead. As noted earlier in this chapter, populations commonly used as "normal" control groups in studies of atypically high exposures have frequently had blood lead levels of 10 to 30 μg/100 ml. Conclusions presented in Step 4 suggest that such "control" lead levels could be from 10- to 1,000-fold higher than natural levels. This observation has fueled speculation that "normal" people might exhibit adverse biological effects of lead if they could be compared to a valid (natural) control population (Patterson 1965, Settle and Patterson 1979).

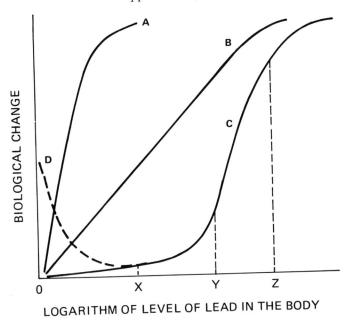

FIGURE 2.10 Possible general forms of the dose–effect curve for biological change associated with lead in the body. Because of a lack of data about effects of low levels of exposure to lead, all three curves are hypothetical, and research is needed to determine which, if any, of the alternatives best fits the true dose–effect relationship (see text for discussion).

TABLE 2.17 Predicted and Measured Ba/Ca and Pb/Ca Ratios in Ancient and Modern Human Skeletons

	Atomic Elemental Ratios	
Material	Ba/Ca	Pb/Ca
Average crustal abundance	3×10^{-3}	6.4×10^{-5}
Predicted in human bones	3×10^{-6}	3×10^{-8}
Measured, Peruvian bones	2.5×10^{-6}	6×10^{-8}
Measured, British bones	7×10^{-6}	2.1×10^{-5}
Measured, American bones	2.9×10^{-6}	3.5×10^{-5}

SOURCE: Data from Ericson et al. (1979).

There is insufficient knowledge at present either to support such speculation or to dismiss it as unfounded. The essential lack of information is ignorance of the shape of the dose–effect and dose–response curves in the region between typical present-day doses and estimated natural doses. As Figure 2.10 shows, several relationships could exist. Curves A and B imply that any dose of lead, perhaps even a naturally occurring exposure, could induce biological changes in direct proportion to exposure. Curve C, on the other hand, suggests a minimal biological response to lead over some range, and a threshold of toxicity at which tolerance to lead is overcome by increasing exposure. Finally, Curve D suggests yet another possibility, that lead might be essential for some biological process, and that biological changes due to deficiency of the element might be observed at very low levels of exposure. All of these possibilities are at present speculative, because biological effects of lead in the very low dose ranges have not yet been measured.

Recently proposals have been made (e.g., Settle and Patterson 1979) concerning the nature of assumptions and policies that should be adopted in the face of ignorance of the biological implications of current exposure to lead. If the assumption is that either Curve A or Curve B represents the true biological relationship, it follows that typical present-day humans may be suffering undetected toxic effects of lead. That hypothesis would demand further evaluation and, if confirmed, could suggest a need for substantial further reduction in typical exposure to lead. On the other hand, acceptance of Curve C implies the existence of either a tolerance capacity or natural protective mechanisms against lead toxicity. If it could be demonstrated that typical exposures to lead do not exceed normal tolerance levels, reductions in exposure might be required only insofar as needed to ensure that there were few or no individuals with exposures above the point of inflection on the curve. Curve D would suggest that an optimal level of exposure, too low to pose toxic hazards but not so low as to create a deficiency condition, might be defined by future research.

There is some evidence that Curve C may be a reasonable approximation of the true function. For instance, it has been suggested that both skeletal sequestration and the localization of lead in nuclear inclusion bodies within cells may serve to isolate the metal from sites of potential physiological effects. The possibility also has been raised that, during 5,000 years of exposures to lead, the human population may have acquired some tolerance or ability to compensate for effects of the element, through adaptation and evolution (J. J. Chisolm, personal communication, 1979).

The scientific basis for these arguments at present is primarily speculative. The hypothesis that observed storage processes serve in protective capacities is unsupported by specific biochemical evidence of differences in toxic effects of lead that can be attributed to the processes. Nevertheless, the hypothesis is one that deserves examination through further research. Tolerance, if it exists, would probably involve homeostatic mechanisms that regulate the compartmentalization of lead within the body. Studies comparing the movement of lead into and out of various physiological pools, particularly bones and blood, in populations with different degrees of exposures could suggest whether adaptive mechanisms exist, and how they regulate the distribution of lead in the body.

If Curve C is assumed to apply, present knowledge cannot indicate where current typical levels of lead in the body fall on the curve. If the present range of ordinary exposures is represented by Segment OX of the curve, typical body burdens might pose a minimal hazard of biological effects. On the other hand, if Segment XZ spans typical present-day body burdens of lead, any natural tolerance that might exist probably would be stressed beyond its protective capacity in some individuals. Segment XY in this case would represent a range in which modest reductions in exposure could bring about significant decreases in the risk of biological effects.

Evidence that a protective mechanism of another sort has been overridden by present-day levels of lead in the environment was discussed in Step 3. Consistent observations in wildlife food chains suggest that organisms at higher trophic levels have progressively smaller relative body burdens of lead, because the element is absorbed only inefficiently from the diet, the chief natural source of exposure. Although this process probably would limit the lead content of humans to low levels under natural conditions of exposure, evidence discussed in Step 4 suggests that present-day exposures result in elevated body burdens in typical Americans (as indicated by skeletal accumulation) that are 2 to 3 orders of magnitude above the natural range. It may therefore be reasonable to infer that protective mechanisms that are adequate over the likely range of natural exposures to lead may be unable to adapt to exposures 100- or 1,000-fold higher.

Present evidence that lead might be an essential element is scanty, and provides no basis for judging where the inflection point in Curve D might fall. Schwarz (1975) maintained rats on a highly purified, low-lead diet, and observed slight impairments of growth in comparison with a lead-fed group. However, Schwarz himself could not successfully repeat the experiment, and similar studies have turned up generally negative evidence. Data from Patterson and others suggest that the present-day lead levels in most organisms are 1 to 2 orders of magnitude higher than natural levels (see Step 3, above). It may therefore be assumed that, even if lead should eventually be found to be essential, there would be no realistic probability of observing a deficiency condition, other than in stringently contamination-free laboratories.

In summary, present knowledge is insufficient to determine whether Curve A, B, C, or D represents the best assumption about biological effects of lead. Even if Curve C or D is chosen, the location of the critical points of inflection relative to the range of typical levels of lead in humans is unknown. This uncertainty makes it difficult to estimate the potential health significance of typical present-day levels of lead in humans. Improved understanding of differences between natural and typical levels of lead in the body and of biological implications of such differences could have an important impact on current and future policy decisions.

Research approaches to improve the basis for estimating natural levels of exposure to lead were discussed earlier in this section. The need for improved knowledge of potential biological effects of typical and lower exposures to lead was discussed in Step 5 of the general exposure case, earlier in this chapter. Only two aspects need emphasis here. First, useful knowledge might be gained by careful assessments of the health status of remote, primitive, present-day populations with very low levels of lead in their bodies. However, the number of confounding variables likely to be present in a cross-cultural epidemiological study is enormous, and would make valid comparisons with Americans all but impossible on some aspects, such as effects on cognitive functions. It would therefore be essential to use a population similar to the group studied in all possible ways (except for lead burdens) as a basis for comparison. Less difficulty would probably be encountered in experimental studies using animals or laboratory preparations. In this case, the primary concern would be control of exogenous lead contamination (in air, dust, animal feeds, water) to guarantee that observations included meaningfully low "control" exposures. Such techniques have already been used in research to examine the potential essentiality of trace elements, and ought to be adaptable to low-level toxicological tests as well.

Elias and Patterson (1979) have raised a significant methodological issue in regard to animal experiments on effects of low doses of lead. Their research suggests that "normal" levels of lead in the bodies of most animals are at least 1 to 2 orders of magnitude greater than natural levels. They argue that such animals would not be suitable as "unexposed" controls for toxicological studies, and that it may be necessary to raise several generations of mice in virtually contamination-free "sanctuaries" in order to produce a strain with very low body burdens that can more reasonably be assumed to be in a natural state with respect to biological effects of lead.

The likelihood that such research would reveal hitherto unsuspected beneficial or toxic effects of average exposures to lead cannot be predicted. However, the implications of a more definitive answer to this question are serious and far-reaching, whether the answer turns out positive or negative. It therefore seems justified to devote some nonnegligible fraction of research support on biological effects of lead to the study of potential biological consequences of very low levels of exposure.

REFERENCES

Alexander, F.W., H.T. Delves, and B.E. Clayton (1973) The uptake and excretion by children of lead and other contaminants. Pages 319–330, Environmental Health Aspects of Lead. Luxembourg: Commission of the European Communities.

Anderson, C. and K.D. Danylchuk (1977) The effect of chronic low level lead intoxication on the haversian remodeling system in dogs. Laboratory Investigation 37(5):466–469.

Angle, C.R. and M.S. McIntire (1979) Airborne lead and children—the Omaha study. Journal of Toxicology and Environmental Health 4(5): (in press).

Barltrop, D. (1978) Absorption of ingested lead by children. Paper presented at Second International Symposium on Environmental Lead Research, sponsored by the International Lead Zinc Research Organization, Inc., and the University of Cincinnati. Cincinnati, Ohio, December 1978.

Barr, M., H. Meinrath, and R. Isherwood (1979) Research into lead pollution. (Letter) The Lancet, June 16, 1979, p. 1289.

Barry, P.S.I. (1978) Distribution and storage of lead in human tissues. Pages 97–150, The Biogeochemistry of Lead in the Environment, Part B, edited by J.O. Nriagu. New York: Elsevier/North Holland Biomedical Press.

Beattie, A.D., M.R. Moore, A. Goldberg, M.J.W. Finlayson, J.F. Graham, E.M. Mackie, J.C. Main, D.A. McLaren, R.M. Murdoch, and G.T. Stewart (1975) Role of chronic low-level lead exposure in the aetiology of mental retardation. The Lancet 1(7907):589–598.

Beckman, L. (1978) The Ronnskar Smelter—occupational and environmental effects in and around a polluting industry in northern Sweden. Ambio 7(5–6):226–231.

Benninger, L.K. (1978) ^{210}Pb balance in Long Island Sound. Geochimica et Cosmochimica Acta 42:1165–1174.

Benninger, L.K., D.M. Lewis, and K.K. Turekian (1975) The use of natural Pb-210 as a heavy metal tracer in the river–estuarine system. Pages 202–210, Marine Chemistry in the Coastal Environment. ACS Symposium Series, No. 18, edited by T.M. Church. Washington, D.C.: American Chemical Society.

Betts, P.R., R. Astley, and D.N. Raine (1973) Lead intoxication in children in Birmingham. British Medical Journal 1:402–406.

Billick, I.H. and V.E. Gray (1978) Lead Based Paint Poisoning Research: Review and Evaluation, 1971–1977. Office of Policy Development and Research. Washington, D.C.: U.S. Department of Housing and Urban Development.

Billick, I.H., A.S. Curran, and D.R. Shier (1979) Relation of pediatric blood levels to lead in gasoline. (Unpublished manuscript)

Boutron, C. (1979) Past and present day tropospheric fallout fluxes of Pb, Cd, Cu, Zn and Ag in Antarctica and Greenland. Geophysical Research Letters 6(3):159–162.

Bull, R.J., S.D. Lutkenhoff, G.E. McCarty, and R.G. Miller (1979) Delays in the postnatal increase of cerebral cytochrome concentrations in lead-exposed rats. Neuropharmacology 18: 83–92.

Burnett, M. (1979) Occurrences and Distributions of Ca, Sr, Ba, and Pb in Marine Food Chains. Ph.D. Dissertation, Division of Geological and Planetary Sciences, California Institute of Technology, Pasadena.

Byers, R.K. and E.E. Lord (1943) Late effects of lead poisoning on mental development. American Journal of Diseases of Children 66:471–494.

Cannon, H.L. (1976) Lead in vegetation. Pages 53–72, Lead in the Environment, edited by T.G. Lovering. U.S. Geological Survey Professional Paper 957. Washington, D.C.: U.S. Department of the Interior.

Cannon, H.L. and B.M. Anderson (1971) The geochemist's involvement in the pollution problem. Pages 153–177, Environmental Geochemistry in Health and Disease. Geological Society of America Memorandum No. 123, Edited by H.L. Cannon and H.C. Hopps. Washington, D.C.: Geological Society of America.

Cannon, H.L. and J.M. Bowles (1962) Contamination of vegetation by tetraethyl lead. Science 137:765–766.

Center for Disease Control (1978) Preventing Lead Poisoning in Young Children. Publication No. 00-2629, U.S. Public Health Service. Atlanta, Ga.: U.S. Department of Health, Education, and Welfare.

Cermak, J.E. and R.S. Thompson (1977) Urban planning. Pages 229-239, Lead in the Environment, edited by W.R. Boggess. Washington, D.C.: National Science Foundation.

Chaiklin, H., J.J. Cook, M.E. Hayes, and V.B. Scanland (1974) Recurrence of lead poisoning in children. Social Work 19(2):196–200.

Chamberlain, A.C. (1966) Transport of *Lycopodium* spores and other small particles to rough surfaces. Proceedings of the Royal Society (London) 296:45–70.

Chamberlain, A.C. (1974) Travel and deposition of lead aerosols. Special Report No. AERE-R 7676, Environmental and Medical Sciences Division, U.K.A.E.A. Research Group. Harwell, England: Atomic Energy Research Establishment.

Chapman, R.E. and J.G. Kowalski (1979a) Guidelines for Cost-Effective Lead Paint Abatement. NBS Technical Note 971, National Bureau of Standards. Washington, D.C.: U.S. Department of Commerce.

Chapman, R.E. and J.G. Kowalski (1979b) Lead Paint Abatement Costs: Some Technical and Theoretical Considerations. NBS Technical Note 979, National Bureau of Standards. Washington, D.C.: U.S. Department of Commerce.

Chisolm, J.J., Jr. (1978) Heme metabolites in blood and urine in relation to lead toxicity and their determination. Advances in Clinical Chemistry 20:225–265.

Chisolm, J.J., Jr. and E. Kaplan (1968) Lead poisoning in childhood—comprehensive management and prevention. Journal of Pediatrics 73:942–950.

Chow, T.J. (1978) Lead in natural waters. Pages 185–218, The Biogeochemistry of Lead in the Environment, Part A, edited by J.O. Nriagu. New York: Elsevier/North Holland Biomedical Press.

Chow, T.J. and C.C. Patterson (1962) The occurrence and significance of lead isotopes in pelagic sediments. Geochimica et Cosmochimica Acta 16:263–308.

Clark, D.R., Jr. (1979) Lead concentrations: Bats vs. terrestrial small mammals collected near a major highway. Environmental Science and Technology 13(3):338–341.

Cole, J.F. (1979) Lead levels and children's psychologic performance. (Letter) New England Journal of Medicine 301(3):161–162.

Coplan, J. (1979) Lead levels and children's psychologic performance. (Letter) New England Journal of Medicine 301(3):162.

Corrin, M.L. and D.F.S. Natusch (1977) Physical and chemical characteristics of environmental lead. Pages 7–31, Lead in the Environment, edited by W.R. Boggess. Washington, D.C.: National Science Foundation.

Council for Agricultural Science and Technology (1976) Application of Sewage Sludge to Cropland: Appraisal of Potential Hazards of the Heavy Metals to Plants and Animals. Report No. 64. Ames, Iowa: Council for Agricultural Science and Technology.

Creason, J.P., D.I. Hammer, A.V. Colucci, L. Priester, and J. Davis (1976) Blood trace metals in military recruits. Southern Medical Journal 69:289–293.

David, O.J., J. Clark, and K. Voeller (1972) Lead and hyperactivity. The Lancet 2:900–903.

Davidson, C.I. (1979) Deposition of particles from turbulent flow in the free atmosphere. Proceedings of the 1979 Annual Meeting of the Fine Particle Society, Philadelphia, Pa., May 1979.

Davidson, C.I. and S.K. Friedlander (1978) A filtration model for aerosol dry deposition: Application to trace metal deposition from the atmosphere. Journal of Geophysical Research 83:2343–2352.

De la Burde, B. and M.S. Choate (1972) Does asymptomatic lead exposure in children have latent sequelae? Journal of Pediatrics 81:1088–1091.

De la Burde, B. and M.S. Choate (1975) Early asymptomatic lead exposure and development at school age. Journal of Pediatrics 87:638–664.

Drill, S., J. Konz, H. Mahar, and M. Morse (1979) The Environmental Lead Problem: An Assessment of Lead in Drinking Water from a Multi-Media Perspective. Office of Drinking Water. EPA-570/9-79-003. Washington, D.C.: U.S. Environmental Protection Agency.

Duce, R.A., G.L. Hoffman, and W.H. Zoller (1975) Atmospheric trace metals at remote northern and southern hemispheric sites: Pollution or natural? Science 187:59–61.

Duce, R.A., G.T. Wallace, and B.J. Ray (1976) Atmospheric trace metals over the New York Bight. National Oceanographic and Atmospheric Administration Technical Report ERL 361-MESA 4. Washington, D.C.: U.S. Department of Commerce.

Durfor, C.N. and E. Becker (1964) Public water supplies of the 100 largest cities in the United States, 1962. U.S. Geological Survey Water Supply Paper 1812. Washington, D.C.: U.S. Government Printing Office.

Elias, R.W. and C.C. Patterson (1979) The toxicological implications of biogeochemical studies of atmospheric lead. Proceedings of the Twelfth Annual Rochester International Conference on Environmental Toxicology. Rochester, N.Y.: University of Rochester. (In press)

Elias, R.W., Y. Hirao, and C.C. Patterson (1975) Impact of present levels of aerosol Pb concentrations on both natural ecosystems and humans. Pages 257–271, Proceedings of the International Conference on Heavy Metals in the Environment, Volume 2, Part 1, edited by T.C. Hutchinson. Toronto: Institute for Environmental Sciences, University of Toronto.

Environmental Defense Fund (1975) Comments by the Environmental Defense Fund on the Environmental Protection Agency's Proposed Interim Primary Drinking Water Standards. Washington, D.C.: The Environmental Defense Fund, Inc.

Ericson, J.E., H. Shirahata, and C.C. Patterson (1979) Skeletal concentrations of lead in ancient Peruvians. New England Journal of Medicine 300(17):946–951.

Ewing, B.B. and J.E. Pearson (1974) Lead in the environment. Advances in Environmental Science and Technology 3:1–126.

Ewing, R.A., M.A. Bell, and G.A. Lutz (1979) The Health and Environmental Impacts of Lead: An Assessment of the Need for Limitations. Office of Toxic Substances. EPA-560/2-79-001. Washington, D.C.: U.S. Environmental Protection Agency.

Fishman, M.J. and J.D. Hem (1976) Lead content of water. Pages 35–41, Lead in the Environment, edited by T.G. Lovering. U.S. Geological Survey Professional Paper 957. Washington, D.C.: U.S. Department of the Interior.

Forbes, R.M. and G.C. Sanderson (1978) Lead toxicity in domestic animals and wildlife. Pages 225–277, The Biogeochemistry of Lead in the Environment, Part B, edited by J.O. Nriagu. New York: Elsevier/North Holland Biomedical Press.

Gale, N.L., M.G. Hardie, J.C. Jennett, and A. Aleti (1972) Transport of trace pollutants in lead mining wastewaters. Pages 95–106, Trace Substances in Environmental Health, Volume VI, edited by D.D. Hemphill. Columbia, Mo.: University of Missouri.

Gibson, J.L. (1904) A plea for painted railings and painted walls of rooms as the source of lead poisoning amongst Queensland children. Australian Medical Gazette, April 1904, p. 149.

Gibson, J.L., W. Love, D. Hardie, P. Bancroft, and A.J. Turner (1892) Notes on lead poisoning as observed among children in Brisbane. Proceedings of the Intercolonial Medical Congress of Australasia, Third Session, p. 76.

Gilfillan, S.C. (1965) Lead poisoning and the fall of Rome. Journal of Occupational Medicine 7:53–60.

Gish, C.D. and R.E. Christensen (1973) Cadmium, nickel, lead and zinc in earthworms from roadside soil. Environmental Science and Technology 7:1060–1062.

Gonick, C. (1978) Investigation of the presence of a lead-binding protein in humans. Paper presented at the Second International Symposium on Environmental Lead Research, sponsored by the International Lead Zinc Research Organization, Inc., and the University of Cincinnati. Cincinnati, Ohio, December 1978.

Graham, P. (1979) Research into lead pollution. (Letter) The Lancet, May 12, 1979, pp. 1024–1025.

Grandjean, P. (1978) Widening perspectives of lead toxicity—a review of health effects of lead exposure in adults. Environmental Research 17:303–321.

Grandjean, P. (1979) Lead content of scalp hairs as an indicator of occupational lead exposure. Pages 311–318, Toxicology and Occupational Medicine, edited by W.B. Deichmann. New York: Elsevier/North Holland Biomedical Press.

Grandjean, P. and B. Holma (1973) A history of lead retention in the Danish population. Environmental Physiology and Biochemistry 3:268–273.

Grandjean, P. and T. Nielson (1979) Organolead compounds: Environmental health aspects. Residue Reviews 72:98–148.

Grandjean, P., O.V. Nielsen, and I.M. Shapiro (1979) Lead retention in ancient Nubian and contemporary populations. Journal of Environmental Pathology and Toxicology 2(3):781–787.

Greichus, Y.A., A. Greichus, B.D. Amman, D.J. Call, D.C.D. Hamman, and R.M. Pott (1977) Insecticides, polychlorinated biphenyls and metals in African lake ecosystems. I. Hartbeespoort Dam, Transvaal and Voelvlei Dam, Cape Province, Republic of South Africa. Archives of Environmental Contamination and Toxicology 6:371–383.

Guinee, V.F. (1972) Lead poisoning. American Journal of Medicine 52(3):283–288.

Hall, D.M. (1979) Lead levels and children's psychologic performance. (Letter) New England Journal of Medicine 301(3):161.

Hall, R.A., E.G. Zook, and G.M. Meaburn (1978) National Marine Fisheries Service Survey of Trace Elements in the Fishery Resource. National Oceanic and Atmospheric Administration Technical Report NMFS SSRF-721. Washington, D.C.: U.S. Department of Commerce.

Hanes, N.B., I.C. Bratina, and L.C. Brown (1979) Lead removal and bacterial growth in home water purifiers. American Water Works Association 1978 Annual Conference Proceedings. Denver, Colo.: American Water Works Association.

Harms, U., H.E. Dresher, and E. Huschenbeth (1977/1978) Further data on heavy metals and organochlorines in marine mammals from German coastal waters. Meeresforschung 26(3/4):153–161.

Harrison, R.M., R. Perry, and D.H. Slater (1975) The contribution of organic lead compounds to total lead levels in urban atmospheres. Pages 1783–1788, Proceedings of the International Symposium on Recent Advances in the Assessment of Health Effects of Environmental Pollution, Volume 3. Luxembourg: Commission of the European Communities.

Hecker, L., H.E. Allen, B.D. Dinman, and J.V. Neel (1974) Heavy metal levels in acculturated and unacculturated populations. Archives of Environmental Health 29:181–185.

Hem, J.D. (1976) Inorganic chemistry of lead in water. Pages 5–11, Lead in the Environment, edited by T.G. Lovering. U.S. Geological Survey Professional Paper 957. Washington, D.C.: U.S. Department of the Interior.

Hine, C.H., H.A. Lewis, J. Northrup, S. Hall, and J.W. Embree (1978) Kidney function in lead workers. Paper presented at the Second International Symposium on Environmental Lead Research, sponsored by the International Lead Zinc Research Organization, Inc., and the University of Cincinnati. Cincinnati, Ohio, December 1978.

Holtzman, R.B. (1978) Application of radiolead to metabolic studies. Pages 37–96, The Biogeochemistry of Lead in the Environment, Part B, edited by J.O. Nriagu. New York: Elsevier/North Holland Biomedical Press.

Hunter, J.M. (1977) The summer disease—an integrative model of the seasonality aspects of childhood lead poisoning. Social Science and Medicine 11:691–703.

Hunter, J.M. (1978) The summer disease—some field evidence on seasonality in childhood lead poisoning. Social Science and Medicine 12:85–94.

Jandl, J.H. (1978) Statement included in Comments of Lead Industries Association, Inc., on the Proposed National Ambient Air Quality Standard for Lead. Testimony presented before the U.S. Environmental Protection Agency, Docket OAQPS 77-1, Washington, D.C., March 17, 1978.

Jaworski, J.F. (1979) The Effects of Lead in the Canadian Environment. Associate Committee on Scientific Criteria for Environmental Quality, Environmental Secretariat. Publication Number NRC 16736. Ottawa, Canada: National Research Council, Canada.

Johnson, D.E., R.J. Prevost, J.B. Tillery, K.T. Kimball, and J.M. Hosenfeld (1978) Epidemiologic Study of the Effects of Automobile Traffic on Blood Lead Levels. Health Effects Research Laboratory, Office of Research and Development. EPA-600/1-78-055. Research Triangle Park, N.C.: U.S. Environmental Protection Agency.

Kennedy, F.D. (1978) The Childhood Lead Poisoning Prevention Program: An Evaluation. Environmental Health Services Division, Center for Disease Control, U.S. Public Health Service, Atlanta, Georgia. (Unpublished manuscript)

Klein, M.C. and M. Schlageter (1975) Non-treatment of screened children with intermediate blood lead levels. Pediatrics 56(2):298–302.

Koeppe, D.E., G.L. Rolfe, and K.A. Reinbold (1977) Environmental Contamination by Lead and Other Heavy Metals, Volume IV, Soil–Water–Air–Plant Studies. Urbana-Champaign, Ill.: Institute for Environmental Studies, University of Illinois.

Kramer, M.S. (1979) Lead levels and children's psychologic performance. (Letter) New England Journal of Medicine 301(3):161.

Krause, G.H.M. and H. Kaiser (1977) Plant response to heavy metals and sulphur dioxide. Environmental Pollution 12:63–71.

Lagerwerff, J.V. (1971) Uptake of cadmium, lead, and zinc from soil and air. Soil Science 111:129–138.

Landrigan, P.J., S.H. Gehlbach, B.F. Rosenblum, J.M. Shoults, R.M. Candelaria, W.M. Barthel, J.A. Liddle, A.L. Smrek, N.W. Staehling, and J.F. Sanders (1975) Epidemic lead absorption near an ore smelter: The role of particulate lead. New England Journal of Medicine 292:123–129.

Lantzy, R.J. and F.T. Mackenzie (1979) Atmospheric trace metals: Global cycles and assessment of man's impact. Geochimica et Cosmochimica Acta 43:511–525.

Layman, E.M., F.K. Millican, R.S. Lourie, and L.Y. Takahishi (1963) Cultural influences and symptom choice: Clay-eating customs in relation to the etiology of pica. Psychological Record 13:249.

Lee, J.A. and J.H. Tallis (1973) Regional and historical aspects of lead pollution in Britain. Nature 245:216–218.

Lepow, M.L., L. Brickman, M. Tillette, S. Markowitz, R. Robine, and J. Kapesh (1975) Investigation into the sources of lead in the environment of urban children. Environmental Research 10:415–426.

Lewis, D.M. (1977) The use of ^{210}Pb as a heavy metal tracer in the Susquehanna River system. Geochimica et Cosmochimica Acta 41:1557–1564.

Lilis, R., A. Fischbein, S. Diamond, H.A. Anderson, I.J. Selikoff, W.E. Blumberg, and J. Eisinger (1977) Lead effects among secondary lead smelter workers with blood lead levels below 80 μg/100 ml. Archives of Environmental Health 32(6):256–266.

Lilis, R., W. Blumberg, J. Valciukas, A. Fischbein, G. Andrews, and I.J. Selikoff (1979) Renal function impairment in secondary lead smelter workers: correlations with zinc protoporphyrin and blood lead levels. Report to the National Institute of Environmental Health Sciences, May 9, 1979. New York: Environmental Sciences Laboratory, Mount Sinai School of Medicine, City University of New York.

Lindberg, S.E. (1979) Mechanisms and Rates of Atmospheric Deposition of Selected Trace Elements and Sulfate to a Deciduous Forest Watershed. Ph.D. Dissertation, Florida State University, Tallahassee; Publication Number 129, Environmental Sciences Division. Oak Ridge, Tenn.: Oak Ridge National Laboratory.

Lynam, D.R. (1979) Lead levels and children's psychologic performance. (Letter) New England Journal of Medicine 301(3):162–163.

Mahaffey, K.R. (1978) Environmental exposure to lead. Pages 1–36, The Biogeochemistry of Lead in the Environment, Part B, edited by J.O. Nriagu. New York: Elsevier/North Holland Biomedical Press.

Mahaffey, K.R. and J.E. Vanderveen (1979) Nutrient–toxicant interactions: Susceptible populations. Environmental Health Perspectives 29:81–87.

Mahaffey, K.R., J.L. Annest, H.E. Barbanos, D. Cox, E. Gunther, R.S. Murphy, and W. Turner (1979) Preliminary Analysis of Blood Lead Concentrations: HANES II, 1976–1978. Paper presented at 13th Annual Conference on Trace Substances in Environmental Health, Columbia, Mo., June 1979.

Maxwell, C.M. and D.W. Nelson (1978) A lead emission factor for reentrained dust from a paved roadway. Office of Air Quality Planning and Standards. EPA-450/3-78-021. Research Triangle Park, N.C.: U.S. Environmental Protection Agency.

McCabe, E.B. (1979) Age and sensitivity to lead toxicity: A review. Environmental Health Perspectives 29:29–33.

McCusker, J. (1979) Longitudinal changes in blood lead level in children and their relationship to season, age, and exposure to paint or plaster. American Journal of Public Health 69(4):348–352.

Millican, F.K. and R.S. Lourie (1970) The child with pica and his family. Pages 333–348, The Child in His Family, edited by E.J. Anthony and C. Koupernik. New York: John Wiley and Sons.

Mok, K.K. and L.E. Smythe (1978) Forms of lead in Sydney city air. Search 9(1–2):49–50.

Moore, M.R. (1979) Prenatal Exposure to Lead. Paper presented at Conference on Low Level Lead Exposure During Childhood: The Clinical Implications of Current Research, June 14–15, 1979, Boston, Massachusetts.

Moore, M.R. and P.A. Meredith (1976) The association of delta-amino-laevulinic acid with the neurological and behavioral effects of lead exposure. Pages 363–371, Trace Substances in Environmental Health, Volume X, edited by D.D. Hemphill. Columbia, Mo.: University of Missouri.

Moore, M.R., P.A. Meredith, W.S. Watson, and B.C. Campbell (1979) The gastrointestinal absorption of 203-lead chloride in man. Paper presented at 13th Annual Conference on Trace Substances in Environmental Health, Columbia, Mo., June 1979.

Murozumi, M., T.J. Chow, and C.C. Patterson (1969) Chemical concentrations of pollutant lead aerosols, terrestrial dusts, and sea salts in Greenland and Antarctic snow strata. Geochimica et Cosmochimica Acta 33:1247–1294.

National Institute for Occupational Safety and Health (1978) Criteria for a Recommended Standard...Occupational Exposure to Inorganic Lead, Revised Criteria—1978. HEW (NIOSH) Publication No. 78-158. Washington, D.C.: U.S. Department of Health, Education, and Welfare.

National Research Council (1972) Lead: Airborne Lead in Perspective. Committee on Biologic Effects of Atmospheric Pollutants, Division of Medical Sciences. Washington, D.C.: National Academy of Sciences.

National Research Council (1976) Recommendations for the Prevention of Lead Poisoning in Children. Committee on Toxicology, Assembly of Life Sciences. Washington, D.C.: National Academy of Sciences.

National Research Council (1977) Drinking Water and Health. Safe Drinking Water Committee, Advisory Center on Toxicology, Assembly of Life Sciences. Washington, D.C.: National Academy of Sciences.

National Research Council (1978a) Geochemistry and the Environment. Volume III: Distribution of Trace Elements Related to the Occurrence of Certain Cancers, Cardiovascular Diseases, and Urolithiasis. A Report of the Workshop at South Seas Plantation, Captiva Island, Florida, October 1974. Subcommittee on the Geochemical Environment in Relation to Health and Disease, U.S. National Committee for Geochemistry, Assembly of Mathematical and Physical Sciences. Washington, D.C.: National Academy of Sciences.

National Research Council (1978b) The Tropospheric Transport of Pollutants and Other Substances to the Oceans. Report of the Workshop on Tropospheric Transport of Pollutants to the Ocean Steering Committee, Ocean Sciences Board, Assembly of Mathematical and Physical Sciences. Washington, D.C.: National Academy of Sciences.

National Research Council (1979) Airborne Particles. Subcommittee on Airborne Particles, Committee on Medical and Biologic Effects of Environmental Pollutants, Assembly of Life Sciences. Baltimore, Md.: University Park Press.

Needleman, H.L. (1979) Lead levels and children's psychologic performance. (Author's reply. Letter to the editor) New England Journal of Medicine 301(3):163.

Needleman, H.L. and A. Leviton (1979) Lead and neurobehavioural deficit in children. (Letter) The Lancet, July 14, 1979, p. 104.

Needleman, H.L., C. Gunnoe, A. Leviton, R. Reed, H. Peresie, C. Maher, and P. Barrett (1979) Deficits in psychologic and classroom performance of children with elevated dentine lead levels. New England Journal of Medicine 300(13):689–695.

Nozaki, Y., J. Thomson, and K.K. Turekian (1976) The distribution of ^{210}Pb and ^{210}Po in the surface waters of the Pacific Ocean. Earth and Planetary Science Letters 32:304–312.

Nriagu, J.O. (1978a) Lead in the atmosphere. Pages 137-184, The Biogeochemistry of Lead in the Environment, Part A, edited by J.O. Nriagu. New York: Elsevier/North Holland Biomedical Press.

Nriagu, J.O. (1978b) Lead in soils, sediments, and major rock types. Pages 15–72, The Biogeochemistry of Lead in the Environment, Part A, edited by J.O. Nriagu. New York: Elsevier/North Holland Biomedical Press.

Nriagu, J.O. (1979) Global inventory of natural and anthropogenic emissions of trace metals to the atmosphere. Nature 279:409–411.

Patterson, C.C. (1965) Contaminated and natural lead environments of man. Archives of Environmental Health 11:344–360.

Patterson, C.C. and D.M. Settle (1976) The reduction of order of magnitude errors in lead analyses of biological materials and natural waters by evaluating and controlling the extent and sources of industrial lead contamination introduced during sample collecting, handling, and analysis. Pages 321–351, Accuracy in Trace Analysis: Sampling, Sample Handling, and Analysis, edited by P. LaFleur. National Bureau of Standards Special Publication 422. Washington, D.C.: U.S. Department of Commerce.

Patterson, J.W. and P. Kodukula (1978) Heavy metals in the Great Lakes. Water Quality Bulletin 3(4):6–7.

Patterson, J.W. and J.E. O'Brien (1979) Control of lead corrosion. American Water Works Association Journal 71(5):264–271.

Perino, J. and C.B. Ernhart (1974) The relation of subclinical lead level to cognitive and sensorimotor impairment in black preschoolers. Journal of Learning Disorders 7:26–30.

Perlstein, M.A. and R. Attala (1966) Neurologic sequelae of plumbism in children. Clinical Pediatrics 5:292–298.

Peterson, P.J. (1978) Lead and vegetation. Pages 355-384, The Biogeochemistry of Lead in the Environment, Part B, edited by J.O. Nriagu. New York: Elsevier/North Holland Biomedical Press.

Piomelli, S. (1979) The effects of lead on heme metabolism. Paper presented at Conference on Low Level Lead Exposure During Childhood: The Clinical Implications of Current Research, June 14–15, 1979, Boston, Massachusetts.

Poole, C., M. Alpers, and L.E. Smythe (1979) Blood lead levels in Papua New Guinea children living in a remote area. (Manuscript submitted for publication)

Posner, H.S., T. Damstra, and J.O. Nriagu (1978) Human health effects of lead. Pages 173–224, The Biogeochemistry of Lead in the Environment, Part B, edited by J.O. Nriagu. New York: Elsevier/North Holland Biomedical Press.

Preer, J.R. and W.G. Rosen (1977) Lead and cadmium content of urban garden vegetables. Pages 399–405, Trace Substances in Environmental Health, Volume XI, edited by D.D. Hemphill. Columbia, Mo.: University of Missouri.

Provenzano, G. (1978) Motor vehicle lead emissions in the United States: An analysis of important determinants, geographic patterns and future trends. Air Pollution Control Association Journal 28(12):1193–1199.

Provenzano, G. (1979) Estimating the benefits of controlling low dose exposure. Paper presented at Conference on Low Level Lead Exposure During Childhood: The Clinical Implications of Current Research, June 14–15, 1979, Boston, Massachusetts.

Pueschel, S.M., L. Kopito, and H. Schwachman (1972) A screening and follow up study of children with an increased lead burden. Journal of the American Medical Association 333:462–466.

Rabinowitz, M. (1972) Plant uptake of soil and atmospheric lead in southern California. Chemosphere 4:175–180.

Rabinowitz, M., G.W. Wetherill, and J. Kopple (1975) Absorption, storage, and excretion of lead by normal humans. Pages 361–368, Trace Substances in Environmental Health, Volume IX, edited by D.D. Hemphill. Columbia, Mo.: University of Missouri.

Repko, J.D. and C.R. Corum (1979) Critical review and evaluation of the neurological and behavioral sequelae of inorganic lead absorption. CRC Critical Reviews in Toxicology 6(2):135–187.

Rice, C., A. Fischbein, R. Lilis, L. Sarkozi, S. Kon, and I.J. Selikoff (1978) Lead contamination in the homes of employees of secondary lead smelters. Environmental Research 15:375–380.

Rickard, D.T. and J.O. Nriagu (1978) Aqueous environmental chemistry of lead. Pages 219–284, The Biogeochemistry of Lead in the Environment, Part A, edited by J.O. Nriagu. New York: Elsevier/North Holland Biomedical Press.

Robbins, J.A. (1978) Geochemical and geophysical applications of radioactive lead. Pages 285–394, The Biogeochemistry of Lead in the Environment, Part A, edited by J.O. Nriagu. New York: Elsevier/North Holland Biomedical Press.

Robinson, E. and R.C. Robbins (1971) Emissions, Concentrations and Fate of Particulate Atmospheric Pollutants. American Petroleum Institute Publication 4076. Menlo Park, Calif.: American Petroleum Institute.

Robinson, J.W., L. Rhodes, and D.K. Wolcott (1975) The determination and identification of molecular lead pollutants in the atmosphere. Analytica Chimica Acta 78:474–480.

Rolfe, G.L. and K.A. Reinbold (1977) Environmental Contamination by Lead and Other Heavy Metals, Volume I, Introduction and Summary. Urbana–Champaign, Ill.: Institute for Environmental Studies, University of Illinois.

Rolfe, G.L., A. Haney, and K.A. Reinbold (1977) Environmental Contamination by Lead and Other Heavy Metals, Volume II, Ecosystem Analysis. Urbana–Champaign, Ill.: Institute for Environmental Studies, University of Illinois.

Ruddock, J.C. (1924) Lead poisoning in children with special reference to pica. Journal of the American Medical Association 82:1682.

Ruhling, A. and G. Tyler (1968) An ecological approach to the lead problem. Botaniska Notiser 121:321–342.

Ryan, J.P. and J.M. Hague (1977) Lead. Mineral Commodity Profiles, MCP-9, Bureau of Mines. Washington, D.C.: U.S. Department of the Interior.

Sachs, H. (1978) Prognosis for children with chronic lead exposure. Paper presented at Second International Symposium on Environmental Lead Research, sponsored by the International Lead Zinc Research Organization, Inc., and the University of Cincinnati. Cincinnati, Ohio, December 1978.

Sayre, J. (1978) Dust lead contribution to lead in children. Paper presented at Second International Symposium on Environmental Lead Research, sponsored by the International Lead Zinc Research Organization, Inc., and the University of Cincinnati. Cincinnati, Ohio, December 1978.

Sayre, J.W. and M.D. Katzel (1979) Household surface lead dust: Its accumulation in vacant homes. Environmental Health Perspectives 29:179–182.

Schaule, B. and C. Patterson (1979) The occurrence of lead in the Northeast Pacific and effects of anthropogenic inputs. In Proceedings of an International Experts Discussion on Lead: Occurrence, Fate, and Pollution in the Marine Environment, edited by M. Branica. Oxford: Pergamon Press. (In press)

Schroeder, H.A. (1974) The Poisons Around Us: Toxic Metals in Food, Air, and Water. Bloomington, Ind.: Indiana University Press.

Schutz, A. (1979) Cadmium and lead. Scandinavian Journal of Gastroenterology 14, Supplement 52:223–231.

Schwarz, K. (1975) Potential essentiality of lead. Archives of Industrial Hygiene and Toxicology 26, Supplement: International Symposium on Environmental Lead Research, pp. 13–28.

Servant, J. and M. Delapart (1979) Lead and Lead-210 in some surface waters of the southwestern part of France. Importance of atmospheric contribution. Environmental Science and Technology 13(1):105–107.

Settle, D.M. and C.C. Patterson (1979) Lead in albacore: Guide to lead pollution in Americans. Science:(in press).

Shapiro, I.M., A. Burke, G. Mitchell, and P. Bloch (1978) X-ray fluorescence analysis of lead in teeth of urban children *in situ*: Correlation between the tooth lead level and the concentration of blood lead and free erythroporphyrins. Environmental Research 17:46–52.

Shier, D.R. and W.G. Hall (1977) Analysis of Housing Data Collected in a Lead-Based Paint Survey in Pittsburgh, Pennsylvania, Part 1. Interagency Report 77-1250, National Bureau of Standards. Washington, D.C.: U.S. Department of Commerce.

Shirahata, H., R.W. Elias, C.C. Patterson, and M. Koide (1979) Chronological variations in concentrations and isotopic compositions of anthropogenic atmospheric lead in sediments of a remote subalpine pond. Geochimica et Cosmochimica Acta 43:(in press).

Siccama, T.G. and W.H. Smith (1978) Lead accumulation in a hardwood forest. Environmental Science and Technology 12(5):593–594.

Silbergeld, E.K. (1979) Role of altered heme synthesis in lead toxicity. Manuscript prepared for use of the Committee on Lead in the Human Environment. (Unpublished)

Silbergeld, E.K. and H.S. Adler (1978) Subcellular mechanisms of lead neurotoxicity. Brain Research 148:451–467.

Solomon, R.L. and D.F.S. Natusch (1977) Environmental Contamination by Lead and Other Heavy Metals. Volume III: Distribution and Characterization of Urban Dusts. Urbana–Champaign, Ill.: Institute for Environmental Studies, University of Illinois.

Stark, A.D., J.W. Meigs, R.H. Fitch, and E.R. DeLouise (1978) Family operational cofactors in the epidemiology of childhood lead poisoning. Archives of Environmental Health 33(5):222–226.

Strong, R.A. (1920) Meningitis, caused by lead poisoning, in a child of nineteen months. Archives of Pediatrics 37:532.

Task Group on the Reference Man (1975) International Commission on Radioactivity. New York: Pergamon Press.

Tepper, L.B. and L.S. Levin (1972) A survey of air and population lead levels in selected American communities. Environmental Quality and Safety, Supplement II:152–195.

Ter Haar, G. (1970) Air as a source of lead in edible crops. Environmental Science and Technology 4(3):226–229.

Ter Haar, G. and R. Aronow (1974) New information on lead in dirt and dust as related to the childhood lead problem. Environmental Health Perspectives 7:83–89.

Tidball, R.R. (1976) Lead in soils. Pages 43-52, Lead in the Environment, edited by T.G. Lovering. U.S. Geological Survey Professional Paper 957. Washington, D.C.: U.S. Department of the Interior.

Tjell, J.C., M.F. Hovmand, and H. Mosbaek (1979) Atmospheric lead pollution of grass grown in a background area in Denmark. Nature 280:425–426.

Turekian, K.K. (1977) The fate of metals in the oceans. Geochimica et Cosmochimica Acta 41:1139–1144.

Turekian, K.K., Y. Nozaki, and L.K. Benninger (1977) Geochemistry of atmospheric radon and radon products. Annual Review of Earth and Planetary Sciences 5:227–255.

Turner, R.R., S.E. Lindberg, and K. Talbot (1977) Dynamics of trace element export from a deciduous watershed, Walker Branch, Tennessee. Pages 661–680, Watershed Research in Eastern North America: A Workshop to Compare Results, Volume 1, edited by D.L. Correll. Edgewater, Md.: Chesapeake Bay Center for Environmental Studies, Smithsonian Institution.

Urban, D. (1976) Statistical Analysis of Blood Lead Levels of Children Surveyed in Pittsburgh, Pennsylvania: Analytical Methodology and Summary Results. National Bureau of Standards. Publication No. 76–1024. Washington, D.C.: U.S. Department of Commerce.

U.S. Bureau of Community Health Services and Center for Disease Control (1979) Joint statement: Lead poisoning in children. Bureau of Community Health Services. Rockville, Md.: U.S. Department of Health, Education, and Welfare.

U.S. Environmental Protection Agency (1977a) Air Quality Criteria for Lead. Office of Research and Development. EPA-600/8-77-017. Washington, D.C.: U.S. Environmental Protection Agency.

U.S. Environmental Protection Agency (1977b) Control Techniques for Lead Air Emissions. Office of Air Quality Planning and Standards. EPA-450/2-77-012. Research Triangle Park, N.C.: U.S. Environmental Protection Agency.

U.S. Environmental Protection Agency (1978) National Ambient Air Quality Standard for Lead. Office of Air, Noise, and Radiation and Office of Air Quality Planning and Standards. Research Triangle Park, N.C.: U.S. Environmental Protection Agency.

U.S. Environmental Protection Agency (1979) Lead: Ambient Water Quality Criteria. Criteria and Standards Division, Office of Water Planning and Standards. Washington, D.C.: U.S. Environmental Protection Agency.

U.S. Occupational Safety and Health Administration (1978) Occupational Exposure to Lead. Book I, Final Standard. Federal Register 43(220), Tuesday, November 14, Part IV, Pages 52952–53014. Book II, Attachments to the Final Standard. Federal Register 43 (225), Tuesday, November 21, Part II, Pages 54353–54616.

Wedding, J.P., R.W. Carlson, J.J. Stukel, and F.A. Bazzaz (1975) Aerosol deposition on plant leaves. Environmental Science and Technology 9(2):151–153.

Wedeen, R.P., D.K. Mallik, V. Batuman, and J.D. Bogden (1978) Geophagic lead nephropathy: Case report. Environmental Research 17(3):409–415.

Wedeen, R.P., D.K. Mallik, and V. Batuman (1979) Detection and treatment of occupational lead nephropathy. Archives of Internal Medicine 139(1):53–59.

Wershaw, R.L. (1976) Organic chemistry of lead in natural water systems. Pages 13–16, Lead in the Environment, edited by T.G. Lovering. U.S. Geological Survey Professional Paper 957. Washington, D.C.: U.S. Department of the Interior.

Wigle, D.T. and E.J. Charlebois (1978) Electric kettles as a source of human lead exposure. Archives of Environmental Health 33(2):72–78.

Wong, P.T.S., B.A. Silverberg, Y.K. Chau, and P.V. Hodson (1978) Lead and the aquatic biota. Pages 279–342, The Biogeochemistry of Lead in the Environment, Part B, edited by J.O. Nriagu. New York: Elsevier/North Holland Biomedical Press.

World Health Organization (1977) Environmental Health Criteria, 3. Lead. Geneva: World Health Organization.

Ziegler, E.E., B.B. Edwards, R.L. Jensen, K.R. Mahaffey, and J.J. Fomon (1978) Absorption and retention of lead by infants. Pediatric Research 12:29–34.

Zielhuis, R.L. (1975a) Dose–response relationships for inorganic lead. I. Biochemical and haematological responses. International Archives of Occupational Health 35:1–18.

Zielhuis, R.L. (1975b) Dose–response relationships for inorganic lead. II. Subjective and functional responses—chronic sequealae—no-response levels. International Archives of Occupational Health 35:19–35.

Zimdahl, R.L. (1976) Entry and movement in vegetation of lead derived from air and soil sources. Journal of the Air Pollution Control Association 26(7):655–660.

Zimdahl, R.L. and P.B. Arvik (1973) Lead in soils and plants: A literature review. Critical Reviews in Environmental Control 3:213–224.

3 Federal Regulatory Activities on Lead in the Human Environment

INTRODUCTION

In this chapter, some aspects of recent decisions about lead in the human environment that have been made by administrative agencies of the federal government are examined. The analysis here is concerned with the relationship between the state of scientific knowledge about lead and its effects on humans, reviewed in Chapter 2, and the scientific basis used by standard-setting agencies to support judgments on critical issues integral to the regulatory process. The purpose of this analysis is to identify major areas of scientific uncertainty that have repeatedly and consistently had major impacts on decision making. The impact of uncertainties on decisions is one prime criterion used in the establishment of priorities for future research (see Chapter 5).

It is not the intent of this chapter to second-guess decisions that have been made, or to criticize agencies for judgments that, under law, they are obligated or constrained to make. As noted in Chapter 1, the information base is never complete enough to eliminate uncertainties or the need for judgment. By identifying areas in which the scientific basis for policy decisions is especially weak, this assessment focuses attention on topics where research could reduce the scope of arbitrary judgments that must be made.

The approach used here is to compare the idealized model decision process, described in Chapter 1, with real decisions by government agencies, proceeding through the process step by step, as in the previous

TABLE 3.1   Recent Decisions by Federal Agencies Pertaining to Lead in the Human Environment

Decision	Agency[a]	Date
Limitation of leachable lead content of glazed ceramic products (7 ppm)	FDA	1971
Phased reduction of allowable lead content of gasoline	EPA	1973
Criteria for health classification of children screened by lead poisoning prevention programs	CDC	1970 1975 1978
Elimination of lead-based paint hazards in HUD-associated housing and federally-owned housing	HUD	1976
Limit of 0.06% lead content in paints, and ban on toys, other articles intended for the use of children, and furniture that bear paints containing more than 0.06% lead	CPSC	1978
National ambient air quality standard for lead	EPA	1978
Standards for occupational exposure to lead	OSHA	1978
National primary drinking water standard for lead (to replace current interim standard)	EPA	Pending
Regulations on lead content of foods	FDA	Pending

[a] Key to abbreviations:
CDC   Center for Disease Control, Department of Health, Education, and Welfare
CPSC   Consumer Product Safety Commission
EPA   Environmental Protection Agency
FDA   Food and Drug Administration, Department of HEW
HUD   Department of Housing and Urban Development
OSHA   Occupational Safety and Health Administration, Department of Labor

chapters. The decisions examined are listed in Table 3.1. None of the agencies followed our model process exactly, but many of the processes included generically similar steps that can be considered under the same headings.

Information about the decision processes followed by various agencies was compiled especially for this study by consultants to the Committee, and is presented as a series of case studies in Appendix C. Sources of the information included public statements by the agencies and other public documents, including legislation, criteria documents, announcements in the *Federal Register*, hearing transcripts, and other records.

It is recognized that subjective values, arguments by affected parties, considerations of a political nature, and other intangible elements play a major part in regulatory decisions, and that public records rarely are explicit in acknowledging the weight given to such factors. This analysis therefore does not assess all factors that contributed to the decisions examined, but concentrates on the available public record of each agency's use of scientific information in the decision-making process.

USE OF SCIENTIFIC INFORMATION AT EACH STEP OF THE DECISION-MAKING PROCESS

Step 1: IDENTIFY SOURCES OF LEAD AND PATHWAYS OF ENVIRONMENTAL TRANSFER

It was concluded in Chapter 2 that the important general and special sources and environmental pathways of exposure to lead are relatively well known in at least a semiquantitative way. As was shown at that point, single sources of exposure dominate all others for a few populations (e.g., workers with occupational exposures, children with pica for paint), but for most children and adults several sources of lead contribute significantly to total exposure. There is considerable uncertainty in quantitative estimates of the contributions of different sources (see Step 3), but the conclusion that many sources are important is well supported.

Agency actions reflect the first conclusion well. One or more agencies have adopted regulations that pertain to lead in the air, water, paint, and housewares, and regulations on lead in foods are pending (see Table 3.1). Among the sources identified in Chapter 2 as likely to contribute significantly to human exposure, only soil is presently not subject to regulations; and EPA is developing standards for lead in sludges, one source of the element in soils (see Appendix C).

However, few of the agencies' actions are based effectively on recognition of the multiple-source nature of most exposures to lead. While statements by the agencies show awareness of the problem, under existing laws no agency has authority to regulate all of the important modes of exposure. Even EPA, which has multimedia responsibilities, operates under several different pieces of enabling legislation that mandate essentially independent approaches to lead in the air, soil, water, pesticides, and solid wastes. While there has been a significant effort to coordinate some regulatory activities by different agencies concerned with lead, the government's approach as a whole has been fragmented and disjointed. Coordination and cooperation among agencies has improved significantly in the last 2 or 3 years, since the creation of the Interagency Regulatory Liaison Group. However, the federal government is still far from having a consistent, balanced, interagency policy on the control of lead in the environment.

Step 2: IDENTIFY SPECIFIC HUMAN POPULATIONS WITH EXPOSURE TO LEAD

Under the various pieces of enabling legislation, some agencies are required to be concerned with relatively specific populations. For instance, OSHA must protect adults with occupational exposures to lead, and the Lead-Based Paint Poisoning Prevention Act requires HUD, CDC, and CPSC to concentrate on hazards of lead to children. Other laws give EPA and FDA broad responsibilities to deal with exposures of the general population (or subsets thereof) to lead through the air, drinking water, soil, or foods.

Where the population of greatest concern has not been identified in the law, the agencies have employed both the epidemiological and the predictive approaches described in Chapter 2 as guides to identify more specifically populations that may require protection from excessive exposure to lead. The EPA air quality criteria document (U.S. EPA 1977a) identifies children and pregnant women as populations at risk, for reasons given in Chapter 2; the FDA has been especially concerned with exposures of children under age 3 to lead in foods (see Appendix C). On the other hand, EPA's water quality criteria document specifies children with pica for soil or paint and adults with occupational exposures as two groups whose exposures to lead are already high, and for whom significant exposure via drinking water would be an important additional risk (U.S. EPA 1979). All of the agencies have focused on subsets of the general population that are believed to be especially sensitive, with the assumption that protection for sensitive groups will also provide protection for the general population.

However, the populations selected for attention are relatively large and diverse; neither urban children, nor pregnant women, nor adults with occupational exposures, nor even children with pica are homogeneous populations. As pointed out in Chapter 2, different subpopulations within such categories are likely to experience risks well above average for the group, because of differences in exposure and differences in individual sensitivity to toxic effects of lead. Current knowledge of factors that make one subset of a population more likely to be at risk than another is qualitative at best, and it is not yet possible to identify with satisfactory specificity groups that require different degrees of protection.

The more specifically agencies have attempted to define the population of greatest concern to them, the more they have been confounded by a lack of adequate information. For example, the target population for HUD's programs to protect against exposure to lead-based paints is primarily young children who live in housing that contains lead paint in a deteriorating condition. But inadequate information about the number of children who live in housing with accessible lead paint and the extent to which those children ingest lead in paint chips or dust and dirt has stymied HUD's attempts to design an effective control strategy for that target population (Billick and Gray 1978).

The lack of specificity in definitions of populations at risk has important implications for all agencies' decisions. If specific populations cannot be identified and control strategies developed for them, more general controls (probably with greater costs to society) may be required. Also, in the absence of specific knowledge of the most sensitive groups, it cannot be determined how much control of exposure is needed. It is therefore not possible to determine whether, for example, the standards adopted by EPA to protect urban children can provide adequate protection for all subsets of the population.

Step 3: ESTIMATE QUANTITATIVELY THE LEVEL OF EXPOSURE TO LEAD BY EACH PATHWAY THAT AFFECTS THE TARGET POPULATION

As discussed in Chapter 2, great uncertainties are associated with quantitative estimates of the degree to which individual sources contribute to total exposure to lead, both for urban children and, to a lesser extent, for the general population. These uncertainties have had profound effects on the decision-making processes in most of the cases examined here. One significant exception was the decision by OSHA, which was justifiably based on the assumption that the workplace environment is the most important source of exposure to lead for the occupational exposure category.

The other agencies, however, have faced substantial obstacles in determining the importance of the one source that is their primary concern—air, water, paint, lead alkyl fuel additives, foods—in terms of total exposure to lead. They have therefore been unable to say with convincing precision how much reduction in exposure can be accomplished by controls over a single source or pathway, or how much reduction is needed over the mode of exposure that is their responsibility.

The judgments of different agencies that have attempted to deal with this uncertainty can be divided into two groups: those that have made only a qualitative assessment of relative exposures, and those (especially in the more recent decisions) that have attempted to develop a quantitative basis for their decisions.

Qualitative Assessments

The agencies that have enacted programs under the Lead-Based Paint Poisoning Prevention Act and its amendments have for the most part relied on qualitative judgments of the contributions of different sources to total exposure to lead. The judgment inherent in the law itself is that paint is the single most important source of exposure to lead for young children, and HUD, CPS, and CDC have developed regulations that reflect that assumption. HUD, for instance, defined "immediate hazards" of lead paint in housing as any paint that was cracked, peeling, or otherwise in a condition that would make it accessible for ingestion by children. The agency did not attempt to include quantitative criteria for the amount of paint that needed to be ingested or the probability that it would be ingested in its definition of hazards. Similarly, the CPSC banned the use of lead-based paints on objects to which children have access, without determining how likely children were to ingest paint from such objects. The lead poisoning prevention programs supported by CDC also have been guided by a qualitative judgment that paint is the primary source of elevated blood lead levels, and CDC-funded programs have been advised in the past to direct their abatement efforts toward the location and removal of paint, often to the exclusion of other potential sources of lead in the child's environment (Steinfeld 1971, CDC 1975). However, CDC's most recent statement advises that abatement measures should consider all likely sources of lead (CDC 1978).

In a similar fashion, EPA based its regulations of the lead content of gasoline on qualitative assessments. The agency concluded that it could not determine quantitatively the contribution of lead in gasoline to total exposure. Instead, EPA based its action on its judgments that inhalation and ingestion of deposited aerosols are important routes of exposure, and that combustion of gasoline is the single most important source of lead in the air and an important source of lead in soil and dust.

Quantitative Assessments

In other decisions, however, EPA, FDA, and OSHA have attempted to define source contributions to total exposure. This choice also is inherent in the pertinent legislation, which requires the agencies to establish numerical standards for permissible concentrations of lead in the ambient air, drinking water, foods, or air in the workplace.

In three of the most recent federal actions on lead—the establishment of an ambient air quality standard by EPA, the issuance of water quality criteria by EPA, and the establishment of limitations on occupational exposures by OSHA—quantitative estimates of the contributions of specific pathways to total exposure have been central, critical concerns. Each of the agencies has had to confront the substantial lack of appropriate data on exposures of specific populations to lead from various sources, described in Chapter 2. Ultimately, neither agency gave much weight to efforts to determine the precise exposures of the population to lead. Instead, both EPA and OSHA placed their major emphasis on empirically derived relationships between the concentration of lead in the air or water and the response of the average blood lead concentration in the target population. The nature of the judgments that EPA and OSHA made in using the empirical data will be examined in Step 4.

Step 4: ESTABLISH THE ASSOCIATION BETWEEN EXPOSURE AND LEAD IN THE BODY FOR THE SPECIFIC POPULATION

Considerable uncertainties about several aspects of the relationships between lead in various environmental media and lead in the body were identified in Chapter 2. For example, the nature and rate of absorption of lead from the lung is poorly understood. Average fractions of dietary lead absorbed are known within approximate bounds for both adults and children, but the range of significant human variation and the influences of numerous factors that cause individual differences in uptake have not been determined quantitatively. The dynamics of distribution of lead within the body and factors that determine the amounts of lead in different physiological pools are poorly understood. Although it is known that blood lead is correlated with exposure, absorption, total body burden, and burden of lead at sites of specific biological effects, neither the functional nature of the relationships nor the factors that control them can be accurately estimated. The average blood lead level, the range and distribution of individual values about the mean, and trends with time have not been well established for most populations.

Quantitative Approaches

Despite these uncertainties, EPA and OSHA have attempted to reach quantitative conclusions about the contributions of specific sources of exposures to body burdens, in order to establish standards for lead in the workplace, ambient air, and drinking water. The approach used in all three cases has been to develop mathematical models of the relationship between lead concentrations in the environment and blood lead concentrations. In each case, the data base that supports such models is small, and neither the exact form of the mathematical function nor the slope of the resulting curve can be determined with great accuracy.

In order to use such empirical models to estimate the reduction in body burden that would follow a given reduction in exposure to lead, the agencies have had to make some unproven assumptions. It is assumed, for instance, that a regression equation relating lead in one environmental medium to lead in blood is an adequate substitute for precise measurements of exposure, absorption, and concentration of lead at physiologically significant sites within the body. It is assumed that empirical relationships derived from a few studies encompass all likely human variations with regard to these parameters, and that the regression equations are valid for the specific populations of concern to the agency setting standards. In addition, in order to determine the fraction of the population that would be protected by standards, EPA and OSHA had to make assumptions about the statistical distribution of blood lead values in the populations at risk.

Sequential chains of assumptions of this sort are necessary to support the choice of any numerical value for an environmental standard. However, there is significant uncertainty in the assumed value for each component of the calculation, and the multiplication of uncertainty factors makes the quantitative basis for the ultimate choice of a standard very uncertain indeed. For example, in setting its ambient air quality standard, EPA determined that its objective was to protect 99.5 percent of children from having blood lead levels above 30 $\mu g/100$ ml. The agency assumed a geometric standard deviation of 1.3 for children's blood lead values, and calculated from that assumption that the geometric mean blood lead level should be 15 $\mu g/100$ ml if less than 0.5 percent were to exceed 30 $\mu g/100$ ml. Then, on the basis of a small number of studies of levels of lead in populations in rural areas, EPA estimated that the contribution of nonair sources to blood lead levels was, on the average, about 10 to 12 $\mu g/100$ ml. EPA concluded, therefore, that if the mean blood lead level was to remain below 15 $\mu g/100$ ml, the contribution of inhaled lead to blood lead could not exceed 3 $\mu g/100$ ml. From its analysis of regressions between blood lead levels and concentrations of lead in ambient air, EPA concluded that the air lead level that would contribute 3 $\mu g/100$ ml to blood lead in children was 1.5 $\mu g/m^3$, and set the standard at that value.

Three critical variables in the above calculations are subject to important uncertainties. The assumed 2-to-1 ratio between lead in air and lead in blood is based on very few data on children, and might easily be 50 percent high or low. The estimate of 10 to 12 $\mu g/100$ ml of lead in blood from nonair sources certainly could be in error by at least ± 3 $\mu g/100$ ml. Finally, the calculated target geometric mean blood lead level of 15 $\mu g/100$ ml is extremely sensitive to the assumed geometric standard deviation. If the value chosen had been 1.5, which is equally supported by the meager available data, the mean blood lead level required to keep 99.5 percent of children below 30 $\mu g/100$ ml would be about 10 $\mu g/100$ ml, and the tolerable exposure to lead in air could be calculated as zero.

It is clear from this example that uncertainties about relationships between lead in the environment and lead in the body make it difficult to defend any specific environmental standard on purely scientific grounds. This example should not cast an unfavorable light on EPA or its ambient air quality standard for lead. Legislative deadlines and court orders combined to force EPA to make arbitrary assumptions that substitute for incomplete knowledge. The action was taken to comply with a court order that the agency meet certain terms of the Clean Air Act, and it must be assumed that both the court and Congress were aware that making such decisions would require some arbitrary judgments by the agency. Clearly, those political and judicial bodies accepted the hazard of errors in judgment by EPA as a smaller risk than the likely results of postponing action because of scientific uncertainties.

The same general approach was used by EPA in setting water quality standards for lead (U.S. EPA 1979) and by OSHA in establishing limits on occupational exposures (U.S. OSHA 1978). The chief advantage of this still-evolving procedure is that it makes it possible to identify very precisely the arbitrary assumptions that have been made, and to focus attention on highly specific needs for better information.

Other Approaches

In contrast to these recent examples, other agencies have taken more qualitative approaches to the question of the contributions of specific sources of exposure to levels of lead in the body. HUD has called attention to the lack of a well-defined relationship between lead-based paint in housing and children's blood lead levels (Billick and Gray 1978); however, as HUD has interpreted the law, regulations have been based on the accessibility of paint to children, and have not dealt with the quantitative steps between exposure and possible biological effects. Similarly, EPA's regulations on lead in gasoline and CPSC's ban on lead in paints simply considered exposure per se to be adequate evidence of a significant risk of biological effects. CDC's program supports local projects that, when they have identified a child with an elevated body burden, attempt to find and eliminate sources of lead in the child's environment, without determining the precise contributions of each to the elevated blood lead level.

If the number of examples considered here is sufficient to establish a trend, the approaches developed by EPA and OSHA will probably be starting points for future standard-setting activities that must consider relationships between lead in the environment and lead in people.

Step 5: ESTABLISH THE ASSOCIATION BETWEEN LEAD IN THE BODY AND
BIOLOGICAL CHANGE IN THE SPECIFIC POPULATION

The extensive and complex body of knowledge of biological effects of lead
in adults, children, laboratory animals, cells, and tissues is summarized in
Chapter 2. Significant uncertainties remain about the effects of typical
levels of exposure to lead on many organs and biochemical functions in
specific populations. However, substantial dose–response data are available for effects of lead in blood on heme synthesis, and the effects of lead
at relatively high blood lead levels on neurological and behavioral functions are well documented. Most other effects in adults and children have
been less studied, and the lowest doses that can produce any effects have
not been conclusively determined (see Chapter 2). In general, there is
better agreement over whether biological changes are associated with
specific blood lead levels than there is over whether or not the changes
observed should be considered adverse effects on health (see Step 6,
below).

Since the purpose of government regulations that limit exposures to
lead in the environment is to protect human health, findings of hazards to
health, supported by dose–effect and dose–response data, would be expected to be part of the basis for regulations and standards. However,
this has not been so in all cases. As noted earlier, qualitative judgments
were the basis for several decisions, and those judgments included determinations that reduction in exposure is justified even in the absence of a
precise estimate of the magnitude or probability of biological effects.
Such rationales were used by EPA in the phased reduction of lead in gasoline, by HUD in requirements for removal of deteriorating lead paint in
specified housing, by CPSC in banning the use of lead-based paint or products accessible to children, and by FDA in establishing an allowable limit
for the lead content of ceramic glazed products.

The more recent decisions—EPA's air and water standards, OSHA's occupational standards, and FDA's pending regulations on foods—have been
explicitly concerned with demonstrating dose–effect and dose–response
relationships. To a significant extent, this orientation reflects the nature
of proof required to meet the terms of the applicable laws. However, the
amount of information available on the biological effects of lead also has
increased significantly in the last 5 years, in large part because the regulatory agencies have sponsored research to improve the basis for setting
standards (see Appendix B).

Each of the agencies that has based its standards on biological evidence
has accepted blood lead measurements as the best available (though not
an ideal) marker of lead in the body. Both EPA and OSHA reviewed the
available evidence of dose–response and dose–effect relationships for rela-

tively high levels of exposure, and attempted to determine the lowest levels of lead in blood associated with specific effects in the target populations. EPA has emphasized the concept of a "critical effect," and has concentrated most of its attention on lead–induced changes in heme synthesis in children. OSHA has been concerned with both higher levels of exposure and potentially longer durations of exposure, and has incorporated considerations of several different kinds of chronic effects on the health of adults into the basis for its standards.

Each agency determined that some biological changes were associated with levels of lead in blood that occur in some members of the populations that concern them. Neither agency reached firm conclusions about the level of lead in blood at which no detectable biological changes would occur. Neither of EPA's criteria documents considered the implications of the difference between present-day levels of exposure of the general population to lead and estimated natural levels (see Chapter 2) in reaching its judgments about what is known of the effects of typical exposures.

Step 6: ESTIMATE THE LIMIT OF NON-DETRIMENTAL BIOLOGICAL CHANGE DUE TO LEAD AND THE ASSOCIATED LEVEL OF LEAD IN THE BODY

Those agencies that have not based their decisions on quantitative dose–effect data (see previous step) have not had to carry out the difficult process of judging the degree of biological change due to lead that they consider detrimental to health. Only four of the cases listed in Table 3.1 have included such judgments, and three agencies (EPA, OSHA, and CDC) have been involved.

EPA's Conclusions

When EPA set the ambient air quality standard for lead, the agency first concluded that its criteria for detrimental levels of lead in the body should be based on the "critical" or most sensitive effect, which it identified as inhibition of heme synthesis. EPA conceded that the elevation of erythrocyte protoporphyrin concentrations and depression of ALAD activity that are observed in some individuals at levels of 10 to 15 $\mu g/100$ ml of lead in blood are not disease conditions, but concluded that the effects are early phases on a continuum of increasing effects associated with rising blood lead levels that ultimately result in a clear-cut condition of impaired health (U.S. EPA 1978). The agency noted that anemia (abnormally low hemoglobin supply) occurs in children whose blood lead levels are above 40 $\mu g/100$ ml, and determined that: "It is a prudent public health practice to exercise corrective action prior to the appearance of clinical symptoms." EPA therefore chose 30 μg/100 ml as the maximum safe blood lead level for individual children, and estimated that the geometric mean blood lead level for the population of children should not exceed 15 μg/100 ml (see Step 4, above). The selection of 15 μg/100 ml for the population mean was based on statistical considerations, and not on EPA's judgment (reached independently) that 15 μg/100 ml is the approximate threshold for elevation of free erythrocyte protoporphyrin (FEP) in children.

EPA used the same approach in its report, *Lead: Ambient Water Quality Criteria* (U.S. EPA 1979), citing its earlier decision on the air quality standard as the chief basis for its decision.

OSHA's Conclusions

OSHA took a stance similar to EPA's, but was more specific and more forceful in enunciating its belief that metabolic and physiological changes associated with lead in the body are sentinels or precursors of disease and should be prevented (U.S. OSHA 1978). OSHA identified physiological changes that it deemed to be the initial stages of continuums of pathophysiological change, and the associated blood lead levels, as follows: inhibition of heme synthesis, <40 μg/100 ml; neurological and behavioral effects, $\geq$40 μg/100 ml; reduced renal clearance, $\geq$40 μg/100 ml; and effects on reproductive functions, $\geq$30 μg/100 ml. With respect to heme synthesis, OSHA concluded that some biochemical changes are observed at blood lead levels as low as 10 μg/100 ml. The agency stated its belief that:

These effects must be viewed as early steps in a continuous disease process which eventually results in lead poisoning. Such effects are of themselves indicative of physiological disruptions of subcellular processes. Therefore, disruption of such processes over a working lifetime must be viewed as material impairment of health. (U.S. OSHA 1978, 54354–54355.)

By using wording of the sort just quoted and by stating explicitly, "EPA or OSHA believes that . . . ," both EPA and OSHA make it clear that there is a great deal of subjective judgment incorporated in their conclusions about what constitutes a detrimental degree of biological change.

CDC's Conclusions

CDC took a position on what constitutes a detrimental level of lead in the body when it issued criteria for use in the blood lead screening programs associated with local projects to prevent childhood lead poisoning. In 1970, the Surgeon General issued a statement defining "undue lead absorption" as a confirmed blood lead level of 40 or more μg/100 ml (Steinfeld 1971). As medical knowledge of the effects of lower levels of lead in the body has improved, the criteria have been revised (CDC 1975, 1978); "undue lead absorption" currently is defined as a blood lead value of 30 or more μg/100 ml, combined with an elevated erythrocyte proto-porphyrin level (see Table 2.3, in Chapter 2). Although the definition of "undue" lead absorption is based on current understanding of the biological effects of lead, CDC's publications have not provided a detailed discussion of the basis for the selection of various action levels shown in Table 2.3. Instead, the agency acknowledges that what constitutes "undue" absorption of lead is a matter of judgment, and explicitly refers to its criteria as "arbitrary definitions" (CDC 1978).

It is notable that each of the agencies has defined a detrimental effect or a detrimental level of lead in blood on the basis of comparisons between small groups with "elevated" body burdens of lead and larger populations of "normal" people, whose average blood lead levels may be between 10 and 20 μg/100 ml. None of the agencies has examined the hypothesis discussed in Chapter 2, that the typical modern body burden of lead may be detrimental per se, since today's "normal" level may be approximately 1 to 3 orders of magnitude higher than a natural body burden. This point has not been seriously considered in any agency's estimation of the minimum amount of absorption of lead that is detrimental to health.

Step 7: IDENTIFY AND DESCRIBE ALTERNATIVE CONTROL STRATEGIES

The different laws concerned with lead in the environment have imposed different requirements on the agencies in terms of the extent to which considerations of control strategies are to be part of the decisions listed in Table 3.1. For instance, the Lead-Based Paint Poisoning Prevention Act makes it HUD's primary responsibility to develop and evaluate abatement techniques to eliminate lead paint hazards; and the same law gives CDC a mandate to support population screening programs, but not to evaluate controls to prevent the occurrence of excessive lead in children's bodies. OSHA, CPSC, EPA, and FDA are mandated to take steps that will protect the public health; the technical and economic feasibility of controls is given different weight in each different piece of legislation.

The same problem noted in Step 1 has had a crucial impact on the agencies' considerations of control strategies. The laws constrain the agencies to deal with a single source or route of exposure at a time. No one agency can examine all the sources of exposure to lead, compare the effects of different combinations of controls on exposure from various sources, and choose the most effective or economical combination of measures. For OSHA, the orientation to a single source of exposure is appropriate; but agencies like HUD, EPA, and FDA, which are concerned with exposures of segments of the general population, all must try to deal with part of a problem, while other agencies deal with the remaining parts. Each agency is aware of the regulatory activities of its sister agencies, and there has been some effective coordination during recent years. However, one of the major coordinating mechanisms, the Interagency Regulatory Liaison Group, does not include HUD or CDC. The federal government has not yet developed a coherent policy that treats lead as a multiple-source pollutant requiring a single, integrated, multi-agency, balanced approach to control. Each agency has pursued its own policies under its own interpretations of its legislative mandates, paying some attention to other agencies' activities where possible.

Impacts of Information Gaps

The efforts of various agencies to develop partial control strategies for lead have been hindered by serious information gaps, discussed in Chapter 2. Technical methods for controlling emissions of lead to the atmosphere (U.S. EPA 1977b) and for detecting and abating lead paint hazards (Billick and Gray 1978) have been developed and evaluated, but much less is known about how to reduce the lead content of many foods, or how to prevent children from ingesting paint or lead-contaminated soil. Although the effectiveness of some control techniques has been estimated in terms of reduced emissions or changes in ambient levels of lead in the environment (U.S. EPA 1977b), the uncertainties described in Steps 3 and 4 above preclude an assessment of the health implications of such changes. Thus, HUD and EPA cannot determine the relative effects of either past or projected removal of lead paint from housing and removal of lead from gasoline in terms of changes in children's blood lead levels. Insofar as a change in blood lead levels has occurred (see Chapter 2), there is at present no way to determine conclusively which agencies' control efforts have contributed most to the change.

An additional area in which information is inadequate is the economic costs and benefits of control measures, or of alternative combinations of measures. Some semiquantitative estimates of direct costs of control are available. EPA examined the costs of compliance with its national ambient air quality standard for lead (U.S. EPA 1977b); CPSC examined costs to industry and consumers of its ban on leaded paints; and HUD estimated costs of different degrees of removal of lead paint from housing (Billick and Gray 1978). However, as noted in Chapter 2, projected benefits of control are much more difficult to estimate in quantitative or economic terms. As a result, no agency has been able to carry out a thorough cost–benefit analysis of control options.

Approaches to Controls Used by Agencies

Some of the cases examined here have followed a procedure similar to the one described in Chapter 1, i.e., identify a wide range of possible control options, and then describe each in sufficient detail to permit a choice. For instance, HUD has made a major effort, as required by law, to identify suitable techniques for removal of paint hazards. EPA has surveyed methods for preventing lead emissions to the atmosphere (U.S. EPA 1977b), and OSHA has assessed the availability of controls for industrial exposure to lead in order to demonstrate that the standards it adopted were feasible (U.S. OSHA 1978). In its pending action on lead in foods, FDA is likely to devote considerable attention to determining the effectiveness of alternative methods for reducing or preventing lead contamination of products. However, none of the agencies in these cases has been required to choose a preferred control approach; that decision has been left largely to state and local governments or private industries. Because none of the standard-setting agencies has been required by law to select the methods to be used to meet its health protection goals, the serious lack of information on the health-related effectiveness, costs, and benefits of controls has not forced the agencies into arbitrary judgments, as occurred in the setting of numerical standards.

In some other cases, however, the legislation (or the agencies' interpretations of it) either required or permitted the selection of a control approach, and the information gaps have resulted in some substantially arbitrary decisions. For instance, HUD had to develop criteria to require removal of lead-based paint from houses under its authority; EPA elected to decide how much and how rapidly the lead content of gasoline should be reduced; and FDA chose to set a limit on the lead content of ceramic glazes. In each case, although a number of alternative options could be identified, the lack of precise information about the effectiveness, costs, and benefits associated with any one set of control conditions seems to have been a serious obstacle to effective comparison of options. In the absence of a credible quantitative basis for such choices, arbitrary judgments and pressures from partisan interests have inevitably appeared to be major determining factors in decisions.

Step 8: APPLY RISK–BENEFIT, COST–BENEFIT, AND OTHER CONSIDERATIONS, COMPARE ALTERNATIVES, AND MAKE A DECISION

At this step of the decision-making process, the agencies collect the information gathered in previous steps, compare risks, costs, and benefits, make trade-offs, and reach judgments about acceptable degrees of risk associated with exposures to lead. Because of differences in the legislation or the agencies' interpretations of their mandates, the factors that have been considered and the weight given to each have varied in the different cases examined here. The basis for each of the individual decisions, as stated by the agencies themselves, is described in some detail in the case studies in Appendix C.

As in previous steps, each agency is faced with acting independently on a small part of a large problem, knowing that other agencies with somewhat different priorities are responsible for dealing with the other parts. Thus, while any definition of an "acceptable" level of lead in air, water, food, paint, or gasoline must be contingent on certain assumptions about the levels present in other media of exposure, no one agency can say what is "acceptable" in all media or regulate all modes of exposure.

Some of the decisions listed in Table 3.1 have been fairly straightforward, at least in contrast to the others. For instance, FDA's limits on leachable lead in glazed ceramic products and CPSC's ban on the use of lead-based paint on toys and other products to which children could be exposed were both based primarily on qualitative judgments of an unreasonable risk of injury, combined with evidence that neither industry nor the public would bear excessive costs as a result of the decisions. Rather arbitrary decisions were made in each case, but the consequences of arbitrariness here do not appear injurious to the public interest.

In most of the other cases, the agencies had to compare and weigh substantial potential hazards to health against significant likely costs to society associated with measures to reduce the hazards. The great uncertainties described throughout this and previous chapters make such comparisons difficult, and place a burden on the agencies to be as explicit as possible about the nature of their judgments and the reasons for them.

EPA's Decisions

EPA has been involved in three of the decisions discussed as examples in this chapter; the basis for the agency's judgments differs somewhat in each case. In requiring the phased reduction of lead in gasoline, EPA admitted candidly that a quantitative relationship between lead in gasoline and public health could not be demonstrated, and based its action on its belief that substantial qualitative evidence of a hazard was sufficient to justify removal of lead from fuels to the greatest extent possible. The degree of and schedule for reduction of lead in gasoline were based on (and have been revised because of) technical and economic considerations that have to do with the suitability of low-lead fuels for vehicles now in use and the ability of refiners to produce low-lead grades of gasoline at a reasonable cost.

EPA initially decided that an ambient air quality standard for lead could not be supported, because of the lack of quantitative information on exposures, contribution of lead in air to body burden, and health effects associated with low levels of lead in the body. However, under court order the agency did eventually set a standard of 1.5 $\mu g/m^3$, averaged over 90 days. The agency had to make numerous unproven assumptions in order to estimate the hazards to health associated with exposure to lead in air (see Step 4). Since the Clean Air Act precludes EPA from making trade-offs between health protection and expected costs of compliance in setting ambient air quality standards, the decision was based solely on the agency's conclusions about the relationship between airborne lead and children's health, with due consideration of a margin of safety. However, EPA did examine the feasibility of meeting the standard, and concluded that all urban areas where the major source of airborne lead is automobile exhaust would attain compliance within a few years because of the phase-down of lead in gasoline. Additional control measures were expected to be required for some point sources, such as smelters, and the agency predicted significant economic impacts on some industries (U.S. EPA 1978).

Although the final National Primary Drinking Water Standard for lead has not been adopted at this writing, EPA's Office of Criteria and Standards has recommended retaining the current interim standard of 50 $\mu g/l$ (U.S. EPA 1979). The basis for this recommendation is a series of calculations similar to those the agency made in setting the air standard. EPA has estimated the contribution of lead in water to lead in blood and defined the maximum increment of lead in water that is consistent with keeping the maximum blood lead level below 30 $\mu g/100$ ml for 99.5 percent of children. Whether the arbitrary assumptions that EPA used in this case will survive the period of public comment is unknown at this point. When EPA promulgates its final standards, the agency will need to consider the technical and economic feasibility of achieving the limits it sets, and strike a balance between health protection and costs.

HUD's and CDC's Decisions

The two primary agencies carrying out the mandates of the Lead-Based Paint Poisoning Prevention Act also have made decisions with substantial implications for both public health and economic costs to society. HUD has concluded, on the basis of its research on the abatement of paint hazards, that the likely costs of removing all lead paint sources from housing are prohibitive. The agency has adopted regulations that require the removal of lead paint hazards—defined as paint in a deteriorating condition—from dwellings that are associated with HUD financing when there is a change of occupants. In establishing the regulations, HUD consciously avoided the use of health criteria to trigger abatement measures. Because of uncertainty within HUD about the extent to which the removal of lead paint would contribute to reduced exposures and lower blood lead levels in children, the agency has been reluctant to pursue or support more aggressive and more costly programs to remove lead paint from the environment of children (see Appendix C).

CDC, in contrast, has been concerned almost exclusively with the hazards of lead to children's health, and has supported programs designed to prevent health damage in children who have excessive blood lead levels. When CDC revised its criteria for classifying children according to the risk of lead-induced health damage, the agency used medical judgment. CDC concluded that children with an abnormal FEP value were at greater risk than children with simply elevated blood lead levels; and an examination of screening data from 180,000 children showed that the number with blood lead above 30 μg/100 ml and an elevated FEP level is about the same as the number with blood lead above 40 μg/100 ml and normal FEP. In CDC's judgment, therefore, screening is more cost-effective (in terms of identifying children in need of remedial attention) if the criteria used are blood lead greater than 30 μg/100 ml coupled with an abnormal FEP value (CDC 1978). However, CDC did not assess the potential broader costs to society likely to follow a redefinition of control objectives to suit maintaining blood lead levels below 30 μg/100 ml. CDC's position, from its public statements, has been that any costs that are required for screening, diagnosis, treatment, follow-up, and source control are necessary and justified by the benefit to public health that these measures provide.

The result of this two-headed decision-making process has been an inability to achieve a national consensus policy on the management of lead paint hazards, and conflicts in goals and approaches that are apparent in statements from HUD, CDC, and others. While the task of controlling exposure to lead-based paint is enormously difficult, it seems extremely unlikely that an appropriate balance of health and feasibility considerations can be achieved with the current division of responsibilities.

OSHA's Decision

In its recent decision on standards for occupational exposure to lead, OSHA was required to balance health protection goals against the expected costs of attaining them. The agency calculated that its adopted standard of 50 μg/m^3 of lead in the air of the workplace would result in a mean blood lead level of about 40 μg/100 ml, and that 99.5 percent of workers would have blood lead values below 60 μg/100 ml. OSHA concluded that a lower average blood lead level was desirable from a health point of view (see Step 6), but judged that a more stringent standard could not be achieved by industry. However, the agency included in its regulations provisions for medical surveillance of workers, and for removal of workers with specified high blood lead levels to areas with lower airborne lead levels. OSHA considered and rejected several alternative approaches, which are discussed in its decision document (U.S. OSHA 1978), and ultimately concluded that the 50 μg/m^3 standard with medical removal provisions "represents the best intersection between maximization of health benefits and feasibility."

FDA's Food Regulations

The FDA's pending regulations on lead in foods are still at an early stage of development, and proposals have not been made public. Clearly, FDA will have to consider the extent to which total exposure to lead constitutes a hazard to health for various populations, the contribution of dietary lead to total absorption of the metal, the degree of control over total exposure that has been achieved by measures adopted by other agencies, the degree of further reduction of total exposure that is desirable, the feasibility of various methods for preventing or reducing lead contamination of foods, and the effectiveness and costs of alternative combinations of measures. The task is obviously as complex and difficult as those undertaken recently by EPA and OSHA, and because of the contribution of dietary lead to total exposure, at least as important.

Summary of Decision Steps

In summary, the decisions reviewed here have varied widely in the nature of trade-offs required and in the degrees to which the agencies have been explicit about their assumptions and have offered a quantitative basis for their actions. There has been a marked trend toward greater reliance on quantitative assessments and explicit judgments in recent decisions. This trend reflects both an improvement in the base of scientific knowledge and an evolution of the art of regulatory decision making over the years encompassed by the cases reviewed here. However, neither the state of knowledge nor the "state-of-the-art" is advanced enough to support a full-scale, explicit comparison of all identifiable costs, risks, and benefits for several alternative policy options, which was described in Chapter 1 as the ideal basis for making decisions about lead in the human environment.

Implementation Plans

The importance of developing sound implementation plans to show how standards can be achieved was stressed in Chapter 1. Implementation has been relatively straightforward in cases that involve product bans or restrictions, such as CPSC's regulations on paints or FDA's standards for ceramic products. Implementation of the other decisions, however, is more complex, and under most of the laws that apply is not the sole responsibility of the standard-setting agency. Except for the small amount of housing that falls under HUD's immediate jurisdiction, most abatement of paint hazards is carried out by local authorities, as are the blood lead screening programs supported by CDC. EPA's air and water quality standards are enforced by the states and by local jurisdictions; the laws are intended to leave some flexibility for solutions to be tailored to local conditions. Because most of EPA's decisions are recent or still pending, implementation plans are still in the developmental stages. OSHA, on the other hand, is responsible for implementing its own standards, and has already set up a schedule for compliance that requires that industries meet the 50 $\mu g/m^3$ standard within 10 years, and establishes interim goals that lead up to full compliance.

Step 9:   EVALUATE THE PROCESS AND THE DECISION

In Chapter 1, the need was stressed for conscientious evaluations of the quality, appropriateness, and sufficiency of data and assumptions at each step of the decision-making process, and the importance of continued evaluation after decisions have been made was emphasized. Post-decision evaluations can assess whether the actions taken have had the expected effects, and may identify opportunities to improve the process of making decisions. It was concluded in Chapter 2 that much of the information needed to conduct effective assessments, including time-series measurements of environmental levels of lead, medical evaluations of the health of populations at whom protective measures are aimed, and appraisals of economic consequences of government actions and private sector responses, is unavailable. Ideally, provisions for obtaining such information should be part of an implementation plan developed to carry out a decision.

Evaluation of the Data Base

Each of the agencies that has summarized scientific information has made judgments at many points that the available data are insufficient; there are far too many examples to cite. However, although the agencies may state that not enough is known on a topic to support a conclusive interpretation, they often have been obligated to make their own interpretations regardless. At the same time, many agencies urge further research on important topics to reduce uncertainty, and some have pursued such research (see Appendix B).

As was also indicated in Chapter 2, there is a widespread lack of data that are appropriate to support some of the specific judgments that have been made. Many cases were noted of extrapolations from biological measurements on one population to assumed effects in other populations, or of the use of environmental data from one site to predict exposures at other locations. Such inferences from possibly inappropriate data may be the best that can be made; however, we believe the agencies should note the added uncertainty that is thereby introduced into the standard-setting process.

For instance, when EPA estimated the contribution of lead in water to lead in blood, the agency commented on the fact that only three studies provided sufficient data to calculate regressions (U.S. EPA 1979). However, the agency did not assess the usefulness of the studies for setting a standard that is intended to protect children, given that only one of the three studies included data on children's blood lead levels. Since it is not known whether children absorb the same fraction of lead ingested in water that adults do, serious questions can be raised about the appropriateness of the use of the data for EPA's stated purpose.

Fundamental questions about the reliability of analytical measurements for lead, especially at low levels of occurrence, are identified in Chapter 2 and Appendix D. The possibility of inaccurate measurement implies uncertainty bounds for most specific sets of data; although the margins of error can be estimated, few agencies have attempted to do so in the cases examined here. An exception is EPA's assessment of the variation in blood lead levels among human populations, where the agency concluded that a significant fraction of the reported differences could be due to measurement variation (U.S. EPA 1977a). The problem of insufficient attention to the valid use of analytical methods is especially acute in estimation of lead concentrations in foods (see Appendix D), and FDA has made improvement of analytical methods a major research priority as it prepares to regulate lead in foods (see Appendix B). A related analytical problem, contamination of samples and reagents, is especially important in studies to estimate the "background" occurrence of lead in the environment. The implications of such contamination errors in terms of the reliability of estimates of pollution effects appear to have received little or no attention from the agencies concerned with making such estimates.

An additional emphasis mentioned in Chapter 1 is the importance of recognizing the cumulative effect of multiple uncertainties on the judgments that ultimately must be made. For understandable reasons, none of the regulatory agencies has been enthusiastic about a frank assessment of the possible margin of error associated with the numerical values they have selected for standards. Given the adversary relationships that exist among regulators, the regulated, and consumer and environmentalist groups, it is probably unrealistic to expect such explicitness from standard-setting bodies. On the other hand, HUD, an agency whose basic mission is not environmental protection, but one that has important responsibility for research on lead hazards, has emphasized the many gaps in current knowledge (Billick and Gray 1978), and has acted less than aggressively to remove lead paints from housing (see Appendix C). Neither of these responses to the problem of uncertainty is particularly satisfactory.

Post-Decision Evaluations

As noted in Chapter 2, many kinds of information needed to conduct post-facto evaluations of decisions are gathered for other purposes, and are at least in theory available for assessments of the consequences of decisions. For example, environmental monitoring data collected to determine compliance with emission standards or ambient standards could be used to assess relationships between specific control measures and trends in exposures. Blood lead data from population screening programs could be correlated with both environmental measurements and indices of control efforts in order to identify factors associated with changes in the health status of populations. In addition, decisions might periodically be reassessed as new research provides better information on topics that required pivotal assumptions when standards were set.

Some agencies discussed here have taken some steps to evaluate their programs, or at least to make such an evaluation more feasible in the future. For instance, the medical surveillance requirements in OSHA's regulations will provide a substantial data base on the effects of the new standards on the health of workers, as well as indicate whether further adjustments of the permissible exposure limitations should be considered. CDC, which is a granting agency rather than a regulatory agency, has sponsored an assessment of the effectiveness of selected lead poisoning prevention efforts and childhood blood lead screening programs that it supports (Kennedy 1978). However, CDC has not taken advantage of the opportunity to compare time-series data on children's blood lead levels in particular urban areas with available data on the levels of lead in the environment. HUD has carried out such an analysis of data for New York

City, and is pursuing similar studies in Louisville, Kentucky, at present (see Appendix B).

For most regulatory agencies, however, the press of new priorities and pending decisions is sufficient to overwhelm the best intentions toward retrospective analysis of decisions. Although the agencies recognize the value of re-examination and correction of the information base where decisions were founded on uncertain evidence, the scientific resources of regulatory agencies are already stretched thin, and there are substantial political and pragmatic disincentives to second-guessing one's own decisions. For the most part, therefore, retrospective evaluations of decisions are a low priority for the agencies, and special efforts to obtain the data required to conduct such assessments have been unusual.

SUMMARY AND DISCUSSION

The decisions reviewed here exhibit some marked differences. Most notably, the nine cases considered can be arranged roughly along a spectrum that proceeds from relatively arbitrary, uncomplicated decisions to efforts to develop an ostensibly objective, complex, quantitative scientific basis for the judgments that agencies have made. The differences can be attributed to a combination of differing legislative mandates, changes with time in the base of available scientific knowledge, and political and social factors. The various influences are not independent, and it is not possible to separate them clearly in order to determine the exact effects of scientific uncertainties on the decisions.

EFFECTS OF LEGISLATION

Some obvious effects of legislative mandates that define the agencies' responsibilities can be identified. First, the different laws treat different sources and routes of human exposure to lead as separate problems, and assign responsibility for dealing with the problems to different agencies. This legislative diversity prevents any agency from effectively dealing with total exposure to lead as an integrated problem, and has resulted in a fragmented, disjointed federal effort. One law—the Lead-Based Paint Poisoning Prevention Act—divides responsibilities for assessment of health impacts and for assessment of control measures between two primary agencies, and no single decision maker is required to compare and weigh benefits to health against costs of control of lead paint hazards.

A second effect of differences in legislation is the extent to which the laws require the agencies to determine numerical limits for exposures to lead. EPA, OSHA, and FDA are required to set numerical standards that almost inevitably require quantitative, explicit approaches to estimation of exposures, doses, and effects.

A third important difference in the enabling acts is the weight given to different factors that must be included in the agencies' assessments. To the extent that the laws omit or exclude consideration of certain factors, such as costs of control, they permit the agencies to avoid extensive efforts to obtain quantitative estimates of those factors.

The various laws were enacted at different times and in different climates of political consensus on environmental protection issues. For example, when Congress adopted the 1970 amendments to the Clean Air Act, it expressed in the law a clear sense that the nation's quest for cleaner air had made insufficient progress up to that point. In that context, Congress reached a difficult decision that primary ambient air quality standards should be based solely on health criteria, and that the economic feasibility of attaining standards should not be allowed to undercut that goal.

Nevertheless, experience suggests that if the initial decision-making process fails to consider all pertinent factors, the decision itself may be imbalanced. For instance, the current oil shortage was largely unforeseen when EPA adopted its regulations to reduce the lead content of gasoline. Recently, the slight effects of the lead regulations on fuel supply prompted a decision to postpone the phase-down of lead in gasoline. This shift in national priorities was made rather hastily, and without extensive public debate or detailed consideration of possible health implications of the postponed reduction of lead emissions.

Obviously, no decision maker can be expected to foresee all possible changes in conditions that might someday affect the perceived correctness of regulatory actions, and judgments of the balance point between conflicting priorities are subject to revision. Nevertheless, we believe that sudden reversals in policy probably could be minimized, and the inconsistent, imbalanced objectives of different agencies could be made significantly more coherent. One major step to this end would be revision of the applicable laws so that each required a similarly comprehensive, systematic consideration of all pertinent aspects of problems as a basis for decisions about lead (or other toxic substances) in the environment.

EFFECTS OF INFORMATION GAPS

Significant gaps in current scientific knowledge have been identified at almost every step of the decision process. The combination of a lack of appropriate data and an insufficient ability to interpret the available evidence prevents reaching scientifically conclusive answers to the following critical questions:

1. The level of lead at specific sites in the body that is "safe";
2. The relationships between forms and amounts of lead in various environmental pools and levels of lead in people;
3. The identity of specific populations at risk, and the magnitude of present risk to those populations;
4. The nature of controls that would effectively reduce risks to specific populations;
5. How much control is necessary, and whether current or proposed standards will achieve "safety"; and
6. The relative costs and benefits to society of alternative combinations of control measures.

Despite the lack of scientific certainty on these vital issues, rational decisions can be made and have been made. The "easier" decisions, those in which hazards to health were obvious and substantial and the expected economic repercussions of actions were small, were made prior to 1970 or in the early years of the past decade. The more recent decisions, however, have required much more difficult choices between relatively imprecise estimates of risk and uncertain, but probably substantial, costs of controls. While qualitative, relatively arbitrary judgments were sufficient for the decisions made a decade ago, today's problems demand a much more deliberate effort to develop an explicit, quantitative basis for decisions.

Policy makers cannot wait for science to abolish uncertainty, and must use their best judgment to interpret the available evidence, answer questions as well as they can, weigh different values, and make social choices. In that context, scientific uncertainty increases the weight given to subjective judgment and the influence of social values and political considerations in the decision. It is possible that judgments that purport to be based on scientific consensus may have been "adjusted" through pressures, negotiations, or gamesmanship until they are compatible with nonscientific concerns, but are no longer scientifically valid, regardless of their political acceptability. To guard against this, explicit statements by the agencies of judgments they have made and the basis for them are essential.

With that preface, the recent trend toward explicit, quantitative statements of the basis for agency decisions is most welcome. However, the still-evolving approach to decisions on lead in the environment has some associated disadvantages that are not inconsequential. One problem is that explicit descriptions of assumptions and methods, including statements of where the evidence is incomplete or inconclusive, reveal the weaknesses in the agencies' scientific arguments. A consequence of this openness may be an increased vulnerability of decisions to challenges by regulated parties or others who are dissatisfied with the outcomes. Aside from this pragmatic disadvantage, there are possible scientific pitfalls. Even when uncertainties are acknowledged, they are rarely given enough weight to prevent a false air of confidence in the accuracy of judgments that have been made. Relatively arbitrary estimates may become the basis for other arbitrary estimates, and so on, until the original uncertain guess begins, simply through repeated use, to take on the characteristics of an established fact.

In our judgment, these negative aspects are outweighed by the advantages of explicit, quantitative approaches to decision making. It is valuable for weaknesses in the basis for a decision to be revealed, as this permits the correction of errors and encourages work toward the reduction of uncertainties. Explicit statements of assumptions show precisely where scientific uncertainties affect the outcome of a decision, and focus attention on research topics that can have substantial import for future policy making. As long as decisions are made within the legal framework of an adversary process and scientific evidence is subject to open discussion and peer review, erroneous or arbitrary scientific judgments will eventually be replaced by more accurate assumptions, in a continuous (if sometimes slow) evolution of knowledge.

SOME BROADER CONCERNS

The assessment of recent regulatory decisions presented in this chapter used the systematic approach described in Chapter 1 as a model, and demonstrated that the decision-making processes used by federal agencies during the last decade have undergone some evolution and improvement. It was noted in Chapter 1 that the question of how the decision-making process can be further improved is also a legitimate topic for inquiry within a properly systematic approach. Assessment of that question, however, requires examining present approaches to the management of lead hazards in a broader historical and political context.

The underlying assumption of laws that created the various authorities under which the federal government regulates exposures to lead is the same in most cases: it is assumed that hazards associated with lead can be identified, assessed, and controlled in a manner that permits society to enjoy the benefits of uses of the metal, and minimizes the attendant hazards. The large role that the federal government has come to play in efforts to identify and manage such hazards is a comparatively recent development; with the exception of the FDA's actions, most of the regulatory activities described in this chapter and Appendix C were carried out under laws enacted after 1970.

A brief look at the history of lead poisoning suggests that, prior to large-scale federal interventions, efforts to manage lead hazards generally were insufficient to prevent serious health damage. For example, industrial toxicologists had identified lead poisoning as a major hazard to the health of workers by the mid-19th century; yet, according to OSHA (1978), present-day exposures to lead remain a serious occupational health hazard, and costly control measures are still needed. Similarly, childhood lead poisoning was positively associated with ingestion of paint in 1892 (see Chapter 2), and by the mid-1920s numerous cases had been reported and the relatively widespread existence of this hazard was recognized. Nevertheless, lead-based paints were widely used for decades, and present and future generations of children will continue to be exposed to hazards associated with residual lead in paints on surfaces in old housing. Finally, general understanding of the toxic properties of lead was available in the 1920s, when lead alkyl fuel additives were introduced; but concern over possible long-term hazards to human health that might result from large-scale dispersion of atmospheric lead did not inhibit the rapid expansion of use of the additives. As a result of these failures to take effective, early preventive actions, urban environments, and to a lesser degree, the global environment, have been contaminated with reservoirs of lead that will remain, for most practical purposes, beyond effective control for the foreseeable future.

This historical perspective raises several questions. An obvious one is, why were opportunities missed to take actions to prevent the serious damage to human lives that lead has produced during the last century? Given reliable medical knowledge of the nature and causes of lead poisoning, why was the disease not eliminated much more rapidly than it has been? Does society's failure to prevent lead poisoning stem from scientific uncertainties? To what extent can the failure be explained by other factors, such as a lack of appropriate institutions and procedures for managing hazards; the beliefs, values, and priorities of society at large and of those in positions of authority; and resistance to change by economic interests? In addition to reasons for past failures, it is appropriate also to ask whether present-day institutions and procedures are adequate to prevent future health damage associated with lead, or with other toxic substances. Is the regulatory approach, and the model decision process used in this report, a sound and effective way to manage such hazards? What is the likelihood that present approaches could fail to prevent major damage to health and to the environment? Can different approaches be conceived that would have a smaller expected rate of failure? If so, what would be the social implications of some different, even radically different, approaches?

The Committee believes that the decision process used in this report is a synthesis of the current "state-of-the-art," but we are open-minded about whether or not this approach is the best that society could devise. Research to examine this question would be valuable. Studies in history, political science, and other disciplines that are concerned with how a society functions should be undertaken to explore the reasons for the prolonged gaps between the appearance of scientific evidence of serious hazards and the effective implementation of preventive measures. Analysis of current institutions and mechanisms should examine whether the influences that delayed satisfactory control of hazards associated with lead remain as serious impediments to present and future control efforts. A careful study of alternative approaches that can produce socially acceptable, sound preventive policies would be useful, and the advantages and disadvantages of such new approaches should be compared with those of the approaches now in favor.

REFERENCES

Billick, I.H. and V.E. Gray (1978) Lead Based Plant Poisoning Research: Review and Evaluation, 1971-1977. Office of Policy Development and Research. Washington, D.C.: U.S. Department of Housing and Urban Development.

Center for Disease Control (1975) Increased Lead Absorption and Lead Poisoning in Young Children. U.S. Public Health Service. Publication Number 00-2629. Atlanta, Ga.: U.S. Department of Health, Education, and Welfare.

Center for Disease Control (1978) Preventing Lead Poisoning in Young Children. U.S. Public Health Service. Publication Number 00-2629. Atlanta, Ga.: U.S. Department of Health, Education, and Welfare.

Kennedy, F.D. (1978) The Childhood Lead Poisoning Prevention Program: An Evaluation. Environmental Health Services Division, Center for Disease Control, U.S. Public Health Service, Atlanta, Ga. (Unpublished manuscript.)

Steinfeld, J.L. (1971) Medical aspects of childhood lead poisoning. Pediatrics 48(3):464-468.

U.S. Environmental Protection Agency (1977a) Air Quality Criteria for Lead. Office of Research and Development. EPA-600/8-77-017. Washington, D.C.: U.S. Environmental Protection Agency.

U.S. Environmental Protection Agency (1977b) Control Techniques for Lead Air Emissions. Office of Air Quality Planning and Standards. EPA-450/2-77-012. Research Triangle Park, N.C.: U.S. Environmental Protection Agency.

U.S. Environmental Protection Agency (1978) National Ambient Air Quality Standard for Lead. Office of Air, Noise, and Radiation and Office of Air Quality Planning and Standards. Research Triangle Park, N.C.: U.S. Environmental Protection Agency.

U.S. Environmental Protection Agency (1979) Lead: Ambient Water Quality Criteria. Criteria and Standards Division, Office of Water Planning and Standards. Washington, D.C.: U.S. Environmental Protection Agency.

U.S. Occupational Safety and Health Administration (1978) Occupational Exposure to Lead. Book I, Final Standard. Federal Register 43(220), Tuesday, November 14, Part IV, 52952–53014. Book II, Attachments to the Final Standard. Federal Register 43(225), Tuesday, November 21, Part II, 54353–54616.

4 Findings

This chapter presents the Committee's findings about the state of scientific knowledge on critical topics related to lead in the human environment, about the use of scientific knowledge in recent federal regulatory decisions on lead, and about the state of federal research programs related to lead.

The findings presented here are of two types. The first kind includes judgments that are primarily scientific, such as whether or not available evidence supports a quantitative conclusion about a relationship between variables, or whether or not estimates used in standard setting rest on well-proven assumptions. Examples are conclusions about levels of lead in the body associated with specific biological changes, or findings about the state of knowledge of contributions of specific sources of lead to total exposure for particular human populations. The second kind of judgment is concerned with the implications of the evidence, and includes subjective scientific, social, and philosophical elements. Examples include perceptions of the degree of urgency associated with hazards to health posed by lead, estimates of the importance of information needs, and conclusions that additional government actions on lead problems are required. On the last, the Committee offers its views as citizens, rather than experts.

LEAD IN THE ENVIRONMENT OF URBAN CHILDREN

HEALTH HAZARDS OF CURRENT EXPOSURES

1. *The evidence is convincing that exposures to levels of lead commonly encountered in urban environments constitute a significant hazard of*

236

detrimental biological effects in children, especially those less than 3 years old. Some small fraction of this population experiences particularly intense exposures and is at severe risk:

a. Reports of death from childhood lead poisoning are currently rare and difficult to verify, and the incidence of confirmed cases of clinical lead poisoning in children has exhibited a continuing decline during the last decade (Chapter 2, Case I, Step 7).

b. Nevertheless, a recent survey indicates that about 0.7 percent of children from 0 to 3 years old in a sample drawn from urban and nonurban populations have blood lead levels that exceed 50 μg/100 ml, and 1.3 percent have levels above 40 μg/100 ml. The risk of adverse biological effects is especially significant for this small fraction of the population. In some urban areas the number of children with excessive exposures may be much higher than the average (Chapter 2, Case I, Step 4).

c. In addition, blood lead screening programs have shown that an unexpectedly large fraction of children have elevated blood lead levels. Recent (1978) data indicate that geometric mean blood lead levels among children less than 4 years old are about 15 to 20 μg/100 ml. On the average, about 6 to 7 percent of children examined meet criteria for undue lead absorption, but screening programs in different cities show that from 3 to 20 percent of children tested fall into this category (Chapter 2, Case I, Step 4).

d. Some recent studies suggest that average blood lead levels of children in some cities are decreasing. It is not yet known whether the trend is a general one, or how much of the observed change may be attributed to improved measurement methods, and how much may be due to decreased exposure to lead. To the extent that exposure has been reduced, the relative importance of specific control measures in contributing to reduced blood lead levels has not yet been established (Chapter 2, Case I, Step 7).

e. The most readily measured biological change that can presently be associated with lead in the body is inhibition of enzymes involved in the biosynthesis of heme. The significance to health of biochemical changes without associated evidence of illness is uncertain, and the question of what degree of inhibition of heme synthesis should be considered a detrimental effect is controversial, both scientifically and in policy debates (Chapter 2, Case I, Steps 5 and 6).

f. Clear evidence of significant inhibition of heme synthesis is associated with blood lead levels of 30 μg/100 ml or more. Recent research suggests that some individuals in a population may exhibit detectable changes in enzyme activity when blood lead levels exceed 15 μg/100 ml (Chapter 2, Case I, Step 5).

g. It is well known that very high doses of lead severely affect the intellectual development of children; the number of cases of clinical lead encephalopathy in recent years is believed to be small. Recent research has associated slightly elevated concentrations of lead in the body with lowered intellectual performance and nonadaptive behavior in young children. However, epidemiological research can not fully exclude the possible influences of confounding variables, and thus cannot prove that the observed effects are caused by excessive exposure to lead. Experiments in animals have demonstrated neurochemical changes, behavioral effects, and learning deficits caused by low-level exposure to lead. Although the available evidence, as a whole, suggests that current exposures to lead may have adverse effects on the intellectual functions of urban children, research on this topic to date has failed to obtain conclusive proof that harm is, or is not, occurring. More study of this question is clearly needed (Chapter 2, Case I, Step 5).

h. At present, techniques for measurement of significant changes in neurological and behavioral functions are less sensitive than those available for measuring effects on heme synthesis. However, as the ability to detect small changes improves, it may become evident that the developing nervous system is the most critical target of lead toxicity (Chapter 2, Case I, Step 5).

ı. The potential interactions among lead, other toxic substances, essential nutrients, genetic differences in susceptibility, and additional stresses that affect urban children are almost completely unknown. It seems likely that such interactions could modify dose–effect relationships for exposure to lead. Further information on this topic is needed (Chapter 2, Case I, Step 5).

SPECIFIC POPULATIONS WITH EXPOSURES

2. *The risk of excessive exposure to and absorption of lead varies significantly within populations, and some children with elevated blood lead levels may be more susceptible to biological changes induced by lead than other children. Current knowledge concerning the reasons for the differences is inadequate:*

a. It is known qualitatively that differences in observed blood lead levels and in sensitivity to effects of lead result from both differences in amounts of lead in the child's immediate environment and differences in characteristics of individual children, such as age, family, cultural surroundings, genetic makeup, socioeconomic status, behavior, nutrition, physiological state, and health status (Chapter 2, Case I, Step 2).

   b. The influence of any of the factors or of combinations of them cannot be estimated quantitatively with current knowledge (Chapter 2, Case I, Step 2).

   c. The lack of better understanding of factors that place individuals at risk limits the ability to define with satisfactory specificity all subsets of urban children that are most exposed or most susceptible. Although some groups at special risk can be readily identified (e.g., children with pica and exposure to lead paint or lead-laden soil), it is uncertain how large such subpopulations are (Chapter 2, Case I, Step 2).

SOURCES OF LEAD IN CHILDREN'S BODIES

   3. *It is well established that urban children are exposed to lead from several sources by many pathways, and the nature of the sources and pathways is known qualitatively. However, the precise contributions of different sources to typical body burdens of lead in urban children have not been determined quantitatively with any degree of confidence*:

   a. Some children are exposed to very intense doses of lead through accidental or deliberate ingestion of soil, dust, or paint chips. In such cases, these sources usually are the predominant avenue of exposure, but uncertainties about these exposures are nevertheless pervasive. Insufficient specific information exists on the amounts, forms, or locations of lead in soil, dust, or paint that are accessible to specific children; the amounts of these substances ingested through normal hand-to-mouth activity or through pica; the number of children who ingest them; and the absorption of lead ingested in such materials (Chapter 2, Case I, Step 3).

   b. All children also are exposed to some lead in the air, foods, and drinking water. The general magnitude of the baseline exposure is understood, but the exposures of individuals are highly variable. The range and distribution of exposures are uncertain, because levels of lead in air, water, and diets to which individual children are exposed have not been extensively documented, and knowledge of the absorption and retention of lead in children is inadequate (Chapter 2, Case I, Step 3).

   c. Empirical correlations between measurements of lead in the body and lead in the air, water, soil, or gasoline are valuable qualitative indicators of source contributions, but they rest on too few data and too many unproven assumptions to be accepted as being quantitatively reliable (Chapter 2, Case I, Step 4).

d. Limited knowledge on these points permits only approximate definitions of the amounts of lead in air, water, paint, gasoline, soil, dust, or foods that constitute hazards. Although such definitions may be expected to improve with further research, policy decisions must be made on the basis of unavoidably imprecise estimates (Chapter 2, Case I, Step 8).

CONTROL TECHNIQUES AND STRATEGIES

4. *Numerous technical and nontechnical measures can reduce exposures of urban children to lead. Some control steps have been implemented already, and additional opportunities for control can be readily identified. However, current knowledge does not permit definitive cost–risk–benefit assessments of most specific measures, and valid quantitative comparisons of control strategies are usually difficult to achieve*:

a. Some measures undertaken primarily for purposes unrelated to control of lead have reduced the amount of lead in the urban environment. Examples include gradual replacement of the housing stock in urban areas, increased use of unleaded gasoline for vehicles with catalytic emission controls, and construction of highways that divert traffic from inner-city areas (Chapter 2, Case 1, Step 7).

b. Specific measures implemented to reduce the likelihood of childhood lead poisoning include population screening, removal of sources of lead from targeted housing units, establishment of a national ambient air quality standard and state implementation plans, reduction of lead contamination of some foods, and public education about hazards of lead poisoning (Chapter 2, Case I, Step 7).

c. No concerted effort has yet been made to determine the net effects of any or all of these control measures on exposure of urban children to lead. It is uncertain what factors have contributed (or how much) to downward trends in blood lead levels noted previously (Chapter 2, Case I, Step 7).

d. Additional control of exposure to lead is needed, because the risk of adverse effects in children, described in (1), is unacceptably high. In all likelihood, future research on biological effects of lead will support the continued progressive lowering of the definition of the level of lead in the body that is considered "detrimental" (Chapter 2, Case I, Step 5).

e. Control measures enacted in recent years have greatly reduced the rate of addition of lead to urban environments, but have not significantly eliminated large reservoirs of the metal, primarily in paints and soils, that remain accessible to children. However, the most effective methods of achieving further reductions in exposures have not been determined in a quantitative way (Chapter 2, Case I, Steps 7 and 8).

f. At least six distinct approaches seem likely to have potential value in reducing hazards associated with lead in the environment of the urban child (Chapter 2, Case I, Step 7):

i. *Regulation*, to limit lead levels in air, water, soil, foods, gasoline and paint; to require the removal of lead paint from housing; to ban products that result in exposure to lead.

ii. *Population screening*, to identify children with elevated blood lead levels and to trigger abatement of sources in the environs of specific children at risk.

iii. *Planning*, including design of transportation systems to reduce traffic density, and zoning to separate point sources from populated areas.

iv. *Technological changes*, including increased reliance on recycled lead, and phasing-out of environmentally damaging uses of the metal.

v. *Social welfare programs*, including urban renewal, health care services and health education, nutritional care, family counseling and child care services, and improvement in the quality of housing.

vi. *Education*, about hazards and possible preventive measures.

g. Control programs to date have emphasized primarily the regulatory approach. Most actions have been concerned with a single medium or source of exposure. Population screening, abatement, and education have been emphasized also, especially in terms of efforts to prevent lead paint poisoning, where regulatory measures are insufficient or impractical (Chapter 2, Case I, Step 7).

h. There is a clear and pressing need for more comprehensive, flexible, and imaginative assessments of strategies for the prevention of exposure to lead. It is especially essential that *combinations* of measures drawn from the six categories in (f) be examined (Chapter 2, Case I, Step 7).

i. Current knowledge permits only crude cost–risk–benefit comparisons of available strategies. Nevertheless, the results can provide useful guidance for some policy decisions (Chapter 2, Case I, Step 7).

j. In order to permit comparison of alternative combinations of control measures, an improved basis for cost–risk–benefit assessment of different strategies is needed. The basis includes many of the information needs noted above.

IMPLICATIONS

5. *The noted uncertainties and lack of consensus about a preferred approach have important implications:*

a. Significant adverse effects on the health of children will continue to occur if indecision about what to do inhibits actions to eliminate exposure to lead.

b. On the other hand, if actions are taken without reasonable assurance that they will have the desired effects, substantial resources may be wasted or used inefficiently.

c. Improvements of the information base for policy decisions can be expected to come about slowly, but the need to make decisions is often more urgent than the advancement of knowledge.

d. Inaction because of uncertainties is unacceptable in the case of lead in the environs of urban children. The attempt to devise improved solutions to the problem is an iterative process. Continued commitment to take appropriate action, combined with a suitably systematic approach to making decisions, offers realistic promise of significant progress.

LEAD IN THE ENVIRONMENT OF THE GENERAL ADULT POPULATION

HEALTH HAZARDS OF CURRENT EXPOSURE

6. *The possibility cannot be excluded that detrimental degrees of biological change are associated with typical levels of lead in the bodies of at least some adults without occupational or other unusual exposures. This hazard is less conclusively established than the hazard to urban children, but is supported by the following conclusions:*

a. Recent data suggest that most adult populations in the United States have mean blood lead levels of about 10 to 20 μg/100 ml. About 3.5 percent of the adult population may have levels above 30 μg/100 ml (Chapter 2, Case II, Step 4).

b. Dose–response relationships for the inhibition of heme synthesis in adults are very similar to those described for children [see finding 1f, above]. The health significance of observed biochemical changes is unknown (Chapter 2, Case II, Step 5).

c. Recent and still relatively tentative findings on populations with occupational exposures to lead suggest that chromosomal abnormalities, toxic effects on the fetus, and interference with male and female reproductive functions may be associated with blood lead levels of 30 to 40 μg/100 ml (Chapter 2, Case II, Step 5).

d. Current estimates of effective levels for lead-induced anemia, subjective complaints, neuromuscular and behavioral effects, and changes in kidney function fall between 40 and 60 μg/100 ml (Chapter 2, Case II, Step 5).

e. Possible associations between lead and cancer, cardiovascular diseases, abnormal skeletal metabolism, and cellular aging have been suggested, but either have not been conclusively demonstrated in humans or cannot presently be described in quantitative dose–effect terms (Chapter 2, Case II, Step 5).

f. This evidence suggests that typical exposures to lead may produce adverse health effects in some members of the general population. There is a narrow margin between typical and probably toxic levels of lead in the body, and undoubtedly the respective ranges overlap to some degree. A clear need exists for better dose–effect and dose–response information on effects that may occur at blood lead levels below 40 μg/100 ml (Chapter 2, Case II, Steps 5 and 6).

g. As in the case of children, the potential interactions among genetic variables, essential nutrients, lead, other toxic substances, and other stresses that affect adults are unknown (Chapter 2, Case II, Step 5).

SPECIFIC POPULATIONS WITH EXPOSURES

7. *Differences in exposure and in genetic, nutritional, physiological, health, and behavioral characteristics of individuals contribute to an uneven distribution of the risk of biological effects of lead among the general population. Knowledge of the influence exerted by any of these factors permits only imprecise identification of specific populations most at risk:*

a. Nevertheless, pregnant women should be considered a group at special risk, because of the likely sensitivity of the fetus to effects of lead (Chapter 2, Case II, Step 5).

b. Further research is likely to identify factors that are associated with elevated exposure to lead or increased susceptibility to its toxicity for additional specific subsets of the general adult population (Chapter 2, Case II, Step 2).

SOURCES OF LEAD IN THE BODIES OF ADULTS

8. *For adults without occupational or other unusual sources of exposure, lead in foods usually is the chief source of lead in the body. Air, tobacco smoke, and drinking water also can contribute significantly to total lead absorption under some conditions. Typical exposures are reasonably well understood qualitatively, but insufficient quantitative information is available to assess the precise origins of exposure*:

a. Levels of lead in air, water, foods, and tobacco; human respiratory volume, dietary patterns, and water consumption; and absorption of lead all vary substantially among populations and individuals. Neither the full range, the statistical distribution, nor recent trends in total exposure to lead have been accurately determined (Chapter 2, Case II, Step 3).

b. Currently available empirical relationships between specific sources of exposure and levels of lead in the body are of limited value for quantitative predictive purposes (Chapter 2, Case II, Step 4).

CONTROL TECHNIQUES AND STRATEGIES

9. *Several measures already in effect and some others that might be implemented could reduce exposures of the general adult population to lead. However, the reduction in risk to health or the cost-effectiveness of alternative combinations of measures or of different degrees of control can be only crudely estimated*:

a. It has not been determined whether measures already taken [see findings (4a) and (4b) above] have had any significant effect on the amount of lead in the bodies of typical adults (Chapter 2, Case II, Step 7).

b. Lead in the diet is the largest currently uncontrolled source of exposure for adults. Improved knowledge is needed on the feasibility and costs of achieving significant reductions in lead levels in foods (Chapter 2, Case II, Step 7).

c. Recent reports indicate that dietary exposures to lead in Scandinavian adults may be up to an order of magnitude lower than exposures of Americans to lead in foods. The reasons for the observed differences have not been determined. Research on this question might indicate the degree of control over dietary exposure that is possible (Chapter 2, Case II, Step 3).

NATURAL CONTRIBUTIONS TO LEAD IN THE ENVIRONMENT AND IN HUMANS

NATURAL AND PERTURBED ECOLOGICAL CYCLES

10. *Accurate estimates of the natural occurrence of lead are needed as a baseline for assessing present-day exposures, especially to lead in the diet. However, present-day levels of lead in the atmosphere and in plants and animals at most sites have been increased by lead from anthropogenic sources and are not true natural levels:*

a. Pretechnological levels of lead in the air, estimated by several geochemical techniques, are roughly 2 orders of magnitude lower than present-day background levels at rural and remote sites in the Northern Hemisphere. The anthropogenic increase is substantially smaller in the Southern Hemisphere (Chapter 2, Case III, Step 3).

b. Deposition of atmospheric lead at typical rural and remote sites may be a source of geochemically significant input of the element to soils and freshwater bodies. The effect of added lead on background levels of the metal in these media cannot be estimated precisely, but it probably is not large (Chapter 2, Case III, Step 3).

c. Atmospheric deposition of anthropogenic lead appears to be the primary source of the element in surface ocean waters, especially remote from continental shores. It has been proposed that this input is responsible for a 10-fold increase in the lead content of the surface layer of the oceans, but the issue has not been resolved (Chapter 2, Case III, Step 3).

d. There is increasing evidence to suggest that deposition of atmospheric lead contributes substantially to background levels of the element in vegetation. However, knowledge is insufficient to indicate conclusively the relative contributions of lead in soil and lead in air to the lead content of plants (Chapter 2, Case III, Step 3).

e. Many aquatic and terrestrial organisms appear to accumulate lead in direct proportion to the widely varying levels in their environments. Proportional lead burdens have been observed to decrease in organisms at higher trophic levels in vertebrate food chains; nevertheless, present-day background lead burdens in some animals today almost certainly are higher than natural levels. Neither the general magnitude of the increase, nor its full extent, nor the range of likely variation among diverse ecosystems can be precisely estimated from available data (Chapter 2, Case III, Step 3).

f. The best available evidence suggests that the lead content of unprocessed foods may be up to 2 orders of magnitude greater than natural background levels, but quantitative estimates of this effect of anthropogenic lead are still subject to great uncertainty (Chapter 2, Case III, Step 3).

g. The most commonly used analytical methods for measuring lead in biological materials are frequently subject to serious errors (Appendix D), and it is likely that the magnitude of anthropogenic effects on lead in foods has seldom been accurately measured (Chapter 2, Case III, Step 3).

h. At some truly remote places (especially in the Southern Hemisphere) the biogeochemical cycle of lead is closer to its natural state than in inhabited regions. It should be possible to observe ecological transfers of lead under much more nearly natural conditions than those studied to date, if such sites can be located and research can be conducted there (Chapter 2, Case III, Step 3).

NATURAL LEVELS OF LEAD IN HUMANS

11. *The levels of lead in present-day Americans probably are 2 to 3 orders of magnitude higher than natural levels of lead in humans:*

a. Exposure/absorption models using some tenuous assumptions produce estimates of absorption of lead under natural conditions that are about 1 to 5 percent of estimated present-day absorption rates (Chapter 2, Case III, Step 4).

b. Some populations in remote areas exhibit mean blood lead levels roughly an order of magnitude lower than those of present-day Americans (Chapter 2, Case III, Step 4).

c. Bones from ancient cultures that made no known use of lead contain about 2 to 3 orders of magnitude less lead than modern American bones (Chapter 2, Case III, Step 4).

d. A few reliable measurements of transfers of lead in wildlife food chains suggest that the natural lead content of human bones may be 2 to 3 orders of magnitude lower than present levels (Chapter 2, Case III, Step 4).

e. Measurements or predictions of natural levels of lead in bones are insufficient to indicate precisely the natural levels of lead in human blood or soft tissues (Chapter 2, Case III, Step 4).

BIOLOGICAL IMPLICATIONS

12. *The biological implications of the historical increase of levels of lead in humans are currently unknown. Speculation that "normal" people may be impaired in undetected ways by present-day levels of lead in*

the body can be neither verified nor dismissed as unfounded without
further research on biological effects of low levels of exposure:

a. It is currently not known whether biological effects of lead are strictly proportional to dose, or whether protective mechanisms or tolerances exist that produce a threshold of toxicity for lead in humans (Chapter 2, Case III, Step 5).

b. Even if some tolerance is assumed, it has not been determined at what level of lead in the body the implied threshold of toxicity lies, or whether commonplace present-day exposures to lead exceed any natural capacity the body might have for adjusting to effects of lead (Chapter 2, Case III, Step 5).

c. The possibility cannot be excluded that very small amounts of lead might be essential to some biological processes, but evidence to date provides virtually no support for this hypothesis (Chapter 2, Case III, Step 5).

THE USE OF SCIENTIFIC KNOWLEDGE IN RECENT GOVERNMENT DECISIONS ABOUT LEAD

INFORMATION USE IN DECISION MAKING

13. *Federal agencies making recent decisions about lead in the environment have had access to extensive assessments and summaries of available scientific knowledge, including information on the uncertainties and limitations of current knowledge. (Appendix A.)*

14. *Decisions by Congress and the courts have required some agencies to establish numerical standards for lead in the environment. In order to do so, the agencies have had to make judgments about relationships among lead in the environment, exposure, lead in the body, and biological effects that go beyond what is generally accepted as conclusively established on the basis of current scientific knowledge:*

a. There has been a recent trend toward development of an explicit, quantitative basis for standards. This approach is desirable, because it focuses attention on arbitrary assumptions and judgments, and identifies critical information needs (Chapter 3).

b. In practical terms, the uncertainties noted earlier make it impossible to determine with confidence whether numerical standards that have been set will result in improvements in health that would justify expected costs of control (Chapter 3).

CONSISTENCY AND COORDINATION OF DECISIONS

15. *The approach by Congress to legislation pertinent to regulation of lead has been incremental, fragmented, and disjointed. The result has been narrowly drawn mandates and inconsistencies in the laws that require federal administrative actions:*

a. Most of the eight major laws that authorize federal regulatory activities on lead are concerned with a single pathway or source of human exposure. No agency has authority to deal with total exposure to lead in a comprehensive, integrated way (Chapter 3, Appendix C).

b. The laws are inconsistent in the degree to which they require or permit all pertinent aspects of decisions, such as costs and benefits of control measures, to be considered (Chapter 3, Appendix C).

c. Under the Lead-Based Paint Poisoning Prevention Act, one agency (HEW) is responsible primarily for protecting children against health hazards of lead, and another agency (HUD) is responsible primarily for assessing the feasibility and costs of abatement of lead paint hazards. No one official is required to weigh the two concerns and determine an acceptable balance between reduced risk and increased costs, given current knowledge. The lack of comprehensive or parallel mandates and the division of efforts have made it unusually difficult to achieve consensus and coordination of appropriate programs to abate lead paint hazards (Chapter 3).

d. There has been some effective recent communication and coordination among different federal agencies concerned with lead in the environment. However, improvements are still needed (Appendix C).

FEDERAL RESEARCH PROGRAMS ON LEAD IN THE ENVIRONMENT

LEVEL OF EFFORT

16. *Federal agencies spent a total of $18 million for research directly concerned with lead, and $63 million for multi-element research that included lead, during the last 3 fiscal years (1977 through 1979) (Appendix B).*

TOPICS INVESTIGATED

17. *Investigations of potential health hazards were overwhelmingly the top priority in research concerned primarily with lead. Multielement*

studies were divided more evenly among several subject areas. Some topics that are pertinent for decision making received little or no support during the 3-year period (Appendix B):

a. Within the research concerned primarily with lead, 67 percent of the $18 million was spent on studies of biological effects; 13 percent was devoted to gathering data on human exposures; and 6 percent was spent on studies of the absorption and pharmacodynamics of lead. Studies of control measures received 10 percent of the funds, and all other topics combined drew less than 4 percent of the total.

b. In the multi-element research category, 53 percent of total expenditures were for studies of the environmental occurrence and cycling of trace elements. Other topics investigated were analytical methods (18.5 percent), biological effects (12.5 percent), and pollution control and abatement (10 percent).

c. Federal support of research on social and economic aspects of the management of lead hazards has been minimal during the last 3 years. There has also been little support for studies of ecological effects of lead, or for research to improve definitions of the natural occurrence and cycling of the element.

AGENCIES INVOLVED

18. *During the last 3 years, at least 21 agencies or sub-agencies of the federal government supported some research that was directly or partially concerned with lead. However, a few agencies accounted for most of the expenditures in both the lead research and multi-element categories (Appendix B):*

a. In the category of research concerned primarily with lead, the leading sources of support during fiscal years 1977 through 1979 were NIEHS, DOE, FDA, EPA, HUD, and HEW (including NIOSH, CDC, and four divisions of NIH, but excluding FDA and NIEHS). NIEHS alone supported 30.5 percent of the government's total.

b. In the multi-element research, the USGS accounted for 47 percent of total expenditures; DOE, BM, NIEHS, EPA, and FDA spent another 46 percent of the total.

c. Other agencies that supported smaller research efforts on specialized topics include FWS, NOAA, NBS, USDA, and NSF. (During the years preceding the period covered by this survey, NSF sponsored a multimillion dollar program of research on lead in the environment. That effort terminated in 1977.)

TRENDS IN LEAD RESEARCH

19. *Within the period 1977 through 1979, federal support of research on lead declined by an estimated 25 percent. This is apparently the descending phase of a peak of activity associated with recent regulatory decisions, and not an erosion of basic support for research on lead. The decline in funding was distributed relatively evenly over subject areas (Appendix B).*

INTERAGENCY COORDINATION OF RESEARCH

20. *Biological topics predominate in lead research, and relatively effective interagency coordinating mechanisms have been developed for toxicological programs. There has therefore been a reasonable balance in government research on health effects of lead. However, improvements in other areas are needed (Appendix B):*

a. Improved coordination of research planning is needed, especially among regulatory agencies. The Interagency Regulatory Liaison Group has made a promising start in that direction, but the effort is too recent to judge its effectiveness.

b. There appears to be an opportunity worth exploring for more effective interaction between regulatory agencies and agencies such as DOE, NOAA, USGS, FWS, and USDA, which support substantial programs of research on topics that might be relevant to regulatory information needs.

5 Recommendations

The Committee's recommendations are divided into two categories. The first group deals with actions that the government could take or should take now to manage hazards associated with lead in the environment. The Committee recognizes that improved information is needed on many major scientific questions, and that some of the gaps in current knowledge may require years of research. Nevertheless, social policy decisions must be made in a timely manner, using the best available evidence, and recognition of the need for better information should not delay essential actions to protect public health and well-being. It is recommended that measures be implemented in ways that permit them to be guided or adjusted by improved knowledge as it becomes available.

The second group of recommendations is concerned with research needs. It consists of a list of topics and suggested research approaches that hold promise for producing information of significant value on questions that are critical to regulatory decisions.

Both the the suggested actions and the research recommendations are broadly defined and may apply to many federal, state, or local government agencies, as well as to private institutions. Specific recommendations for HUD, the agency that sponsored this study, are presented separately.

RECOMMENDED ACTIONS

The Committee believes that measures to reduce or prevent exposure to lead cannot wait until research has resolved the many uncertainties

251

described in this report. Incomplete knowledge on many topics has pre-cluded our conducting even a crude cost–risk–benefit analysis of options. Nevertheless, on the basis of both the state of scientific knowledge and our own value judgments, the Committee feels the following actions would be reasonable and prudent:

• *Improved institutional mechanisms should be developed for dealing with the many aspects of lead in the environment in an integrated, systematic, coordinated, consistent manner.*

1. Since the current disjointed approach is primarily attributable to the laws under which present government programs are carried out, Congress will necessarily be a principal actor in achieving improvements. Congress should: (a) Consider whether the diverse and inconsistent laws that provide for control of lead hazards might be rewritten into a single, comprehensive statute. Such a law could require the coordinated consideration of all aspects of environmental exposures to toxic agents, and apply the same requirements for assessing risks, costs, and benefits to all components of multimedia problems. Lead appears to be an excellent prototype for an assessment of the feasibility, advantages, and disadvantages of pursuing this goal. (b) Consider the creation of more formal and comprehensive coordination mechanisms than those that now exist, such as the Interagency Regulatory Liaison Group (IRLG). (c) Consider designating a "primary agency" for actions on specific aspects of problems, and requiring active participation of agencies concerned with other aspects of the same problems. (d) Consider an amendment to the Lead-based Paint Poisoning Prevention Act that would place authority for decisions about the control of lead paint hazards under a single, health-oriented, regulatory agency.

2. Without need of Congressional action, the following steps can be taken immediately: (a) HUD and CDC should be included in all IRLG activities that are concerned with lead. (b) Agencies that conduct research on aspects of environmental exposure to and effects of lead should undertake to develop a common research agenda. (This has begun already, through the IRLG Task Force on Metals of the Research Planning Work Group, but needs to be expanded to include agencies not now part of IRLG, such as HUD, HEW, CDC, and the Departments of Energy, Interior, and Commerce.) (c) Joint support of research of value to several agencies, such as economic and technical assessments of alternative strategies for reducing total exposure to lead, would be desirable.

• *Childhood blood lead screening should be continued and expanded to include a broader sample of the population at risk.*

1. Although childhood blood lead screening programs appear to be effective in identifying and protecting many individual children at risk, many cities do not have screening programs, and less than 30 percent of the population believed to be at greatest risk is examined annually. An expansion of this effort (subject to 3, below) is needed.

2. It has become clear that the problem of elevated exposure to lead is not restricted to children in deteriorating inner-city housing, but is more ubiquitous. As the definition of an acceptable level of lead in the body has been lowered, the population potentially at risk has expanded. Screening programs should encompass any children in the susceptible age group who might reasonably be expected to be exposed to significant amounts of lead.

3. Insofar as possible, new lead screening efforts should be undertaken within more comprehensive health care, and existing lead programs integrated into multifaceted health services.

• *Efforts to abate lead hazards for children with elevated blood lead levels should be continued or expanded at the local level. Increased federal funding might be made available to support such hazard abatement.*

1. In cities with established, effective screening and abatement programs, efforts should continue as long as undue exposure to lead remains a significant public health problem. New or more effective efforts are needed in other cities that have not yet begun or have only recently begun lead poisoning prevention programs.

2. Insofar as possible, abatement of lead hazards should be integrated with more comprehensive housing rehabilitation programs.

3. It is essential that evaluative procedures be incorporated in whatever programs are undertaken, so that a firm basis can be developed and made available to others for judging the effectiveness of alternative approaches to hazard abatement.

4. Lack of funds has imposed an important constraint on expansion of abatement efforts in the past. Since abatement of sources of lead is essential to control efforts, additional support, including federal support, is needed.

• *More extensive efforts should be made to identify specific sources of potentially excessive exposure of urban children to lead.*

1. At least a crude inventory of the occurrence of potential lead hazards should be compiled. At minimum, the information should be made available to people at risk of exposure, and to local authorities responsible for decisions about abatement measures.

2. Specific information needs include: (a) identification of housing units that contain lead-based paint on surfaces, especially paint in deteriorating condition; (b) identification of areas in which lead concentrations in drinking water exceed permissible standards; (c) identification of sites at which the soil is heavily contaminated with lead; and (d) determination of lead concentrations in outdoor and indoor atmospheres in residential areas near sources of lead emissions.

• *A serious effort should be made to reduce the baseline level of exposure to lead for the general population of the United States.*
1. Such action is needed both to decrease the risk of adverse effects in people with average exposures and to reduce the baseline of lead intake to which special exposures are added for urban children, the occupationally exposed, and others.
2. As an obvious initial focus for implementing this recommendation, the effort now under way by the FDA to reduce lead levels in foods deserves strong support.
3. Additional opportunities should be sought to make technological changes that could reduce human exposures to lead, such as elimination of lead-soldered food containers.

• *Public information and education programs should continue, with emphasis on the multisource nature of exposures to lead and on actions individuals can take to reduce personal risks of exposure.*
1. Examples of such actions include more alert adult supervision of children to prevent ingestion of paint, soil, or dust; avoiding eating home-grown vegetables from gardens near streets with heavy traffic; and contacting appropriate local agencies for assistance in detecting or eliminating potential sources of exposure around the home.

• *The accuracy, reliability, and usefulness of measurements and monitoring data for lead in the environment and in people must be substantially upgraded.*
1. Increased effort should be made to conduct monitoring in meaningful ways. For example, measurements of airborne lead should be based on particle-size distribution, not just total lead; and more emphasis is needed on the specific properties of lead present, such as chemical and physical form or isotopic ratios.
2. Reliable, consistent long-term data are needed on such critical variables as environmental levels of lead and lead in the bodies of young children.

3. All laboratories participating in analyses for lead should maintain stringent quality assurance measures, and should be required to participate regularly in interlaboratory comparison programs.

GENERAL RECOMMENDATIONS FOR RESEARCH

To improve the base of knowledge for regulatory decisions on lead, better scientific understanding is needed about a wide range of topics. Some improvement can be achieved through relatively straightforward data gathering. Other topics, however, will require problem-oriented, multidisciplinary investigation, and some questions may demand more fundamental research.

The topics listed encompass many scientific disciplines and investigative approaches. Since the problems addressed are interrelated, subject areas overlap, and a single research program might easily pursue more than one topic listed. The research needs presented here are balanced among biological effects of lead, environmental sources of exposure, and technical and social assessments of control measures. While research on health hazards associated with lead in the environment will require continuing strong support, there is also a need for both better balance and more attention to several additional topics than have been evident in recent federal research programs on lead.

The recommended studies are not focused on the specific needs of any one agency, but rather form a broad base of information needed to deal with total exposure to lead in an integrated manner. Specific recommendations for HUD's Lead-Based Paint Poisoning Prevention Research Program are presented separately later in this chapter.

The Committee's judgment of the relative importance of different research needs is indicated by ratings of high, medium, or low priority. The assignment of priorities was based in part on a subjective assessment of the importance of specific information needs for decision making; no formal sensitivity analysis was performed. In addition, the feasibility of obtaining needed knowledge carried some weight in our assessment of priorities. The order of topics on the list is not intended to reflect the order of priority.

TOPICS FOR RESEARCH

The Committee recommends that research be conducted on the following topics:

● *Effects of typical levels of lead in the body on the health of children and adults.*

Improved understanding is needed of dose–effect and dose–response relationships for known and suspected biological effects of lead in humans. Priority in studies concerning children should be given to examining the health consequences of subtle biochemical and physiological changes, especially those that may affect the development of central nervous system functions. Studies on adult populations need to examine a number of potential effects, especially those on genetic, reproductive, and renal functions. Where ethical or practical constraints limit research on human subjects (especially children), emphasis should be given to pursuit of appropriate animal studies.

The needed research includes:

1. Epidemiological studies of populations, including biochemical and functional tests on individuals, representing the full range of currently typical exposures to lead.

2. Toxicological research on effects of lead, at doses corresponding to commonplace exposures, on biochemical and physiological functions of cells and animals, with special emphasis on the delineation of biological changes that may be precursors of pathophysiological processes.

3. Pharmacodynamic investigations of the absorption, distribution, storage, mobilization, excretion, and homeostatic regulation of lead in humans.

4. Studies to define more precisely the nature and extent of heightened susceptibility to lead toxicity during the pre- and perinatal periods and the first few years of life, especially in terms of the developing nervous system and behavior.

5. Studies to define more precisely the relationships between timing of doses and effects, and especially the relative hazards of single or infrequent high exposures compared to chronic, lower levels of exposure to lead.

6. Investigations to improve understanding of the relationships between lead in blood, dentine, hair, or other accessible tissues and concentrations of lead at physiologically significant sites.

7. Investigations of interactions among lead, other environmental contaminants, physiological stresses, genetic and ethnic differences, and essential nutrients.

Within this subject area topics 1 through 5 should have high priority, and 6 and 7 should have medium priority.

● *Factors that contribute to risk in adults and children.*

Systematic investigations are needed to provide more definitive assessments of the importance of specific factors in placing an individual or a class of individuals at risk of (a) excessive exposure to lead or (b) biological effects of typical levels of lead in the body. Research should examine the relative significance of levels of lead in specific environmental pools (e.g., soil, air, water, dust, foods, and paint); other physical environmental variables; social, cultural, ethnic, and family factors; individual behavior patterns; and individual differences in age, sex, physiology, nutritional state, or health.

The needed research includes:

1. Careful, systematic investigations of relationships between measured levels of lead in the body and a comprehensive checklist of variables, using both statistical/correlation and case/control epidemiological methods.

2. Investigations of specific factors, such as age, pica, dietary patterns, or exposure to paint, to determine with more precision the nature of their contributions to hazards associated with lead.

Both topics should have medium priority.

● *Fractional contributions of different environmental sources to lead in the body for specific populations of children and adults.*

No single approach can provide conclusive evidence on this critical topic. Improved knowledge will require coordinated investigations using many approaches, including:

1. Studies to examine empirical multiple statistical regressions among indices of lead in the body (e.g., blood lead, dentine lead) and measured levels of lead in the air, water, foods, soil, paint, dust, and other possible contributing sources.

2. Extensive data gathering on the levels and chemical/physical properties of lead in specific foods, water supplies, gasoline, soils, dusts, and paints and in people; on dietary and liquid consumption patterns and soil, dust, or paint ingestion tendencies of individuals and groups; and on relationships between ingestion and excretion of lead in various source materials.

3. Careful measurements of specific transfers, such as deposition of aerosol lead on edible crops, absorption of solder lead into canned foods, weathering of lead paints, or absorption of inhaled or ingested lead.

4. More effective use of distinctive physical and chemical characteris-

tics of the forms of lead in different environmental pools (e.g., chemical form, isotopic ratios, elemental composition of source materials, particle size, and density), which could serve to identify the origins of lead in studies described in 2 and 3.

5. Improvement of models to estimate specific processes that are difficult to measure directly.

6. Measurements of environmental transfers and contributions of different sources to total exposure to lead in remote, pretechnological populations, or others with very low exposures.

7. Continued development of general models of source contributions, environmental mass-balance estimates, and other frameworks for integrating the information.

Within this subject area, topics 1, 2, and 7 should have high priority; 3 and 4 should have medium priority; and 5 and 6 should have low priority. Regression analysis (topic 1) is severely limited as a basis for defining causal relationships, but the hypotheses thus generated provide valuable guides for more precise methods of study. Although topic 6 would involve research with substantial methodological difficulties that would produce only limited amounts of new knowledge, such studies are nevertheless somewhat urgent, since the remaining number of human populations that are truly unaffected by the influences of civilization is dwindling.

- *Time-series data on levels of lead in the body for specific subsets of the population of the United States.*

Information is needed on trends in blood lead levels and other indexes of lead in the body, and better definitions of the statistical distribution of individual values in specific populations are essential for standard-setting purposes. This topic should have high priority.

- *Cost–risk–benefit comparisons of alternative combinations of control measures and different degrees of reduction of total exposure.*

Until better answers to the questions listed above are available, definitive cost–risk–benefit comparisons of control strategies will be difficult to achieve. Nevertheless, the effort is worthwhile. Information needs to support such analysis include:

1. Quantitative measures of the effectiveness of various control measures that have already been implemented, including both regulatory actions and medical surveillance and therapy, based on demonstrations of causality such as those listed in previous recommendations.

2. Improved estimates in economic or other terms of the costs and benefits of specific actions or combinations of actions that have already been adopted.

3. Comparable assessments of the potential effectiveness, costs, and benefits of new and innovative approaches to control of exposure to lead, especially combinations of different methods.

4. Improvements in certain technical aspects of control measures, such as control of corrosiveness in water supplies, or prevention of lead contamination of foods during processing.

5. Explorations of the social, technological, and economic ramifications of the elimination of or substitution of other materials for major uses of lead in the economy.

6. Studies in the social and behavioral sciences to improve the basis for defining an "acceptable" degree of risk, specific in terms of health hazards associated with lead.

7. Analysis of existing legal and institutional factors to determine the most effective approaches for dealing with total exposure to lead in an integrated, coordinated fashion.

Within this subject area, topics 1 and 7 should have high priority; 2, 3, 4, and 6 should have medium priority; and 5 should have low priority.

● *Natural and perturbed ecological cycles of lead.*

Improved understanding is needed of the natural biogeochemical cycle of lead, of specific transfers of the element on various scales, and of the effects on natural processes of lead introduced by human activities. Specific important topics include:

1. Improved measurements of critical geochemical processes and transfer rates, such as deposition of atmospheric lead, leaching of soil lead, and transfer of lead from land masses to the oceans.

2. Studies to determine mechanisms and rates of critical biological processes, such as uptake by plants of lead from the atmosphere, water, soils, and sediments; biotransformation of lead; and the transfer of lead in wildlife and domestic food chains.

3. Improvement of the basis for estimating the magnitude of the historical increase in typical human exposures to lead above natural baseline levels, including studies of remote, pretechnological human populations.

4. Potential for bioaccumulation and toxicity of lead in domestic animals, wildlife, and other organisms of significant ecological, aesthetic, or economic importance.

Research on these topics is generally of a more fundamental nature than that on most of the other topics listed here; consequently, its relevance for immediate policy decisions is more limited. However, some of the research may be of vital importance for long-term policy choices, and such fundamental research should have relatively high priority over the long run.

• *Improved methods for the detection and accurate measurement of small amounts of lead in the environment and in biological samples.*

The inability to measure lead accurately at low concentrations has often been the limiting factor in the definition of problems and the conduct of research. Improved answers to the questions outlined above will require improved measurement techniques, including:

1. Better definition of the unique chemical and physical characteristics of lead in various environmental pools, and increased attention to the usefulness of specific aspects of these properties in identifying sources and measuring transfer processes.

2. More sensitive and accurate techniques for the determination of amounts and forms of lead in foods.

3. Additional markers of levels of lead in the body, to augment information provided by blood lead or dentine lead measurements.

4. Improved and more sensitive portable instruments for *in situ* determination of lead in paints, soils, dusts and other materials.

5. Effective development and dissemination of techniques for preventing lead contamination of samples, equipment, and reagents.

6. Improved standard reference materials for lead in environmental samples and biological fluids and tissues.

Within this subject area, topics 1,5, and 6 should have high priority, and topics 2 through 4 should have medium priority.

SPECIFIC RECOMMENDATIONS FOR HUD'S LEAD-BASED PAINT POISONING PREVENTION RESEARCH PROGRAM

The first recommended action, above, calls for substantially improved coordination of federal regulatory and research programs concerned with lead in the environment. Recommendations for HUD are based on a concept of an appropriate role for the agency within a balanced, multi-agency research effort. At the heart of that concept are a belief that each agency should concentrate on what it does best and the recognition that effective resolution of some questions will probably require the joint efforts of several agencies with complementary legislative mandates, interests, and strengths.

In that context, it is recommended that HUD concentrate its research efforts on better defining the nature and magnitude of sources of lead in and around housing and the urban environment, and on assessments of innovative strategies for the control of exposure to lead from such sources. Studies of the relationships between sources of lead and the lead in people are vital, but should be conducted in a comprehensive manner by agencies with greater expertise and resources to support costly, sophisticated metabolic and epidemiological research. (The primary agencies in health-related research listed above probably should be NIEHS and EPA, with HUD, FDA, and others contributing to individual projects.)

We recommend the following topics as specific items for HUD's Lead-based Paint Poisoning Prevention research agenda:

- *Sources of lead in the urban environment.*

1. Careful determinations should be made of specific chemical and physical characteristics of lead in paint, soil, dust, drinking water, indoor air, and outdoor air near residences. Information of this sort would provide essential knowledge of possibly unique properties of different pools of lead that could supply vital clues to the origins of lead in people.

2. Continued and expanded efforts are required to determine the extent and seriousness of potential exposure to housing-related sources of lead. At least a crude national inventory is needed that can indicate the number of housing units with lead-based paint on surfaces or with lead plumbing, and the typical distribution of lead levels in house dust, soil, and street dust near housing units.

3. Studies of the weathering of lead paints should be carried out to determine rates of transfer to soil and dust pools.

Topics 1 and 2 should have high priority, and 3 relatively low priority.

- *Control techniques and strategies.*

1. In our judgment, research to improve technical methods for the removal of paint hazards has reached a point of diminishing returns. Marginal improvements in the technical and economic feasibility of paint removal or barrier techniques can certainly be envisioned, and better information is needed on the most appropriate combinations of methods for specific local conditions.

2. However, development of improved understanding of paint hazard abatement techniques needs to be pursued within a broad, systematic context. In order to know how vigorously removal of paint should be pursued, it is also important to know the importance of paint as a source of lead in children's bodies, the degree to which abatement of paint hazards in housing would reduce body burdens of lead, the costs of such abate-

ment, and the most cost-effective combination of approaches to reduce total exposure to lead.

It is therefore recommended that the Lead-Based Paint Poisoning Prevention Research Program emphasize studies of the following kinds:

(A) Additional studies to demonstrate and evaluate the effectiveness, technical feasibility, and costs of the best presently available methods for removal of lead paints, under a variety of field conditions.

(B) Studies to determine the relative usefulness of technical and non-technical approaches to reducing exposures to lead in housing.

Local lead poisoning prevention programs have employed diverse efforts to educate the public about lead paint hazards, to identify hazards to specific children, to abate sources of lead in some cases, and to provide follow-up attention and counseling by health professionals in some cases. Careful studies should be conducted to determine the costs and effectiveness of individual elements in such programs, and especially of various combinations of approaches.

(C) Economic assessments of policy alternatives, including several possible combinations of actions by government agencies.

Scenarios assuming different degrees of removal of lead from air, water, and food, and varying degrees of removal of lead-based paints and soils from housing should be developed. An attempt could then be made to project the effects of combinations of actions on levels of lead in people, and the value to society of both averted health damages and costs of control measures. The initial results of such analysis would be crude, and great care would be required to develop an appropriate set of assumptions. Nevertheless, the effort could produce a "first-iteration" guide to cost-effective strategies for control of total exposure to lead, and highly focused information needed to narrow the range of policy choices.

Research on these topics should be a high priority for several agencies, and probably should be conducted as a collaborative effort among HUD, CDC, EPA, and FDA.

FEASIBILITY OF RESEARCH AND LEVELS OF EFFORT

Many of the recommended studies on both the list of general topics for research and the items singled out for HUD's attention require only that readily available methods be applied to new or additional information-gathering tasks. The resources required to identify factors that contribute to risk, to obtain time-series data on human body burdens of lead, or to compile an inventory of lead sources in the nation's housing can therefore be estimated in a relatively straightforward manner.

On the other hand, research on biological effects of low levels of exposure to lead, some studies of geochemical and ecological transfers of the element, and economic assessments of the social costs and benefits of alternative control strategies would draw on research disciplines in which investigative methods are still evolving. For such studies, it is much more difficult to predict the time and resources likely to be required to achieve substantial advances in knowledge.

Some of the questions rated high in priority would require expensive research. For instance, gathering data to support multiple regression analyses of sources of lead in people would be costly. Toxicological studies are inherently expensive, and more so when precise measurements of small differences in exposure and of subtle biological changes are required. The sophisticated analytical techniques required to obtain definitive information on the specific chemical and physical forms of lead in different environmental pools have frequently been rejected in the past on grounds of cost.

On many of the topics identified here, to defer research because it is expensive would be penny-wise and pound-foolish. On questions that are critical for decision making about lead, answers of significant value may require the most powerful and precise available research techniques. A few definitive measurements may be worth more than thousands of imprecise or ambiguous ones.

However, despite these considerations, it is not necessarily true that the level of expenditures on research about lead should be greatly increased. The systematic approach inherent in this report offers a mechanism for continuing assessment of the state of knowledge relative to information needs for policy making, and for isolating critical topics on which substantial expenditures of resources are justified. Judgments have been offered here about the critical topics, as indicated by designations of high priority items on the lists of research problems. Obviously, the list and priority ratings will require periodic review and revision in the context of coordinated interagency research planning efforts.

The federal government has spent about $6 million a year for research on lead during the last 3 years, and about $21 million annually for more general studies of environmental trace substances that included lead. HUD has spent about $1 million per year since 1971 on lead-based paint poisoning prevention research, but less than that in the last 3 years.

In order to obtain useful answers to decision-related questions, both HUD and the government as a whole might need to make a modest increase of effort in lead research. A rapid increase is neither practical, considering the number of other research priorities that compete with lead for available resources, nor especially wise, since the result of rapidly increased funding could be a proliferation of mediocre research. The most important considerations are that increased efforts be focused selectively on specific, critical problem areas, and that a concerted effort be made to support high-quality work based on the most definitive investigative methods available.

An Alternative Perspective— Lead Pollution in the Human Environment: Origin, Extent, and Significance*

CLAIR C. PATTERSON

*Two members of the Committee, Cliff Davidson and Jerome Nriagu write:

As fellow members of the Committee on Lead in the Human Environment we endorse most of the issues presented in this alternative perspective. We would have liked to have collaborated with Patterson, but joint authorship was not feasible. The decision to prepare this alternative perspective came late in the period of our deliberations. The exchange of ideas and the working out of statements would have required many more months than the brief period made available to Patterson by the National Academy of Sciences because of the time constraints of the contract with the U.S. Department of Housing and Urban Development. We therefore write this statement to indicate our general support of the important ideas presented here.

Preface

This report uses a fresh perspective, different from traditional approaches used in the past, to address the charge to the Committee on Lead in the Human Environment. Historical material relating to the development of lead technology not previously summarized in the literature is given here. The review presented here regarding natural occurrences of lead is that of the majority of investigators who are working in this field, who conceived the lines of research that are being pursued, and who have obtained the acceptable data relating to this subject. This report does not present information concerning the occurrences of lead in urban environments because this subject has been thoroughly reviewed in other reports that are cited in the following text.

This report was written in collaboration with D. M. Settle, California Institute of Technology, Pasadena, and R. W. Elias, Virginia Polytechnic Institute and State University, Blacksburg, and it includes summaries of studies in the process of preparation and publication that have been carried out by the three of us with the following coworkers: M. Burnett, B. Schaule, R. Aines, and G. Kolbasuk, California Institute of Technology, Pasadena; C. Davidson, Carnegie-Mellon University, Pittsburgh; T. Hinkley, U.S. Geological Survey, Denver; Y. Hirao, Aoyama Gakuin University, Tokyo; M. Koide, University of California at San Diego; L. Newbern, Virginia Polytechnic Institute and State University, Blacksburg; J. Erickson, Harvard University; and H. Shirahata and K. Fujii, Muroran Institute of Technology, Muroran, Japan. Names of additional coworkers at these and other universities are given in published studies that are cited in the following text.

CLAIR C. PATTERSON

Contents

268

Introduction

Sometime in the near future it probably will be shown that the older urban areas of the United States have been rendered more or less uninhabitable by the millions of tons of poisonous industrial lead residues that have accumulated in cities during the past century. Babies are more susceptible to the hazards presented by these lead residues than are adults because they place objects and their hands in their mouths more frequently, much of their time is spent on or near surfaces which contain high concentrations of lead residues so that handled objects and their hands become highly contaminated with these lead deposits, they breathe air that contains higher than ordinary concentrations of reentrained lead dusts because of their proximity to sources of these dusts, their excessive requirements for calcium elevate their absorption of lead from intestines to much higher fractions than those characteristic of older humans, and their immature developing cells are more susceptible to damage from lead than are mature cells. Extrapolating from present data, there is some basis for believing that it will be shown in the future that significant irreversible deleterious effects to the central nervous systems of some ten thousand inner-city babies are being caused each year in the United States by exposures to industrial lead [1]. Extrapolating from present information, it also seems probable, from the viewpoint of cellular biochemistry, that it will be shown in the future that average American adults experience a variety of significant physiological and intellectual dysfunctions caused by long-term chronic lead insult to their bodies and minds which results from excess exposures to industrial lead that are five hundred-fold above natural levels of lead exposure, and that such dysfunctions on this massive scale may have significantly influenced the course of American history.

The U.S. Department of Housing and Urban Development, which requested this report and which is responsible to some extent for regulating the occurrence of lead in dwellings, wished to know whether contributions of lead from house paints to lead exposures experienced by inner-city babies are outweighed by, or were more significant than lead contributions from leaded gasolines, because they have some jurisdiction over the former but not the latter. Although HUD had already obtained evidence which indicated that leaded gasolines do make substantial contributions of lead to inner-city babies [2], a report issued according to engineering perspectives and traditions of the past would not provide specific guidance that would enable HUD or the Congress to significantly reduce within a short time, by regulatory action or statute, lead poisoning among inner-city babies. One cause for this is that some types of the residual sources of industrial lead, such as urban soils, building paints and putties, water distribution systems, and kitchen wares, are highly intractable and can be dealt with on a significant scale only at the cost of many tens of billions of dollars for each of the various types of sources. Another cause for inaction on a traditional engineering basis is that not enough information is available now to allow overwhelmingly forceful statements to be made concerning the relative proportions of lead contributed to inner-city babies by different sources such as leaded gasoline exhausts, leaded paints, leaded materials in water systems and kitchen utensils, lead in foods, etc. Another major cause for delay is a lack of knowledge that would permit extremely strong statements to be made about the ill effects caused by lead exposures now being received by inner-city babies.

In the face of this situation, I tried to do something positive by describing a new approach that might lead to corrective action. My view is that sufficient information is available to indicate that steps should be initiated now to reduce and eventually halt the mining and smelting of lead and the manufacturing of leaded products within the shortest possible time, that the manufacturing of some leaded products be halted forthwith, and that immediate steps should be taken to clean up existing lead residues and render them nonhazardous. Traditional engineering views avoid this issue. Instead, such views imply that the mining and smelting of lead and the dispersal of manufactured lead products can be safely carried out under proper controls, and that the real problem is to find out exactly where the lead is going and exactly which types of exposures are harmful, so that the proper type of controls can be instituted.

Most engineers in all fields are appalled by the prospect of dismantling, on the basis of evidence that has not been buttressed in minute detail by medical engineering observations, such a costly and enormous industrial enterprise with which many engineers have or have had professional or educational associations and which permeates every facet of the lives of all Americans. On the other hand, I believe that the traditional premise held by engineers and their protagonists will foster unwarranted delay of corrective action, and might also promote considerations, by means of cost/benefit analyses, of the relative merits of engineering solutions that would ultimately prove to be more inhumane than the existing situation.

The analysis presented here shows clearly what had not been recognized until very recently: that the mining and smelting of lead and dispersal of manufactured leaded products within the human environment is actually a monumental crime committed by humanity against itself. Although this is not an unusual occurrence, this particular tragedy is unique in that it has a genesis which is visibly linked to developments in engineering technology throughout the last ten thousand years, and which is amenable to study in simple terms. This may be valuable because these developments can also be directly related to human social problems. Further study of this subject may yield insight into broad aspects of many social problems created by developments in engineering technology.

The analysis presented here shows why it is important to seek solutions to these problems through basic research rather than simply to enlarge applied science and engineering efforts. Recommendations are made to initiate studies of the biochemistry of lead in laboratory sanctuaries which exclude industrial lead contamination with the expectation that knowledge will be obtained which will relate to the issue whether to terminate the mining and smelting of lead. The long history of lead technology shows that people's past attempts to solve problems created by lead poisoning by means of applied engineering methods have all failed. New approaches are needed which should include organized guidance from those sectors in human emotions which heretofore have had little influence. To this end it is recommended that support be strengthened and enlarged for scholarly research into the origins of *H.s.sapiens* and into factors which influenced the development, during the past forty thousand years, of both engineering technology and those humane activities, which, if given an opportunity, might properly guide the development of engineering technology along lines better suited to the best interests of *H.s.sapiens* than has been the case until now.

REFERENCES

1. Needleman, H.L., C. Gunnoe, A. Leviton, R. Reed, H. Peresie, C. Maher, and P. Burrett (1979) Deficits in psychologic and classroom performance of children with elevated dentine lead levels. *New England Journal of Medicine 300*, 689–695.
2. Billick, I.H. and V.E. Gray (1978) Lead Based Paint Poisoning Research: Review and Evaluation, 1971–1977. Office of Policy Development and Research—Washington, D.C.: U.S. Department of Housing and Urban Development. Billick, I.H., A.S. Curran and D.R. Shier (1979) Relation of pediatric blood levels to lead in gasoline (submitted to *Science*).

Origin of
Lead Pollution from
Developments in
Engineering Technology

INTRODUCTION

Lead is a metallic element that occurs naturally in extremely small concentrations, but it is highly toxic in a slow-acting manner, and small amounts can destroy human lives through irreversible degradation of mental abilities and general well-being without necessarily killing people immediately by means of acute poisoning effects nor causing the victims to be conscious of dysfunctions within themselves. The relationship between natural and toxic occurrences is illustrated in Figure 1 where the amount of natural lead in a prehistoric human on the left is represented by a single dot, and where by comparison the two thousand dots in the modern human on the right represent the approximate minimum amount of industrial lead that has been found to cause obvious lead poisoning defined in long-standing classical terms in a large proportion of a group of people. Between these two persons is a representation of the average American containing 500 dots, which by the same comparison depict the average amount of industrial lead pollution contained in Americans today. It should be understood that it is probable that this person is also poisoned with lead but in more subtle ways that have not yet been disclosed. In all three figures most of the lead is contained in the skeleton, where it has a prolonged residence time. Calcium is continuously added and subtracted from the skeleton. About half of the total daily input of calcium to the blood originates from the skeleton, and from this same reservoir lead is also reintroduced to the rest of the body, along with cal-

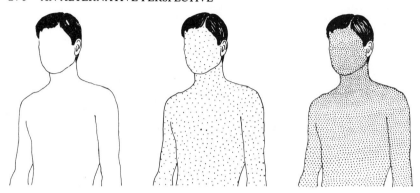

FIGURE 1   Comparison of relative amounts of lead in people: natural amount found in prehistoric people on the left; average amount found in present-day Americans in the middle; and minimum amount which will cause classical lead poisoning in a significant fraction of a group of people on the right. Each dot represents a unit of lead equivalent to 3×10^{-4} g Pb/70 kg person, based on a prehistoric natural skeletal value Pb/Ca (atomic) $= 6 \times 10^{-8}$ at age 45, reference [1].

cium, to maintain levels of lead in the body related to those in the skeleton. This is not an abstract scientific matter that has little relation to everyday life, but is a description of a real situation which exists now and applies to most people in the United States and other industrialized countries. Not much can be done to remove this excessive amount of highly toxic slow-acting industrial poison from the bodies of living Americans. The question is whether we will take steps now to remedy this situation so as to reduce the concentrations of this poison in the bodies of our progeny and thereby probably lessen the incidence of intellectual dysfunctions, diseases, and genetic disorders among them.

Although it is not known with certainty how long the difference between the amounts of lead in the figure on the left and the figure in the middle has existed within American people, there are indications that it represents a long-standing situation among Americans, and one which has existed for thousands of years in most people within industrialized and earlier civilizations in the Old World. Analyses of lead in bones of both Romans and people who lived during medieval times [2] show quite clearly that the situation depicted in Figure 1 is if anything a conservative description of past conditions. After 1850 and until 1925, world medical opinion held that there was no industrial lead in the figure in the middle [3] and that in accordance with logical assumption its lead content was equivalent to that portrayed by the figure on the left. In 1933 it was discovered that the figure in the middle did indeed contain the amount of lead portrayed in Figure 1 [4]. World medical opinion thereupon shifted to the belief that the lead content of the figure on the left was equivalent to the amount portrayed by the figure in the middle. This mistake arose because industrial lead in the middle figure was thought to originate from natural rather than from industrial sources. In 1965 it was proposed on the basis of theoretical considerations that the amount of lead in the figure on the left did actually represent natural lead in humans [5], but it has taken fourteen years of basic research to prove this to be so.

The response by present-day administrators in regulatory agencies, doctors in applied medicine, environmental engineers, and most people preparing prestigious government reports on lead in the environment, who had assumed, on the basis of the premise originating from the 1933 discoveries, that the person on the left was supposed to look like the person in the middle, when confronted with the knowledge depicted in Figure 1, has been either to deny that the situation exists or to say that no action can be taken to change this situation until this marked difference in body lead concentrations between the person on the left and the one in the middle has been shown to be harmful [6]. Biochemical considerations suggest that this difference is much too large not to be harmful [7]. However, the research which must be carried out to verify this will probably prove time consuming because it is difficult to study animal controls within environments totally free of industrial lead contamination.

In the meantime we are confronted with the question of whether or not it is acceptable from a humanitarian point of view to wait until such knowledge becomes available. Studies of the lengthy history of the development of the technology of lead indicate that the mining and smelting of lead should be terminated on the basis of humanitarian considerations because the past record of engineering attempts at control consists of a series of causally related failures, each with more seriously detrimental consequences to public health than those of its precursor, ending today in a situation that appears to constitute a near-catastrophic hazard.

INFLUENCE OF CHANGING ENVIRONMENTAL CIRCUMSTANCES ON THE DEVELOPMENT OF ENGINEERING TECHNOLOGY

The past century is but a small segment of the six thousand year history of lead technology. Environmentalists and industrialists tend to have a limited perspective regarding current problems caused by lead technology and fail to appreciate that valuable information can be gained from studies of the antecedents of lead technology. They regard ancient procedures in metallurgy, such as those depicted in Egyptian, Greek, and Roman stelae, as being unrelated to current problems, but this is not true. The germ plasm which characterizes *H.s.sapiens* has been alive for some forty thousand years [8] so that all humans have collectively participated in those past deeds through this immortal device and none can claim isolation from developments in engineering technology carried out by their ancestors. Archaeologists working in the field of pyrotechnology have reported the results of their studies of early technological developments of lead metallurgy and their findings have been summarized in reviews [9]. A contemporary summary of medieval and ancient lead mining and smelting techniques has been written and translated [10] and reports have been published of the development and use of lead smelting techniques, and of lead production during the last century [11].

However, this information concerning lead has not yet been summarized in a manner that discusses factors which brought about developments in engineering technology which led to the production and use of lead, and the effects that this technology has had on the evolution of human cultures during the past ten thousand years. In this section a tentative interpretive summary is given of the subject, prepared from both published and unpublished studies of many investigators. This synthesis is an approximation made up of specific interpretations selected from alternative interpretations that exist for each of the major points that comprise this story of lead technology, and it is highly susceptible to modification. Citations to alternative literature are not given because most of those studies were made without knowledge of any unified history of lead technology, and such studies must be restated to consider such a history in order for them to be applicable. It does not follow that this story is rendered false by the existence of such alternative interpretations, rather this holistic synthesis may lend strength to some interpretations and not to others.

A semiquantitative summary of world lead production during the last six thousand years is depicted in Figure 2. Annual productions are plotted on a logarithmic scale, which compresses the top of the graph downward, so that on a linear scale it is actually a million times higher (about ten kilometers) above the bottom than appears in the displayed form of the graph. This figure may be usefully called the poison index of engineering technology during the past six thousand years, because lead is highly toxic to humans in small quantities and changes in its production have been intimately related to many vital developments in engineering technology.

The beginning of man's involvement with lead and its problems goes further back in time than that shown in Figure 2 to some ten thousand

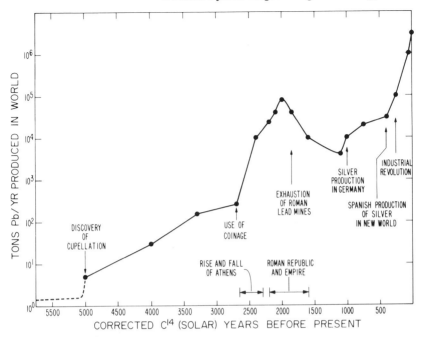

FIGURE 2 World lead production during the last 5500 years, reference [6]. This figure may be called the poison index of engineering technology during this period because lead is highly toxic to humans in small quantities and changes in its production have been intimately related to many vital developments in engineering technology.

years ago when the climate during the last glacial period suddenly changed and the glaciers retreated [13]. Distributions of plants and animals were altered and humans reacted to this stress where domesticable plants and animals occurred by becoming sedentary, and in such new situations they developed the new technologies of agriculture, animal husbandry, and urban living [14]. In these sedentary cultures food supplies stabilized and increased, population densities increased, and social structures became more complicated.

It was under these circumstances that the hammering and use of native copper began more than nine thousand years ago in the Old World [15]. The later appearance in the archaeological record about seven thousand years ago of cast copper objects produced by reduction smelting of oxidized copper ores coincides with the appearance of high temperature glazes on ceramics. This suggests that the discovery of smelting was related to the production of high temperature glazes in two-chambered kilns which had a reducing atmosphere in the upper chamber [16]. It is believed that the development of two-chambered high temperature kilns and high-temperature fired ceramics grew from a need for radiant heating ovens to bake the wheat that was being cultivated in sedentary societies. During the next thousand years metallurgists learned how to deliberately regulate impurities of smelted copper and this culminated in the discovery and use of bronze [17], a marvellously useful tin or arsenic copper alloy which quickly supplanted stone tools and weapons and equipped armies that built and defended empires. All of the above metallurgical developments took place within a period of about three thousand years.

The same sequence of metallurgical developments, starting with the hammering of native gold and proceeding through reduction smelting of oxidized ores and the development of alloys to the discovery of bronze, was repeated later during a thirty five hundred year interval by a different group of people in South America [18]. There are differences between the development of bronze in the Old and New Worlds. Consecutive steps in the later development in South America lagged five thousand years behind those in the earlier one, and the development of metallurgy in the New World was related largely to religious ceremony, rather than to the utilitarian purposes which characterized early metallurgical developments in the Old World. Furthermore, since the domesticated grain in the New World was corn, not wheat, radiant heating ovens and high temperature ceramics and glazes were not developed, yet reduction smelting of oxidized copper ores was independently discovered there. Despite these differences, the developments which led to the independent discoveries of bronze may have been triggered separately in each case by a more or less similar set of environmental circumstances. The highly complex pattern of human population responses which resulted from this supposedly fixed stimulus is remarkable for its ability to have been repeated with such little change, independent of differences in time, place, and gene pool. Although *H.s.sapiens* used crafted ornaments made of animal parts, this hominid species showed no inclination to hammer or use native copper during its thirty thousand year existence before the glaciers melted and sedentary cultures evolved [19]. Both of the above observations support the view that the development of metallurgical technology resulted from involuntary, consecutive reactions by human populations to changes in their environment in a feedback manner without conscious human control being a factor in guiding the direction of that development. This is an example of the implacable drive to carry out developments in engineering technology that is embedded in *H.s.sapiens* by two billion years of evolution. The power of humanitarian emotions to guide this development along proper channels evolved only forty thousand years ago and seems fragile by comparison.

Beginning at about six thousand years ago, lead metal was probably produced during the following thousand year interval as a by-product of smelting mixtures of native silver, which occurred only in very sparse quantities, and silver chloride ores in charcoal furnaces [17]. Lead was an impurity in the halide ores (which had the appearance of a variety of native silver) and would separate as a metal in this process; however, this by-product constituted only a small fraction of the silver that was obtained mainly by gathering native silver during this period.

The formation of empires defended by armies in the Old World created such a demand for bronze that it stimulated the discovery of much more complex and difficult techniques for smelting copper sulfide ores and the mining of these ores [20], which were more abundant than the oxide ores of copper used in reduction smelting. The use of these new techniques led to the discovery five thousand years ago that lead containing a small amount of silver could be smelted from lead sulfide ores which usually contain traces of silver sulfide, and that the silver could be isolated from the smelted lead-silver alloy by a second smelting process, called cupellation, involving the re-oxidation of the lead but not the silver [21]. This discovery of cupellation marks the time at which world lead production truly began. The desire for silver was the principal stimulus for lead production until recent times. Lead mined and smelted for itself has constituted a significant portion of total lead production only during the past century. Until several centuries ago, about four hundred tons of lead in oxide form were obtained as a smelted by-product for each ton of silver produced by cupellation. This by-product lead oxide was for the most part again reduced to the metal form (now free of silver) by a third smelting process for subsequent multiple uses of lead.

During the two thousand years that followed the first production of silver from lead ores in the Old World, great disparities on a regional basis arose among the occurrences of populations, food supplies, raw materials, and crafted goods, which generated a powerful incentive to discover how goods could be produced and distributed by means other than tribal craftsmen, barter, piracy, and pillage. During this period the development of knowledge concerning weights and measures, analytical methods for testing precious and base metals, and knowledge concerning the abundances and distributions of precious and base metal ores [22] led finally to the discovery and use of silver coinage about twenty six hundred years ago [23]. Although a causal relationship between the production of silver from lead, its use in coinage, and the growth of Classic Greek culture has not yet been established, such a relationship may exist. Shortly after societies in the eastern Mediterranean began to use silver coinage (Athens possessed the largest lead-silver deposits known at that time) they were transformed into powerful dominating federations which fostered our present social structures, business interrelationships, and ethics. This illustrates the deep-rooted association which probably exists between the technology of lead and our social institutions.

Stimulated by the successful use of silver coinage, world lead production rose abruptly to about ten thousand tons per year during the Classic Greek period, as shown in Figure 2. Lead was widely used in alloys, building construction, pigments, cosmetics, sapa, and to sheath ships, gutters, and cisterns. Sapa was an ingredient prepared by slowly simmering sweet grape juice with spices and herbs for days in covered pure-lead kettles. It contained several thousand ppm lead (in part as finely divided solids) and was added to green wine to keep it from souring while it aged [24]. It acted as a bactericide, although this wasn't known at the time. These widespread uses of lead undoubtedly elevated skeletal concentrations of lead in humans well above natural levels in this region at this time.

The decline of Athenian power about twenty three hundred years ago coincided with the exhaustion of lead-silver ore from her lead mines. The Roman Republic, after her defeat of Carthage, exploited with a vengeance lead-silver deposits in Spain that had been under Punic control. This dramatically increased world production of silver and lead more than a century before the Christian Era began. At the height of Roman power and influence, lead production may have amounted to some eighty thousand tons per year, as shown in Figure 2. The rate of Roman lead and silver production far exceeded that of any earlier culture, and the huge quantities of silver that were produced probably served as a cornerstone for Roman financial power which was a factor in the creation of this great empire. Among the many uses of lead appropriated by the Romans from the Greeks was the unfortunate practice of preparing sapa and adding it to green wine. This may have been one of the major causes for elevation of skeletal concentrations of lead in Romans to levels far above natural ones. Analyses of Roman bones from this period indicate that people in the lower economic classes may have had twice as much lead in their bodies as typical Americans today, while wealthy Romans may have had about four times as much [24]. These data suggest that classical forms of lead poisoning probably affected most upper-class Romans in ancient times. This seems incredible, but these findings do tend to confirm theories regarding the origin of the general insanity and sterility which appears to have affected many rulers of the Empire [24]. Although this factor, appropriately enough, probably contributed to the dissolution of the Roman Empire, exhaustion of lead-silver mines throughout the Empire following more than three centuries of intensive mining was another cause of the Empire's downfall. When the mines gave out, economic chaos followed upon the disappearance of Roman silver stocks [25]. These stocks were reduced by inadvertent, irrecoverable losses such as shipwrecks, hoards rendered inaccessible through catastrophe, and losses through mishandling of coin that were imperceptible to the Romans on a national scale, but which nevertheless had an appreciable effect over a period of time. It is estimated that the total loss rates were about 2% per year, which meant that silver stocks would be reduced to one-tenth of their original mass within a little more than a century unless they were sustained by continued mine production to supplant the loss. Thus, several thousand years ago lead was a crucial factor in the glory, madness, and downfall of one of the greatest empires in history.

Lead production declined to only a few thousand tons per year during medieval times, and continued at these low rates during this thousand year interval. Mining and smelting operations, which still employed Roman engineering techniques, were carried out by groups of independent entrepreneurs rather than by slave labor in massive national enterprises.

When Europeans invaded the Americas, the Spaniards exploited silver and lead deposits in Mexico and Peru. As shown in Figure 2, outputs from these sources increased world lead production to such high levels they rivaled those achieved earlier by the Romans. The forty thousand tons of silver which the Spaniards transferred from the New World to Europe during the period from about 1550 to 1750 helped to ruin the status of Spain as a major world power through the suppression of local industry by sustained major purchases of foreign goods [25]. However, the introduction of this great mass of Spanish silver into the European economy undoubtedly helped to initiate the Industrial Revolution. After this time, as shown in Figure 2, world lead production increased to levels above a million tons per year, where it has remained for nearly a century.

It appears that each of the three major upward surges in the poison index of engineering technology during the past twenty five hundred years was associated with social developments which had profound effects on some characteristics of succeeding civilizations. Modern industry has roots which extend through the Industrial Revolution to the Spanish Empire of the sixteenth century. Modern law and business organization have roots which extend back to Roman times. Modern governmental structure, ethics and business relations have lineages which extend back to Classic Greek culture.

FAILURE OF APPLIED ENGINEERING METHODS TO ALLEVIATE LEAD POISONING

It can be shown that the past record of attempts to alleviate the lead poisoning in human populations by applied engineering solutions have always failed, and have usually created a more dangerous situation than the one which had existed before. Some ancient physicians were apparently aware of cause and effect relationships between lead and the more acute forms of its poisonous effects on metallurgical craftsmen [26], and in such cases they probably tried to separate their patients from those sources of lead obviously related to the poisonous effects. In those days, the engineering approach used to solve these problems created by lead poisoning was to confine the poisonous effects of lead to slaves, mainly in mines and smelteries. This greatly worsened the situation for human populations as a whole by allowing lead production on a large scale to become a traditional enterprise in succeeding human cultures.

In the case of sapa, its poisonous effects went unrecognized throughout Greek and early Medieval times, even though it later became understood that lead was the active ingredient in sapa which acted to keep wine from souring. During Medieval times this knowledge resulted in the discarding of the preparation and use of sapa according to ancient tradition for the direct addition of lead oxide or acetate to wine to prevent its souring [27]. During the seventeenth century it became so commonly recognized that such practices resulted in lead poisonings that an applied engineering solution to this problem was formulated, which was to enact laws prohibiting these procedures, but this attempt failed. Even though the occasionally identified violators of these laws were severely punished, this adulteration of wine by lead continued until Pasteur discovered bacteria (a basic scientific discovery) after which time sulfur dioxide was widely used in place of lead (an applied engineering solution).

By 1850 physicians had correctly diagnosed and accurately described classical lead poisoning by carefully studying clinical cases of lead poisoning among industrial workers [28]. The engineering approach to the solution of this problem at that time was to control the sources of lead in the factories which were poisoning the workers. Obvious benefits to the health of industrial workers resulted from such corrective measures. These benefits, in association with the manner in which lead poisoning became widely recognized in the medical community, served to characterize lead poisoning as an occupational hazard rather than a consequence of an environmental poison. It was at this crucial time in the development of lead technology that the scales were tipped against humanity by its bemusement with applied engineering and its failure to appreciate that the large scale mining and dispersal of a highly toxic metal among humans was intrinsically wrong. As a result lead industries were endowed at this time with the "divine right" to mine and smelt lead and introduce it into human environments on an unrestricted scale.

During the early part of this century responsibility for instituting and enforcing measures to protect the health of workers in lead industries, such as smelteries and paint and battery factories, was transferred to public agencies [29]. This was done because it appeared to be an effective way to achieve humanitarian goals. These applied engineering attempts to reduce the incidence of recognized lead poisoning among human populations masqueraded as humanitarian actions. But in fact they were not because they fostered the increased production of lead which is responsible for a major portion of the intractable poisonous lead residues now present in urban areas.

The greatest failure of applied engineering approaches to control the incidence of lead poisoning resulting from industrially produced lead among human populations is connected with the manufacture and burning of lead alkyls. During the 1920's an unofficial decision was made by the U.S. Public Health Service to permit the manufacture and burning of lead alkyls [30]. This came about because the government more or less officially assumed the right to institute new measures that were to be taken in the manufacture of lead alkyls to protect the health of workers in lead alkyl factories, to require that stringent controls for the protection of the public were to be used during the transport of lead alkyls from factories to refineries, and to require that warning labels be affixed to gasoline pumps. It was assumed, on the basis of inadequate tests of animals exposed to leaded gasoline exhausts from engines, that no harm would come to humans from such exhausts [30]. This tragically misguided decision has bestowed upon the earth a heritage of lead polluted atmospheres, oceans, continents, cities, and people.

The new generation of government regulatory agencies formed in the United States after World War II has attempted to solve newly disclosed problems related to industrial lead, such as adverse effects by lead on catalytic converters in auto exhaust systems and lead poisoning among inner-city babies, by using applied engineering controls in the tradition of the past as described above. Although a reduction of the concentration of industrial lead in gasoline may solve the problem of interference with catalytic converters, it does not necessarily solve the problem of environmental pollution from the burning of lead alkyls. The partial reduction of lead in automotive fuels can be offset by increases in the rate of burning of automotive fuels so that the overall burning rate of lead alkyls may not be reduced to desirable levels. Control criteria [31] relating to atmospheric lead concentrations have been formulated in a context of ignorance concerning the true extent of industrial lead pollution in the human environment, as is shown in Section 4 of this report.

A characteristic feature of all the engineering problem-solving approaches described above is that they have been applied without consideration of consequences upon the truly human aspects of human lives. This defect has been a major cause of their failures. Lead technology has been intimately linked with the overall development of engineering technology during the past ten thousand years, and evidence suggests that people were never in conscious control of this overall development to see that it received guidance from truly humanitarian considerations. The defect appears therefore to be closely related to this involuntary development feature of engineering technology. In view of the increasing severity of the hazards which have resulted from successive failures of engineering approaches in solving lead poisoning problems, it appears that attempts to institute conscious human control guided by humanitarian principles over developments in lead technology in place of engineering approaches are warranted.

Although it now is or in the near future it will become clear that steps should be taken to reduce and eventually halt the mining and smelting of lead and the manufacture of leaded products, this action, if taken within the traditional context of applied engineering, may have disastrous consequences. The historical record suggests, instead, that intervention with regard to the best interests of *H.s.sapiens* by conscious human control in the overall development of engineering technology should originate from the category of those emotional actions that uniquely characterize *H.s.sapiens* from all other organisms on this earth, if not our galaxy, instead of from the category of emotional actions that generated engineering technology and which have a more direct lineage to the two billion year involuntary struggle by organisms within the earth's biosphere to modify their environments through self-gratification responses to physical-need stimuli.

REFERENCES

1. *Air Quality Criteria for Lead* (1977), EPA-600/8-77-017, U.S. Environmental Protection Agency, Washington, D.C. Settle, D.M. and C.C. Patterson (1979) Lead in albacore: guide to pollution in Americans. Accepted for publication in *Science*. Elias, R.W. and C.C. Patterson (1979) The toxicological implications of biogeochemical studies of atmospheric lead. Proceedings of the Twelfth Annual Rochester International Conference on Environmental Toxicity, Rochester, N.Y. (To be published). Ericson, J.E., H. Shirahata, and C.C. Patterson (1979) Skeletal concentrations of lead in ancient Peruvians. *The New England Journal of Medicine 300*, 946–951.

2. Gilfillan, S.C. *Rome's Ruin by Lead Poison.* Book to be published. Gilfillan, S.C. (1965) Lead poisoning and the fall of Rome. *Journal of Occupational Medicine 7,* 53–60. Mackie, A., A. Townsend and H.A. Waldren (1975) Lead concentrations in bones from Roman York. *Journal of the Archaeological Society 2,* 235–237. Jawarowski, Z. (1968) Stable lead in fossil ice and bones. *Nature 217,* 152–153.

3. Aub, J.C., L. Fairhall, A. Minot, and P. Reznikoff (1925) Lead poisoning. *Medicine 4,* 1.

4. Kehoe, R.A., F. Thamann, and J. Cholak (1933) Normal absorption and excretion of lead in people. *Journal of Industrial Hygiene 15,* 257.

5. Patterson, C.C. (1965) Contaminated and natural environments of man. *Archives of Environmental Health 11,* 344–360.

6. Settle, D.M. and C.C. Patterson (1979) in Reference [1].

7. Elias, R.W. and C.C. Patterson (1979) in Reference [1].

8. *Human Evolution: Biosocial Perspectives* (1978), edited by S.L. Washburn and E.R. McCowan. London: Benjamin/Cummings.

9. A representative but not exhaustive list of studies includes: Tylecote, R.F. (1962) *Metallurgy in Archaeology.* London: Edward Arnold Publishers. Forbes, R.J. (1964) *Studies in Ancient Technology,* Vol. 7–9. Leiden: Brill. Aitchison, L. (1960) *A History of Metals.* New York: Interscience. Rickard, T.A. (1932) *Man and Metals.* New York: Interscience. Root, W.C. (1949) The metallurgy of the southern coast of Peru. *American Antiquity 15,* 10–37.

10. Agricola, G. (1556) *De Re Metallica.* Translated (1912) by H.C. Hoover and L.H. Hoover in *The Mining Magazine,* London. Reprinted (1950) New York: Dover Publications.

11. U.S. Bureau of Mines, *Minerals Yearbook* 1923–1975. Smith, L.A. (1925) Summarized data of lead production. U.S. Bureau of Mines, Economic Paper 5; Hixon, H.W. (1898) *Notes on Lead and Copper Smelting and Copper Converting.* New York: The Scientific Publishing Company. Robinson, I.M. (1978) Lead as a factor in the world economy. *The Biogeochemistry of Lead in the Environment, Part A,* edited by J.O. Nriagu. New York: Elsevier/North Holland Biomedical Press. Kesler, S.E. (1978) Economic lead deposits. *The Biogeochemistry of Lead in the Environment, Part A,* edited by J.O. Nriagu. New York: Elsevier/North Holland Biomedical Press.

12. Settle, D.M. and C.C. Patterson (1979) in Reference [1].

13. Strahler, A.N. (1971) *The Earth Sciences.* New York: Harper and Row.

14. Butler, K.W. (1971) *Environment and Archeology: An Ecological Approach to Prehistory,* 2nd Ed. Chicago: Aldine Atherton.

15. Hole, F. and K.V. Flannery (1968) The prehistory of Southwestern Iran: a preliminary report, *Prehistoric Society Proceedings 33,* 147–206. Braidwood, R.J. (1967) *Prehistoric Man,* 7th Edition. New York: Morrow.

16. Coughlan, H.H. (1967) Notes on the prehistoric metallurgy of copper and bronze in the Old World. *Occasional Papers on Technology 4* (Pitt Rivers Museum). Oxford: Oxford University Press. Also Aitchison, L. (1960) in Reference [9].

17. Patterson, Clair C. (1971) Native copper, silver, and gold accessible to early metallurgists. *American Antiquity 36,* 286–381.

18. 'Grossman, J.W. (1972) An ancient gold worker's tool kit: the earliest metal technology in Peru. *Archaeology 25,* 270–279. Patterson, C.C. (1971) in Reference [17], and unpublished studies.

19. Butzer, K.W. (1971) in Reference [14]. Clark, G. (1961) *World Prehistory.* Cambridge: Cambridge University Press. Bibby, G. (1960) *Testimony of the Spade.* New York: A. Knopf. Breul, A.H. (1952) *Four Hundred Centuries of Cave Art,* translated by M.E. Boyle. Paris: Montignoe. Graziosi, P. (1960) *Paleolithic Art.* New York: McGraw Hill. Maringer, J. (1960) *The God of Prehistoric Man.* New York: A. Knopf.

20. Tylecote, R.F. (1962) and Forbes, R.J. (1964) in Reference [9].
21. Forbes, R.J. (1964) and Aitchison, L. (1960) in Reference [9]. Patterson, C.C. (1971) in Reference [17]. Wagner, G.A., W. Gentner, and H. Gropengeisser (1979) Evidence for third millenium lead–silver mining on Siphnos Island (Cyclades), *Naturwissenschaften 66*, 157–158.
22. Partington, J.R. (1935) *Origins and Developments of Applied Chemistry*.
23. Seltman, G.T. (1955) *Greek Coins*, 2nd Edition. New York: Methuen. Hill, G.F. (1964) *Ancient Greek and Roman Coins*. Chicago: reprinted by Argonaut.
24. Gilfillan, S.C. (1965) and unpublished book in Reference [2], Gilfillan, S.C. and C.C. Patterson, unpublished studies.
25. Patterson, C.C. (1972) Silver stocks and losses in ancient and medieval times. *Economic History Review 25*, 205–235.
26. Stevenson, L.G. (1949) *A History of Lead Poisoning*, Ph.D. Dissertation, Johns Hopkins University.
27. Gochel, D.E. (1697) De vini audi per acetum lithargyri, cum maximo bibentium damno dulcificatione. *Miscellanea Curiosa*, Decuriae III, 81–85.
28. Tanquerel des Planches, L. (1839) *Traite des maladies de plomb ou Saturnines* I–II. Paris.
29. Hamilton, Alice (1934) *Industrial Toxicology*. New York: Hoeber. Hamilton, A. and H.L. Hardy (1949) *Industrial Toxicology*. New York: Harper and Bros.
30. Advisory Committee on Tetraethyl Lead. *Public health aspects of increasing tetraethyl lead content in motor fuel*. PHS Publication No. 712. 1959. Washington, D.C.: U.S. Public Health Service.
31. *Air Quality Criteria for Lead* (1977), EPA-600/8-77-017, U.S. Environmental Protection Agency, Washington, D.C.

Disclosure of Extreme
Lead Pollution of Americans
by Research in
the Pure Sciences

INTRODUCTION

As shown in the previous section, human environments within urbanized regions have been polluted with lead for thousands of years. As will be shown in the next section, the earth's atmosphere, biosphere, and oceans became generally polluted on a hemispheric basis with lead during the last century as a result of great increases in lead smelting activities combined with the burning of immense quantities of leaded automotive fuels, so that today extreme excesses of lead occur in nearly all Americans. Although these effects have existed for a long time, and analyses for lead in plants, animals, and other substances have been carried out in thousands of laboratories for nearly a century, the existence of this intense pollution effect became recognized only within the last decade. It had been overlooked because industrial lead contamination added to samples before and during analyses was mistakenly believed to be "normal" lead in the samples.

This situation changed when investigators using isotopic compositions of oceanic leads to study the magmatic history of the earth's crust found that much more lead seemed to be entering the oceans now from rivers than had been leaving the oceans via sediments in the ancient past [1]. The difference could be explained on a mass inventory basis as originating from industrial sources such as leaded gasoline exhausts, and this suggested that industrial emissions of lead might be interfering with natural cycles of lead in the oceans on a global scale. Investigators then changed their research aims and used the special analytical technique of isotope dilution mass spectrometry (IDMS), that had been previously developed in the field of geochronology for measurements of lead-uranium ages of microscopic minerals in rocks, to track down the meaning of this clue by looking for anthropogenic perturbations of natural geochemical and biochemical lead cycles.

These later studies carried out by a number of investigators within an academic environment during the past seventeen years show in quantitative terms how lead used to cycle naturally through plants and animals in the earth's biosphere. These investigations show that enormous differences exist between present-day flows of lead through air, plants, and animals and those that had occurred during prehistoric times. The key to the success of these later investigations of lead was that elaborate techniques were used to reduce, control, and measure industrial lead contamination added to samples before and during analysis [2].

The history of the development and use of the IDMS method described in this section shows that the discovery of the true extent of lead pollution resulted from scholarly research in pure sciences that was carried out in the face of hindrance and disregard from funding agencies and investigators in fields of applied science and engineering. This experience is in accord with the existence of a chronic conflict between basic scientific research on the one hand and applied science and engineering on the other, whereby the institutionalized activities of the latter are continually threatened with revolution by the former. Although human emotions involved in science have been clearly and certainly provided with an opportunity to function in the hierarchy of social structures created by developments in engineering technology during the past thousand years, and science makes explicit use of instruments provided by engineering technology, the human emotions which determine the activity called science, like art, music, literature, and religion seem to belong to a species of intellectual activity which grew as a branch from the main stem of hominid intellectual evolution forty thousand years ago [3], so that such intellectual activities appear to be quite separate from those which caused the development of engineering technology itself, the latter seeming to have a more direct, rather than a branched, lineage within the main stem of hominid intellectual evolution. Although this point of view is speculative and alternative explanations regarding this dispute between the pure and applied sciences have been put forth [3a], there does seem to be an unresolvable difference between the human emotions which separately determine actions in science on the one hand and in engineering technology on the other. There is a real hostility to guidance from humanitarian emotions within applied science and engineering that makes it *unwise to en-*

large and strengthen applied science and engineering at the dispropor-
tionate expense of basic science because proper formulation of solutions
to human social problems created by developments in engineering tech-
nology will in consequence be seriously hindered or prevented.

ANALYTICAL METHODS FOR LEAD

In the early years of this century gravimetric and sulfide-color analytical methods were used to study the occurrences of lead. In basic scientific research these methods were confined mainly to studies of natural and artificial inorganic minerals, soils, and sediments, with little application to waters, plants, and animals, while major uses were in industry and medicine. Because of the insensitivities of these methods and the belief that lead poisoning was an industrial hazard, general medical opinion at this time held that lead did not "normally" occur in humans, but was present in them only as a result of improper use of industrial lead [4].

During later years especially those between World Wars I and II, emission spectrographic, electrogravimetric, X-ray fluorescence, and spectrophotometric methods combined with various separation and isolation techniques were developed for identifying and measuring for analytical purposes small, nearly invisible quantities of metals, including lead. These more sensitive and accurate methods were used to some small extent in basic scientific studies of lead in waters, plants, and animals, but most lead studies in the field of basic science at this time were still confined to inorganic systems. The major uses of these analytical methods for lead were in industry and medicine. The spectrophotometric method was used by investigators in the field of industrial medicine to overturn older medical views about the "normal" occurrence of lead in humans by demonstrating the ubiquitous occurrence of lead in "normal" human blood, foods, and excreta [5]. As a consequence, general medical opinion then changed so as to mistakenly regard typical occurrences of lead in foods and people as "normal," when actually such occurrences originated mainly from industrial lead pollution. They failed to question the exceedingly small factors of only three to five which separated levels of lead observed in poisoned people from levels of lead in typical people.

After World War II, emission and plasma emission spectrometric and spectrographic, anodic stripping and pulse-polarographic electrometric, flame-flameless-plasma source atomic absorption, energy dispersive-refractive X-ray fluorescence, proton induced X-ray emission, and spark source mass spectrographic methods were developed for identifying and measuring for analytical purposes microquantities of metals, including lead. The development and proliferation of these analytical techniques for metals was driven mainly by industrial and medical needs, but a strong demand to use these methods for analysis of toxic metals, such as copper, zinc, cadmium, arsenic, mercury, chromium, nickel, and lead, was generated in addition by the enormous growth of public agencies who wished to monitor the environmental occurrences of these metals. On the basis of proportions of use among various fields, it is estimated that basic research in the physical sciences still serves only as a minor segment of the total use of these methods for studies of lead, although this distinction between applied studies and basic research has been obscured by an exponential growth of the gathering for monitoring purposes of lead data relating to air, water, sediments, plants, and animals, sponsored by various new and enlarged public agencies.

There is now available in the world literature a great mass of data relating to lead concentrations in air, water, and plant and animal tissues determined by all of the analytical methods listed above (except IDMS), largely as a result of applied science and engineering studies carried out during the past four decades. Most of these applied science lead data for samples from nonurban regions are erroneous, involving reported values ranging from ten-fold to a thousand-fold greater than actual lead concentrations. In few, if any, of these data are the proportions of natural lead, which range from 1/2 to 1/100th of actual total lead in the nonurban samples, correctly identified and reported. A small portion of the lead concentration data for nonurban samples reported in the literature are not in serious error, and although the major share of such data were obtained by the ultra-clean IDMS analytical method, some of it originates from flameless atomic absorption, pulse polarographic–anodic stripping and plasma emission spectrometric analytical methods.

DEVELOPMENT OF IDMS FOR GEOCHRONOMETRIC PURPOSES

The breakthrough to an awareness of the true state of affairs in this situation came with the use of solid source thermal ionization high resolution isotope dilution mass spectrometric analyses combined with ultra-clean sample collection, handling, and analysis techniques. This IDMS method for lead (not to be confused with spark source IDMS) involves the adding of a known trace quantity of a pure lead isotope (five different ones are available for this purpose) to the four lead isotopes already contained in a weighed sample, and homogenizing the isotopic mixture by acid decomposition and dissolution. The mixture of tracer and sample lead isotopes is chemically isolated by micro techniques, and the ratio of the tracer lead isotope to a sample lead isotope is determined in a solid source thermal ionization high resolution mass spectrometer. From the observed ratio and the weights of tracer isotope and sample material, the concentration of lead in the sample can be calculated. Although the quality of its data output for lead is unsurpassed, this analytical method is so exceedingly cumbersome and expensive compared to other methods in terms of quantity of lead concentration data produced by a given amount of expense and effort, it has never been widely used by investigators among various nations in either the pure or applied sciences. The amount of lead concentration data produced by this method and published in the world literature is so minute in comparison with the total amount produced by other methods that many analysts in the world today are unaware that the method exists. It is not mentioned in the analytical sections of any of the prestigious reports published concerning lead in the environment [6].

Before World War II the geochronometric history of the earth had been sketched out in an approximate fashion using uranium-lead ages derived from gravimetric and mass spectrometric analysis of gram quantities of macropegmatitic uranium, thorium, and lead minerals, whereby the parent/daughter ratios in the radioactive minerals were determined gravimetrically, and the isotopic compositions of the leads were determined by mass spectrometric analysis of milligram quantities of lead halide salts heated in furnace sources. The rare occurrence of these ore-type minerals in the geologic environment was a matter of considerable frustration to stratigraphers who needed to know ages of many rocks, so they pressed strongly for age dating techniques which could be applied to ubiquitous minerals in common rocks. This need was fulfilled by the solid source thermal ionization high resolution mass spectrometer, which was developed during World War II [7] to study microgram quantities of solid fission and transuranic products formed in nuclear reactors. After the war this instrument was used in geology to study the occurrences of microgram amounts of uranium, lead, thorium, potassium, rubidium, and strontium in microscopically small radioactive minerals that had been separated by grinding and heavy liquid processes from common rocks. This procedure allowed the ages of formation of most common igneous rocks to be determined, and when it was applied first to U/Pb, K/Ar (using gas source mass spectrometers) and Sr/Rb radioactive decay schemes, and later to other such schemes in ubiquitous microscopic minerals, it brought about a revolution in geology by providing a vast number of igneous rock ages and chemical tracer data relating to magmatic reactions. As a consequence the age of the earth and solar system and details in the history of igneous development in the earth, moon, and meteorites after that time have been delineated by a number of investigators in different nations working in the fields of geochronology, nuclear geochemistry, and cosmochemistry.

This analytical method applied to lead is uniquely suited to the challenge of providing correct answers in the midst of overwhelming lead contamination. It can measure very small amounts of lead contamination with less ambiguity and more accuracy than any other method, because the mass spectrometer signal is unusually free of false positive and negative effects and the isotopic pattern of the lead contamination signal, when lead contamination is being explicitly investigated, provides a unique double-check on its own identity not available to any other method, and in some cases it can be distinguished from sample lead during the analysis of samples. There are no comparisons with standards or working curves used in this method, so there are no complications introduced by contamination of standards, which greatly simplifies contamination measurements. Contamination contributions from different sources are determined by trial and error measurements of supposedly only one unknown parameter within a series of differently postulated arrangements of variables that are assumed to be known but are actually unknown. Since errors in these assumptions are universal, and are revealed and eliminated only by repeated trials of different arrangements of the assumed variables, the complexities of assumptions and trial repetitions become unwieldy and unproductive if the standards also contain lead contamination that must be determined, reduced, and controlled. During the early stages of development of the IDMS method for geochronometry, lack of proper lead contamination control became known immediately, either by measured ages that didn't fit patterns that had been established by earlier macropegmatitic studies, or by the obliteration of radiogenic lead from macrominerals by nonradiogenic lead contamination. As a result, continuous striving to reduce contamination became institutionalized as a traditional part of the method, and developments in clean and ultra-clean laboratory techniques in various laboratories during the thirty years since the method was first used for geochronometry have reduced lead contamination during analysis more than a thousand-fold. This was accompanied by a corresponding thousand-fold increase in sensitivity for lead through improvements in surface ionization techniques by various investigators in different nations.

Today lead contamination is excluded from ultra-clean laboratories used for IDMS studies of lead and some other trace metals in a manner analogous to the exclusion of pathogens from bone surgeries. The interiors of the laboratories are constructed of plastic; they are sealed and pressurized with ultra-clean air; entrances are air-locked; investigators wear clean shoes, gowns, caps, and plastic gloves (sometimes washed with acids before use); reagents and containers are purified and cleaned of lead and other metals by elaborate procedures within these laboratories; the introduction of lead and other metal contamination from numerous sources is constantly monitored; and approximately half of all activities in these laboratories is devoted to purification and cleaning of reagents and containers, monitoring lead and other metal contamination, and modifying and improving lead and other contamination control procedures. Although the quality of the lead data produced by these laboratories is exceedingly high, the quantity of it is quite small.

In clean laboratories used for ordinary geochronometric purposes, lead contamination levels have been generally reduced so that microgram (μg, 10^{-6} gm) to submicrogram quantities of lead in igneous minerals can be studied without significant interference from contamination. In those few ultra-clean laboratories where lead in lunar rocks and single microcrystals is studied for nuclear geochemical and cosmochemical purposes, contamination controls are far more stringent, so that nanogram (ng, 10^{-9} gm) and subnanogram quantities of lead in igneous minerals can be isotopically studied in these laboratories without serious interference from lead contamination. A few clean and ultra-clean laboratories have also been recently developed in the United States and other nations for trace metal studies in chemical oceanography and geochemistry of polar snows, aerosols, and sediments. Although great improvements in the analyses of trace metals other than lead have been achieved in these latter laboratories so as to yield significant advances in scientific knowledge, it has not yet been demonstrated that problems of lead analysis at the nanogram level have been successfully dealt with in all of these latter laboratories.

APPLICATION OF ULTRA-CLEAN IDMS TO LEAD POLLUTION STUDIES

At present there are only a few ultra-clean laboratories in which concentrations and isotopic compositions of nanogram amounts of lead in nonurban plant and animal tissues and waters are being accurately determined with absolute reliability without serious interference from lead contamination. Although proper reduction and control of lead contamination is costly and time-consuming, it is a prerequisite for virtually all accurate analyses of such nonurban substances. For example, the stemwood of trees, which characterize the main mass of the earth's biosphere, contains only 1 to 3 ng of lead per gram of wood [8], while the flesh of wild terrestrial carnivores contains only 5 to 10 ng of lead per gram of tissue [8], and remote streams contain only 5 to 50 ng lead per kilogram of water [8]. Determinations of lead in such materials can be reliably made only when lead contamination has been separately determined for all sources, each of which may individually contribute from 5 to 200 picograms (10^{-12} gm) of lead, and which sum to an accurately known few tenths of a nanogram. This level of contamination is very much smaller and much better understood than the typical, poorly determined and vaguely understood, "lead blanks" of 50 to 10,000 nanograms per analysis that are reported from laboratories where most lead analyses are presently being carried out.

This excessive lead contamination in most laboratories prevents analysts in them from analysing lead correctly in any but highly contaminated materials from urban regions. In nearly all cases where laboratories using ultra-clean IDMS methods have carried out parallel analyses of plant and animal materials, waters, and air for lead that had also been analysed in laboratories that used conventional, high data output methods for lead analysis, serious errors are revealed. Nearly all of the thousands of lead analyses in plants, animals and sediments reported in the U.S. Bureau of Land Management Baseline Study of Outer Continental Shelf Regions are probably wrong [9]. All of the many reported analyses of lead in old stemwood of trees are erroneously high by a factor of 1000 [8]. Despite more than forty years of study and measurement of the occurrence of lead in open ocean waters, it has been found that all previous analyses of lead in such waters are wrong [10], most by three orders of magnitude, and correct lead analyses in open ocean waters have been reported in only one recent study [11]. All of the lead concentrations in the atmosphere at remote locations reported by the Health and Safety Laboratory of the U.S. Department of Energy [12] are erroneously high.

This section deals with only a portion of the reliable analyses of lead in nonurban materials that have been made or reported in the literature by a number of investigators at various universities and research institutes in different countries. Reliable studies of lead in nonurban substances, such as [13], have been carried out in clean laboratories using both the IDMS and flameless atomic absorption methods, and some reliable studies of lead in urban samples have been carried out using the IDMS method, such as [14].

As mentioned at the beginning of this section, the research interests of some investigators using ultra-clean IDMS analytical techniques were focused on studies of lead in air, plants, and animals by the discovery that industrial lead emissions might be perturbing the natural occurrence of lead in the oceans. This effect could be caused on a global scale by transport of industrial lead emissions through the atmosphere. If this is happening now, the atmospheric concentrations of lead on a hemispheric basis must have been less in earlier times. This matter was investigated by measuring the occurrence of lead in Arctic snow strata of different ages to see if concentrations of atmospheric lead in the Northern Hemisphere increased with time [15]. At the same time studies of the occurrences of lead in seawater were initiated to determine possible effects of industrial lead contamination in the oceans [16]. These new research aims also led to development of the concept of biopurification of calcium with respect to lead in nutritive calcium pathways [17]. In order to check the validity of this concept, biogeochemical studies of inputs and outputs and occurrences of lead and calcium and the other metals were initiated in a remote ecosystem [18]. The results and significance of all the above studies are discussed in Section 4.

CONTRAST OF RESPONSES OF FUNDING AGENCIES AND INVESTIGATORS IN FIELDS OF PURE AND APPLIED SCIENCES TO IDMS BIOGEOCHEMICAL STUDIES

Funding. There was a marked contrast in attitude toward the funding of this new type research between the National Science Foundation (NSF), which provides most of the support for basic research in the pure sciences, and that of U.S. agencies supporting applied science and engineering. The following example is used to illustrate what happens when there is a conflict of interests between investigators in basic research and funding agencies and is not meant to be accusatory. In the case of Caltech the NSF undertook support of this research, despite some resistance by peer reviewers in the pure sciences to agree to fund work which seemed related to applied studies of pollution. Earlier, when the research interests of this group were concerned with nuclear geochemistry of lead in igneous systems, the work was sponsored by the Rockefeller Foundation, the U.S. Atomic Energy Commission (AEC), and the American Petroleum Institute (API). Although the latter were both mission-oriented agencies, they had supported this basic research for a decade because it helped to develop knowledge which had logical relationships with potential economic occurrences of uranium and the characterization of sedimentary strata (useful in oil exploration). The API terminated its support because there was a conflict of interest between the new proposed research aims and the industrial activities of the API membership. The AEC terminated its support because these new proposed research aims were no longer related to their applied science programs. The U.S. Public Health Service (precursor to the Environmental Protection Agency) refused to fund this new research, except for a small grant during the initial phase of the Arctic snow studies, in part because the proposals received negative peer reviews which originated from industrial influences, and also because the proposed research aims were not in accord with the applied science missions of the agency at that time.

These same agencies were stimulated by public controversy in the United States which arose from the publication of a geochemical review published at this time which criticized existing views concerning lead pollution [17]. This was one identifiable factor which in part caused the API and some U.S. and foreign lead industries to greatly enlarge their support of applied science and engineering investigations of the environmental occurrences of lead with the intent of demonstrating the benign character of the lead pollution situation, and U.S. and foreign mission-oriented public agencies concerned with public health to greatly expand their support of surveillance studies, carried out according to traditional views, of lead in the human environment. It is unfortunate that some of this large combined funding activity in the applied sciences was not directed to the expansion of basic research in ultra-clean IDMS laboratories. Laboratories using conventional analytical methods for the determination of lead that were funded produced an immense amount of data which are now embedded in the world literature. These data concerning the occurrences of lead in nonurban materials have been compromised by failure to properly account for lead contamination, and are misleading.

Interactions with Pure Sciences.   IDMS data reported during the last ten years about the occurrences of lead in air, snow, and water had a beneficial influence on the work of some investigators in the pure sciences through interlaboratory experimentation and exchange of ideas and information. Although these other investigators seldom use the IDMS method for lead, they have come to depend on it for cross-checking their lead data.

Published IDMS data concerning the occurrences of lead and other trace metals in polar snows [15] initiated controversy among geochemists in a number of countries about the quality of previously published trace metal data in polar snows. This was followed by a marked improvement in contamination control along the lines used in ultra-clean laboratories during later firn and ice collections and analyses by investigators using analytical methods other than IDMS. This was a factor which helped to bring about new reports of trace metal concentrations other than lead (actually macro metal constituents of sea salts and silicate dusts) that were consistently much lower than those reported earlier. These data showed systematic patterns of metal concentrations which enabled investigators to clearly recognize on a chemical basis the different occurrences of sea salts and silicate dusts in polar snows. For example, they abandoned earlier ideas that sea salts were chemically fractionated by gross amounts [19], and they discovered that concentrations of atmospheric silicate dusts during interglacial times in the Pleistocene were lower than during periods of glacial advance [20]. The IDMS data for metals in polar snows was also a factor which helped stimulate a reevaluation of the occurrences of other heavy metals and sulfate in polar snow strata [21]. The transfer to other laboratories of these new techniques for contamination control during analyses for lead in polar snow is more difficult than is the case for other metals because problems concerning lead contamination are far more intractable to solution. Duplication of previously published IDMS lead work in polar snows has been attempted in two pure science research laboratories where conscientious attempts were made to reduce and control lead contamination and where atomic absorption analytical methods were used. Investigators in one laboratory reported an observed decline in lead concentration levels going back in time in Arctic firn and ice only to concentration levels found in 1900 with no further decline observed [20]. Investigators in the other laboratory reported they were unable to observe any decline in lead concentrations in going back in time in Antarctic firn [23]. Various indications discussed in the next section suggest that problems of lead contamination in the analysis of old firn and ice strata have not yet been successfully dealt with in these two laboratories.

During the nineteen sixties investigators using ultra-clean IDMS techniques observed an unusual shape for the vertical distribution profile of common lead in the oceans, which suggested that perturbations by industrial lead emissions were occurring in the oceans on a hemispheric scale [16]. It was not known at this time that these observed lead concentrations exceeded true concentrations by an order of magnitude because water sample collectors, although carefully cleaned, were being contaminated by lead effluents from research vessels as they were lowered through surface waters surrounding the ships. Nevertheless these early IDMS studies showed only several hundred nanograms lead per kilogram of surface water, decreasing to about 30 nanograms lead per kilogram in deep waters, while most values for lead in seawater reported in the world literature ranged from 5,000 to 10,000 nanograms lead per kilogram seawater. At this same time the IDMS method was applied to studies of barium concentrations in seawater [24], which stimulated the proliferation of the application of IDMS to studies of barium [25]. Contamination control for barium is a relatively minor problem. The lead findings initiated interlaboratory calibration experiments concerning lead in seawater among some investigators in pure science from various countries. It was later found that the earlier IDMS data were in positive error by about a factor of ten due to sample collector contamination, and that anodic stripping and atomic absorption analytical methods in current use yielded lead concentrations that were in error by ten-fold to one hundred-fold above concentrations standardized by the ultra-clean IDMS method [10]. These findings were a significant factor in helping to institute new contamination control techniques during sample collection and analysis in chemical oceanography, and they also helped promote the construction of clean and ultra-clean laboratories at a number of academic institutions in various countries. New data on the occurrences of copper, zinc, and cadmium in seawater obtained by using these new clean techniques now exhibit a systematic character that had been previously lacking, and which is now amenable to interpretation [26]. Although interuniversity cooperative work has demonstrated that investigators in some laboratories can now properly collect and analyse surface samples of near shore estuarine seawaters that contain relatively high concentrations of lead (about 50 nanograms lead per kilogram of water), at present there are only a very few laboratories which appear to have the potential for correctly analysing lead in deep ocean water. The extreme difficulty of controlling lead contamination is illustrated by the fact that after more than six years of collaborative effort among many laboratories in various countries it still cannot be said definitely that proper contamination control procedures for lead have been instituted in many clean laboratories so that all types of seawaters can be reliably collected and accurately analysed for lead in them.

A new seawater sampler which protects itself against effluents from ships has been used to collect uncontaminated seawater samples which has allowed reliable and accurate profiles of lead concentrations to be determined in the oceans at several locations. These new measurements (which show the same vertical distribution profile shape as before but at lower concentrations of 1 to 20 nanograms lead per kilogram water in the North Pacific and 6 to 35 nanograms lead per kilogram water in the North Atlantic) suggest that industrial lead emissions are indeed perturbing the natural occurrences of lead in the oceans of the Northern Hemisphere [11]. The data will be discussed in Section 4.

In recent years aerosol chemists in the pure sciences have found that the concentrations of some heavy metals including lead are very much greater in aerosols from remote areas than might be expected if the aerosols were derived solely from crustal rock and soil dusts [27]. Initially these investigators ascribed the observed excess lead to natural sources such as volcanoes, bursting bubbles in the ocean, and forest emissions, but lead in Arctic snow data showed that this excess lead in atmospheric silicate aerosols exhibited an increase with time to high levels during the last century, which indicates that the excess lead is of anthropogenic origin. This situation led to cooperative multi-university investigations funded by NSF of the problem of the origin of excess lead and other metals in atmospheric aerosols in remote regions. Investigators in several universities in this consortium have improved their contamination control procedures for lead to such an extent that they can now correctly determine lead at extremely low concentrations in the atmosphere using analytical methods other than IDMS, so that it is now possible for these laboratories to correctly measure excess lead in aerosols that is not erroneously high due to artifact contamination [28] which effect had previously characterized much of the published data. Preliminary results from these cooperative studies suggest that sea surface bubble emission of lead may not be as important as first thought, and that volcano emissions are insignificant sources of excess lead. All new preliminary findings from this consortium are consistent with the model that the true origin of excess lead in aerosols is anthropogenic.

The accuracy and reliability of new lead data in nonurban substances provided by the ultra-clean IDMS analytical method have enhanced the significance of data concerning the geochemical occurrences of ^{210}Pb. The new data for common lead show that its atmospheric source function is now similar to that for ^{210}Pb, but was different in earlier times. It is now recognized that the excess input of industrial lead to the oceans occurs through the atmosphere [11] and that older data concerning common lead concentrations in river waters were erroneously high. ^{210}Pb investigations have shown that the transfer of lead from rivers through estuarine environments to the oceans is an exceedingly complex process [29] and that it will be necessary to use knowledge provided by ^{210}Pb studies to determine the inputs of common lead from rivers to oceans during prehistoric times. The reliability of estimates of the atmospheric input fluxes of common lead to the oceans can be increased greatly by considering associations with measured atmospheric fluxes of ^{210}Pb to the oceans [11]. ^{210}Pb dating techniques for sediments [30] have enabled reliable measurements to be made of chronological changes in lead concentrations and isotopic compositions in marine and lake sediments.

Involvement of archaeologists in ultra-clean laboratory studies of lead in ancient bones has produced new ideas for further research into human origins and ancient activities. Their involvement in trace element studies of ancient pyrotechnology carried out under clean conditions has yielded a better understanding of the development of ancient metallurgy.

Interaction with Applied Science and Engineering. In these fields, because of their utilitarian and institutionalized nature, there are always two types of opposing groups: those who defend the *status quo* of any situation, and those who wish to alter it. Doctors in the applied science of medicine, who were inclined to alter accepted medical opinion regarding lead pollution, fostered and enriched research in the field of lead biogeochemistry. The editor of a medical journal [31] and two professors of medicine [32] encouraged the preparation of a critical geochemical review of lead pollution which focused new research on natural occurrences of lead in the biosphere. In addition, pure science studies of the occurrences of lead in ancient teeth and bones resulted partly from interaction with doctors engaged in applied science studies of relationships between concentrations of lead in teeth and the health of urban children [33], and with a sociologist interested in relations between the concentrations of lead in Roman bones and the downfall of Rome [34]. An environmental engineering scientist [34a] was among those who helped create the circumstances that led to this report.

On the other hand, doctors in the applied sciences of industrial medicine, public health, toxicology, pharmacology, and other fields allied with industrial interests have actively tried to keep the new findings concerning the natural biogeochemistry of lead from altering established medical opinion about lead pollution. Some persons in these applied sciences attempted to disprove the new findings by making pragmatic measurements of lead in blood of extant primitives without recourse to basic research which showed lead levels similar to those in city dwellers [35]. Later pragmatic measurements of lead in blood of people by investigators unassociated with industry have since refuted the findings of the earlier blood measurements by showing that these people have very low levels of lead in their blood [36]. Some participated in more subtle ways as members of prestigious committees who issued reports concerning lead in the environment. They mobilized the full weight of their professional authority behind toxicological orthodoxy to denounce the new ideas regarding the natural occurrences of lead [37]. Although the 1972 National Academy of Sciences NRC Report on Lead prominently displayed a graph depicting the increase in lead concentrations with time in Arctic snow, the authors ignored the implication of these data and went on to deny, in their summary of the extent of environmental pollution by lead, that there was any appreciable general perturbation by industrial lead on biologic systems [38]. This same industrial influence is reflected in summaries of major reports issued by the U.S. Environmental Protection Agency and the United Nations World Health Organization five years later. Despite the publication of more data concerning the biogeochemistry of natural lead after 1972 showing the wide extent of lead pollution, these 1977 reports repeat the statement that the impact of man-made pollution is not perceptible except around smelters, in the immediate vicinity of roads carrying heavy traffic, and in densely populated areas [39]. This steadfast refusal by persons in the applied sciences who are influenced by their relationships with industry to recognize the true extent of anthropogenic perturbation of natural lead levels in the environment, and to alter general medical opinion accordingly, serves to greatly minimize, in public opinion, the apparent total lead pollution effect in American people by tacitly elevating the accepted general background level of lead in all organisms.

The NRC report on Lead in the Human Environment continues this tradition by attempting to show that natural levels of lead in various substances cover wide ranges [40]. In that report it is claimed that the upper limits of "background" ranges of lead are defined by the voluminous lead data in the literature that has been provided by conventional analytical methods for lead to which credence is given because its quantity is so vast, although most of it is in error by factors that range from ten-fold to a thousand-fold. On the other hand, it is claimed that the lower limits of "background" lead levels obtained by ultra-clean IDMS techiques must be considered with reservation because there is so little of it, and because it has not yet been confirmed by generally accepted analytical methods for lead, the latter event not only being impossible at present, but improbable for years to come.

Existing standard reference materials of muscle and plant tissue provided by the National Bureau of Standards for lead are unsuitable and misleading for lead standardization purposes in analytical laboratories, because these materials contain one hundred to ten thousand times more lead than is proper for standards representing nonurban samples. The Bureau was asked to prepare standards that would properly evaluate the abilities of laboratories to determine lead concentrations correctly in scientifically significant samples. They refused on the supposition that most analysts believe such standards are irrelevant to their practical everyday analytical requirements, and that most analysts would not analyze them. Although such refusals by analysts would be based on false premises, because these so-called "practical" requirements ignore the presence of excessive lead contamination which makes such "practical" analytical exercises meaningless, this is actually a strong factor which does prevent the Bureau from preparing such standards.

Many of the potential users of these standards are analysts in surveillance laboratories of government agencies. Interactions between pure scientists and analysts and administrators in several government agencies concerning lead analyses of environmental samples have been nonproductive. Analyses of lead concentrations by IDMS in parallel field samples of marine animals together with interlaboratory calibration experiments carried out with analysts in a National Marine Fisheries Laboratory (NMF) supported by the National Oceanic and Atmospheric Administration showed that there was excessive lead contamination in the NMF laboratory during sample collection and analysis. Despite this discovery, that laboratory subsequently issued a document reporting large quantities of lead concentration data characterized by these excessive errors [40a]. Since the U.S. Food and Drug Administration had funded the analytical work reported in this document, administrators in that agency were asked to consider ways to upgrade the laboratories they supported so that more acceptable lead data would be provided. The administrators refused to consider such action on the grounds that mandates directing their activities restricted their attention to lead concentration levels that were related to "practical" health problems. This demonstration (that circular reasoning dictates some policies in some government agencies) shows that administrators in the National Bureau of Standards are correct in their evaluation of the situation.

In another case, discussions were held by IDMS analysts with analysts in the Health and Safety Laboratory of the U.S. Department of Energy concerning lead concentrations that had been determined by both groups in parallel field samples of remote air. Comparison of these data showed that excessive lead contamination rendered the Health and Safety Laboratory data for remote air samples valueless. This laboratory rejected offers to carry out cooperative work that might improve the quality of its lead data in remote air samples, and later issued a document reporting large quantities of lead concentration data characterized by these excessive errors [12].

The new IDMS findings show that stream waters in remote regions contain only 5 to 50 nanograms lead per kilogram, yet the U.S. Environmental Protection Agency's *Quality Criteria for Water* document states that the natural concentrations of lead in fresh waters range from 1000 to 10,000 nanograms lead per kilogram. This view originates from the fact that excessive lead contamination in most laboratories prohibits analyses of lead concentrations in water below levels of about 1000 nanograms lead per kilogram water. When directors in the EPA were asked to consider ways to upgrade their surveillance laboratories so that they could analyse lead in fresh waters at the nanogram per kilogram level, the directors refused to consider this action on the ground that mandates directing their activities restricted their attention to lead concentration levels that were related to "practical" health problems.

IDMS findings concerning lead which to date constitute the most reliable studies available of the relative proportions of lead absorbed into systemic blood by humans from food and air [41], have been ignored by government agencies that should not have done so. The reason for this seems to be that this work undermines a large but meaningless exercise currently being carried out in surveillance work supported by some government agencies. This IDMS work is the only one which correctly delineates complex relationships among lead in food, air, blood, and bones which had been incorrectly simplified by nonexplicit assumptions in a relationship that attempted to correlate lead in air with lead in blood, first set forth in 1965 [17] and later abandoned by the author, but picked up [42] and now widely used by the EPA and other agencies to report demonstrably incorrect engineering relationships between blood and air in prestigious reports [6]. In another case, the IDMS method was being used to measure changes in isotopic compositions of lead in urban aerosols with time [43]. Such data are of profound importance to the surveillance of lead in the environment because they delineate the relative significance of different sources of industrial lead introduced to the atmosphere. This research was terminated prematurely by the EPA on the grounds that it was irrelevant to their missions. Since there are no trustworthy archives of dated atmospheric filters, important information has been irretrievably lost as a consequence of this decision.

REFERENCES

1. Chow, T.J. and C.C. Patterson (1962) The occurrence and significance of lead isotopes in pelagic sediments. *Geochimica et Cosmochimica Acta 26*, 263–308.
2. Patterson, C.C. and D.M. Settle (1976) The reduction of order of magnitude errors in lead analyses of biological materials and natural waters by evaluating and controlling the extent and sources of industrial lead contamination introduced during sample collection and analysis. Pages 321–351, Accuracy in Trace Analysis: Sampling, Sample Handling, Analysis, edited by P. La Fleur. National Bureau of Standards Special Publication *422*, Washington, D.C.
3. Leakey, R.E. and R. Lewin (1977) *Origins*. New York: E.P. Dutton. 3a. Robbins, D. and R. Johnston (1976) The role of cognitive and occupational differentiation in scientific controversies, *Social Studies of Science 6*, 349–368.
4. Aub, J.C., L. Fairhall, A. Minot and P. Reznikoff (1925) Lead poisoning, *Medicine 4*, 1.
5. Kehoe, R.A., F. Thamann and J. Cholak (1933) Normal absorption and excretion of lead in people, *Journal of Industrial Hygiene 15*, 257.
6. NAS-NRC *Airborne Lead in Perspective* (1972) Washington, D.C.: National Academy of Sciences. World Health Organization, Geneva (1977). *Environmental Health Criteria 3, Lead*, Section 1, 13–14. *Air Quality Criteria for Lead* (1977), EPA-600/8-77-017, U.S. Environmental Protection Agency, Washington, D.C.
7. Hayden, R.J., J.H. Reynolds and M.G. Inghram (1949) Reactions induced by slow neutron irradiation of Europium. *Physical Reviews 75*, 1500–1507.
8. List of published work and summary of new work given in Settle, D.M. and C.C. Patterson (1979) Lead in albacore: guide to lead pollution in Americans. Accepted for publication in *Science*.

9. Patterson, C.C., D.M. Settle, B.K. Schaule and M.W. Burnett (1976) *Baseline Studies of the Outer Continental Shelf* (Bureau of Land Management Contract #696-16, Washington), Vol. 3, Report 4.4.

10. Participants of the standardization of lead in seawater workshop (12 authors) (1974) Interlaboratory lead analyses of standardized samples of seawater. *Marine Chemistry 2*, 69–84. Participants of the lead in seawater workshop (12 authors) (1976) Comparison determinations of lead by investigators analysing individual samples of seawater in both their home laboratory and in an isotope dilution standardization laboratory. *Marine Chemistry 4*, 389–392. Patterson, C.C. (1974) Lead in seawater workshop, Meeting Report, *Science 183*, 553.

11. Schaule, B. and C. Patterson (1979, in press) The occurrence of lead in the Northeast Pacific and effects of anthropogenic inputs. *Proceedings of an International Experts Discussion on Lead: Occurrence, Fate, and Pollution in the Marine Environment.* Oxford: Pergamon Press. Schaule, B. and C.C. Patterson, Lead concentrations in the Northeast Pacific Ocean: evidence for global anthropogenic perturbations (unpublished manuscript).

12. Feeley, H.W., L.E. Toonkel, and R.J. Larsen (1978) Radionuclides and trace metals in surface air. *Environmental Quarterly*, Environmental Measurements Laboratory *EML-356*, Appendix B, pages 173–185.

13. Chow, T.J., J.L. Earl and C.B. Snyder (1972) Lead concentrations in air, White Mountain, California, *Science 178*, 401–402. Duce, R.A., G.L. Hoffman, B.J. Roy, I.S. Fletcher, G.T. Wallace, J.L. Fasching, S.R. Piotrowicz, P.R. Walsh, E.J. Hoffman, J.M. Miller and J.L. Hefter (1976) Trace metals in the marine environment. Pages 40–77, *Marine Pollutant Transfer* edited by H.L. Windom and R.A. Duce. Lexington, Mass.: Heath. Chow, T.J., J.L. Earl and C.F. Bennett (1969) Lead aerosols in marine atmosphere. *Environmental Science and Technology 3*, 737. Martin, J.H., K.W. Bruland and W.W. Broenkow (1976) Cadmium and mercury transfer in a coastal marine ecosystem. Pages 135–184, *Marine Pollutant Transfer* edited by H. Windom and R. Duce. Lexington, Mass.: Heath. Martin, J. and G. Knauer (1973) The elemental composition of plankton. *Geochimica et Cosmochimica Acta 37*, 1639.

14. Chow, T.J., C.B. Snyder and J.L. Earl (1975) Isotope ratios of lead as pollutant source indicators. United Nations FAO and International Atomic Energy Association Symposium, Vienna, Austria (IAEA-SM-191/4). Proceedings pages 95–108. Rabinowitz, M.B., G.W. Wetherill and J.D. Kopple (1977) Magnitude of lead intake from respiration by normal man. *Journal of Laboratory and Clinical Medicine 90*, 238–248.

15. Murozumi, M., T.J. Chow and C.C. Patterson (1969) Chemical concentrations of pollutant lead aerosols, terrestrial dusts and sea salt in Greenland and Antarctic snow strata. *Geochimica et Cosmochimica Acta 33*, 1247–1294.

16. Tatsumoto, M. and C.C. Patterson (1963) The concentration of common lead in seawater. Pages 74–89, *Earth Science and Meteoritics* edited by Geiss and Goldberg. Amsterdam: North Holland. Tatsumoto, M. and C.C. Patterson (1963) Concentrations of common lead in some Atlantic and Mediterranean waters and in snow. *Nature 199*, 350–352. Chow, T.J. and C.C. Patterson (1966) Concentration profiles of barium and lead in Atlantic waters off Bermuda. *Earth and Planetary Science Letters 1*, 397–400.

17. Patterson, C.C. (1965) Contaminated and natural lead environments of man. *Archives of Environmental Health 11*, 344–360.

18. Hirao, Y. and C.C. Patterson (1974) Lead aerosol pollution in the High Sierra overrides natural mechanisms which exclude lead from a food chain. *Science 184*, 989–992. Elias, R., Y. Hirao and C.C. Patterson (1975) Impact of present levels of

aerosol Pb concentrations in both natural ecosystems and humans. Pages 257–272. *International Conference on Heavy Metals in the Environment*, Toronto, Ontario, Canada.

19. Boutron, C. (1979) Alkali and alkaline earth enrichments in aerosols deposited in Antarctic snows. *Atmospheric Environment 13*, 919–924.

20. Cragin, J.H., M.M. Herron, C.C. Langway, Jr. and G. Klonda (1977) Interhemispheric comparisons of changes in the composition of atmospheric precipitation during the late Cenozoic era. In *Polar Oceans* edited by M. Dunbar, Proceedings of a Conference on Polar Oceans, Montreal, May, 1974. Organized by ICSU/SCOR/SCAR.

21. Koide, M., E.D. Goldberg, M.M. Herron, and C.C. Langway (1977) Transuranic depositional history in South Greenland firn layers. *Nature 269*, 137–139. Weiss, H.V., M. Koide, and E.D. Goldberg (1971) Mercury in a Greenland Ice Sheet: evidence of recent input by man. *Science 174*, 692–694.

22. Herron, M., C. Langway, N. Weiss and J. Cragin (1977) Atmospheric trace metals and sulfate in the Greenland ice sheet. *Geochimica et Cosmochimica Acta 41*, 915–920.

23. Boutron, C. (1979) Past and present day tropospheric fallout fluxes of Pb, Cd, Cu, Zn and Ag in Antarctica and Greenland. *Geophysical Research Letters 6*, 159–162.

24. Chow, T.J. and E.D. Goldberg (1960) On the marine geochemistry of barium. *Geochimica et Cosmochimica Acta 20*, 192.

25. Chan, L.H., D. Drummond, J. Edmond and B. Grant (1977) On the barium data from the GEOSECS expedition. *Deep Sea Research 24*, 613–645. Bernat, M., T. Church and C. Allegre (1972) Barium and strontium concentrations in Pacific and Mediterranean sea water profiles by isotope dilution mass spectrometry. *Earth and Planetary Science Letters 16*, 75–80.

26. Bruland, K.W., C. Knauer and J.H. Martin (1978) Zinc in north-east Pacific water. *Nature 271*, 741–743. Moore, R.M. and J.D. Burton (1976) Concentrations of dissolved copper in the eastern Atlantic Ocean 23°N to 47°N. *Nature 264*, 241–243. Bender, M.L. and C. Gagner (1976) Dissolved copper, nickel, and cadmium in the Sargasso Sea. *Journal of Marine Research 34*, 327. Boyle, E.A., F. Sclater, and J.M. Edmond (1977) The distribution of dissolved copper in the Pacific. *Earth and Planetary Sciences Letters 37*, 38–54. Boyle, E.A., F. Sclater and J.M. Edmond (1976) On the marine geochemistry of cadmium. *Nature 263*, 42. Martin, J.H., K.W. Bruland and W.W. Broenkow (1976) in Reference [13].

27. Duce, R.A., G.L. Hoffman and W.H. Zoller (1975) Atmospheric trace metals at remote northern and southern hemispheric sites: pollution or natural? *Science 187*, 59–61.

28. University of Rhode Island, GSO. Unpublished work.

29. Benninger, L.K. (1978) ^{210}Pb balance in Long Island Sound. *Geochimica et Cosmochimica Acta 42*, 1165–1174. McCaffrey, R.J. A Record of the Accumulation of Sediment and Trace Metals in a Connecticut, U.S.A., Salt Marsh. Ph.D. Thesis, Yale University.

30. Goldberg, E.D. (1963) Geochronology with lead-210 in radioactive dating. *Vienna International Atomic Energy Agency*, 391–402.

31. Boucot, Katherine, R., Editor, *Archives of Environmental Health*.

32. Harriet Hardy, Massachusetts Institute of Technology. Henry Schroeder, Dartmouth College.

33. Shapiro, I.M., G. Mitchell, I. Davidson, and S.H. Katz (1975) The lead content of teeth: evidence establishing new minimal levels of exposure in a living preindustrialized human population. *Archives of Environmental Health 30*, 483–486. Grandjean, P., O.V. Nielson and I.M. Shapiro (1979) Lead retention in ancient Nubians and con-

temporary populations. *Journal of Environmental Pathology and Toxicology 2*, 781–787. Needleman, H.L., C. Gunnoe, A. Leviton, R. Reed, H. Peresie, C. Maher and P. Barrett (1979) Deficits in psychologic and classroom performance of children with elevated dentine lead levels. *New England Journal of Medicine 300*, 689–695.

34. Gilfillan, S.C., *Rome's Ruin by Lead Poison*. Book to be published. Gilfillan, S.C. (1965) Lead poisoning and the fall of Rome. *Journal of Occupational Medicine 7*, 53–60.

34a. Morgan, James, California Institute of Technology.

35. Goldwater, L.J. and A.W. Hoover (1967) An international study of "normal" levels of lead in blood and urine. *Archives of Environmental Health 15*, 60–63.

36. Hecker, L., H.E. Allen, B.D. Dirman and J.V. Neel (1974) Heavy metal levels in acculturated and unacculturated populations. *Archives of Environmental Health 29*, 181–185. Piomelli, Sergio. Blood lead levels in urban and remote populations (Unpublished manuscript. Reported to EPA March 1979. Contract #DA-8-1686J). Poole, C., M. Alpers and L.E. Smythe (1979) Blood lead levels in Papua New Guinea children living in a remote area. Submitted for publication in *Archives of Environmental Health*.

37. Statement by toxicologists (1968) Diagnosis of inorganic lead poisoning: a statement, *British Medical Journal 4*, 501.

38. National Academy of Sciences-National Research Council *Airborne Lead in Perspective* (1972) in Reference [6].

39. World Health Organization, Geneva (1977) in Reference [6] and Air Quality Criteria for Lead (1977) in Reference [6].

40. See Chapter 1–4, National Academy of Sciences-National Research Council *Lead in the Human Environment* (1979). Washington, D.C.: National Academy of Sciences.

40a. Hall, R.A., E.G. Zook, G.M. Meaburn, NOAA Technical Report NMFS SSSRF 721 (U.S. Department of Commerce, National Oceanographic and Atmospheric Administration, Washington).

41. Rabinowitz, M.B., G.W. Wetherill and J.D. Kopple (1977) in Reference [14].

42. Goldsmith, J.R. and A.C. Hexter (1967) Respiratory exposure to lead epidemiological experimental dose–response relationships. *Science 158*, 132–134.

43. Chow, T.J., C.B. Snyder and J.L. Earl (1975) in Reference [14].

Comparisons of Past and Present Occurrences of Lead in the Global Environment and in Humans

INTRODUCTION

There are three different kinds of lead contamination associated with natural lead in any substance analysed for lead in a laboratory. Industrial lead is added as environmental contamination to natural lead in materials *in situ*. A second type of lead contamination is added to the substance by the investigator when he collects and handles the material. A third type of lead contamination is added as laboratory contamination from reagents, containers and air during analysis to this mixture of leads in the material. In urban regions environmental lead contamination for such things as air, precipitation, dusts, and vegetation predominates over the laboratory and collection types of lead contamination, as shown in Figure 3, so that most published analytical data for such substances are generally not in serious error. However, the proportion of natural lead in these substances is a very small fraction of the total.

In remote regions environmental contamination effects are several orders of magnitude smaller than in urban regions. Under these circumstances laboratory contamination and collection contamination effects, typical of those found in most laboratories where lead analyses are routinely performed by conventional methods, greatly outweigh environmental contamination effects, as shown in Figure 3. It is therefore difficult to determine environmental lead correctly in remote regions. Examples of such errors are the excessive amounts of lead reported to be associated with aerosols in remote regions, the contamination of seawater

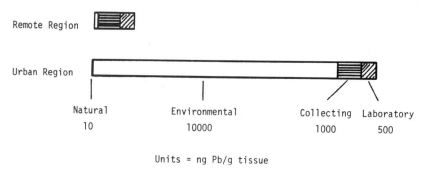

Units = ng Pb/g tissue

FIGURE 3   Relative amounts of industrial lead contamination (environmental, collecting, and laboratory) and natural lead found in an urban and a remote leaf. This same relationship holds for other substances. The amounts depicted above are typical of those found in most laboratories where lead analyses are routinely performed by conventional methods.

samples by effluents from ships, and failure to correctly analyse lead in old tree stem wood and in fresh tuna. These examples are discussed in the following text. Even after collection and laboratory types of lead contamination have been greatly reduced by means of clean laboratory techniques, proper evaluation and control of laboratory lead contamination during analysis remains a difficult problem. For example, the failure of some investigators to reduce their controlled levels of lead contamination below 50 picograms Pb/g ice has prevented them from observing a decline of environmental lead contamination to levels of 1 picogram Pb/g ice in ancient polar snows.

Even if the total amount of environmental lead contamination plus natural lead in a substance from a remote region has been correctly determined, the problem remains of distinguishing between these two different kinds of lead. This cannot be done pragmatically because there are no substances in the atmosphere, hydrosphere, or biosphere that are not contaminated with industrial lead to some degree, so that the proportion of natural lead in the total found in any substance must be determined indirectly from reconstructions of natural conditions based on biogeochemical models.

The great mass of published lead data for nonurban materials is a potpourri of undefined mixtures of the four above kinds of lead (natural, environmental lead contamination, collection and handling contamination, and laboratory contamination). Most of these data are rendered meaningless because of this effect. It is pointless to consider their significance unless the levels of each of the three different kinds of lead contamination are known in them with some degree of certainty, and the occurrence of the samples in their ecosystems are defined sufficiently as to give them scientific significance.

NATURAL LEAD CONCENTRATIONS IN AIR

The estimated natural concentration of lead in air over land areas likely to have been inhabited by humans in prehistoric times is about 0.04 ng Pb/m³. The major sources of natural lead in air are believed to be wind-blown soil, organic emissions from plant foliage, seasalt spray, smoke from forest fires, and emissions of lead-rich aerosols from volcanoes. At present, atmospheric lead originating from anthropogenic sources generally outweighs atmospheric lead originating from natural sources, so that the natural component of atmospheric lead cannot be measured directly. Approaches which are used to estimate natural backgrounds of lead in the atmosphere over continents in prehistoric times are: (1) studies of serial records of changes of lead concentrations with time in silicate dusts accumulated in polar snow and water laid sediments; (2) serial records of changes of isotopic compositions of lead with time in water laid sediments; (3) calculation of atmospheric lead concentrations from observed concentrations of atmospheric dusts; and (4) use of mass inventories of natural lead emissions to the atmosphere.

Serial Records of Changes of Lead Concentrations with Time in Silicate Dusts. Lead concentrations in soils are about 10 ppm and, if windblown dust from soils is the major source of lead in the atmosphere, the Pb/Si, Pb/Al, and Pb/(Ca + K) ratios should approximate those in soils, but they do not in the earth's atmosphere today. Lead is observed to be enriched about a hundred-fold above these values in aerosols collected on filters and washed out by rain in remote regions of the oceans and continents in the Northern Hemisphere. These enrichments refer to concentrations of lead within aerosols (chemical compositions of aerosols) independent of the amounts of aerosols themselves in the atmosphere. Some unusually large excesses of lead reported in present-day atmospheric silicate dusts are erroneous because of prevalence of artifact lead contamination [1], and similar excesses of lead have been erroneously reported for the same reason in dusts in ancient snows [2]. Despite such errors, reliable measurements have been made which do show the existence of excess lead in present-day atmospheric silicate dusts contained in the air at remote locations [3]. It must be ascertained whether this excess lead originates from natural or anthropogenic sources. If the excess is observed to increase with time over the last few centuries, it must be anthropogenic and natural concentrations of atmospheric lead can therefore be estimated from typical concentrations of silicate dusts in the atmosphere. These chemical enrichments of lead are observed to decrease to crustal concentrations in going back in time in snow and sediment strata. The chronological record of Pb/(Ca + K) in dated North Greenland ice strata shows that this ratio approximated crustal compositions in the atmosphere three thousand years ago, was about ten-fold above crustal abundances two hundred fifty years ago, rose to about fifty-fold excess by the early 1900's, and rose further to two hundred-fold excess by 1965 [4]. Recently, other investigators reported that they could not confirm the decrease in Pb/(Ca + K) ratios in Greenland ice strata for times earlier than 1900, but their lead data are not trustworthy at these low concentrations because they attempted to clean dirty ice cores whose surfaces were contaminated 10^6-fold above lead concentrations in the ice, and their analytical sensitivities and blanks did not permit reliable measurements below about 50×10^{-12} g Pb/g ice [5]. However lead concentrations at levels of $\leq 1 \times 10^{-12}$ g Pb/g ice actually occur in ancient ice. The concentrations of lead in Antarctic snow strata, uncontaminated by local leaded exhaust emissions, appear to increase from $< 1 \times 10^{-12}$ g Pb/g ice to $< 50 \times 10^{-12}$ g Pb/g ice in going from early to recent times, but that increase is poorly defined because the overall concentrations of lead in Antarctic snows are an order of magnitude less than they are in the Arctic, where they increase from $< 1 \times 10^{-12}$ g Pb/g ice to 200×10^{-12} g Pb/g ice [4]. Natural concentrations of lead in Antarctic snows are probably less than those in the Arctic because they contain less soil dust. Anthropogenic additions of lead in Antarctic snows are less because most industrial emissions of anthropogenic lead to the atmosphere are confined to the Northern Hemisphere. Another investigator has claimed that concentrations of lead in Antarctic snows do not increase with time, and that increases in Arctic snows are insignificant [6]. Examination of details of contamination control and analytical procedures reported by this investigator indicates that lead contamination probably was not properly reduced and controlled below levels of about 50×10^{-12} g Pb/g ice during analysis [7].

The historical record of reliable measurements of lead in polar snows indicates that there was no excess of lead above average crustal concentrations in silicate dusts during prehistoric times, and that the excess which is observed today grew with time in approximate accordance with increased rates of emission of industrial lead to the atmosphere.

It is generally agreed that concentrations of lead in urban atmospheres and runoff waters are excessive due to anthropogenic emissions and this can result in pollution of the upper layers of nearby water laid sediments by local emissions of industrial lead in urban regions. However, it has generally been believed that excess amounts of industrial lead in the atmosphere at remote locations are too small to cause measurable effects in the upper layers of water laid sediments in these regions. Setting aside the record of lead in sediments from urban regions, recent additions of excess industrial lead to the atmosphere in remote regions have been observed to exert measurable effects in upper layers of terrestrial sediments and in atmospheric deposition fluxes in open oceans. It has been found that lead concentrations in the organic fraction of sediments in a remote pond in the California High Sierra increased four-fold during the past century [8]. This change corresponded to a ten-fold increase in lead concentrations in air above the pond drainage during that same interval. The record in pond sediments could not show decreases in atmospheric lead concentrations in earlier times because it was obscured by natural lead in the sediments. Deep ocean sediments in the North Pacific record a deposition of authigenic (originally soluble) lead in ancient times at the rate of 2 ng Pb/cm^2 yr, coupled with a simultaneous deposition of 1 ng Pb/cm^2 yr silicate lead in particles with typical crustal composition [9]. This can be compared with a present-day atmospheric input to the North Pacific Ocean above the sediments of about 60 ng Pb/cm^2 yr nonsilicate lead coupled with 0.5 ng Pb/cm^2 yr silicate lead [10]. The increased atmospheric input of excess lead is computed from present-day relationships between concentrations of common lead and ^{210}Pb in surface waters of the ocean and the input of ^{210}Pb to the oceans. Both the marine and terrestrial sedimentary records in remote regions far from local urban contamination indicate that the excess of lead associated with silicate dusts in remote atmospheres was less in earlier times than it is today, which is concordant with observations in polar snows.

Serial Records of Changes of Lead Isotopic Compositions with Time. Changes in isotopic compositions of leads deposited in marine and pond sediments can be used to show that the minimum increase in excess lead in atmospheric silicate dusts in remote areas has been more than an order of magnitude in recent centuries. The isotopic compositions of lead in soils of major fluvial drainage basins emptying into the world's oceans are characteristically different among the various basins, and it is found that in ancient times these isotopically different leads were deposited in deep ocean sediments in regions adjacent to each drainage basin instead of being isotopically homogenized by mixing before deposition. This isotopic pattern of lead in deep ocean sediments requires that atmospheric inputs of lead to the oceans must have been insignificant in ancient times because leads of different isotopic compositions in wind-blown dust would have been homogenized by mixing in the atmosphere. This oceanic isotopic lead in sediments pattern restricts mixed atmospheric lead inputs to such a low level that it requires that at least 90%

of the one hundred-fold chemical excess of lead above crustal compositions in tropospheric aerosols in marine air today must be of recent (industrial) origin. Today, isotopic compositions of industrial atmospheric leads over land differ from isotopic compositions of the excess lead deposited in ancient sediments, but the isotopic composition of the excess lead deposited from the atmosphere in recent upper sediments in a remote pond in North America is the same as that of industrial lead in the atmosphere [8]. This isotopic effect can account for about 90% of the chemical excess of lead above crustal compositions observed today in atmospheric aerosols. Fluctuations in lead isotopic compositions prevent a closer accounting by this method.

Calculation of Natural Atmospheric Lead Concentrations from Observed Concentrations of Atmospheric Dusts. The average concentration of lead in igneous rocks at the earth's surface is about 12 ppm [9]. Typical soils generated from these rocks will contain about the same amount of lead. The concentrations of soil dusts are smaller in Antarctic atmospheres compared to Arctic air, and concentrations of dusts are smaller in marine atmospheres than in those over the continents. Natural levels of silicate dusts in continental air at midlatitudes may be about 5 $\mu g/m^3$ [11]. The calculated natural concentration of lead in the atmosphere over continents in prehistoric times originating from dusts was about 0.06 ng Pb/m^3.

Natural Atmospheric Lead Concentrations from Mass Inventories of Natural Lead Emissions. The mass inventory of major annual lead emissions to the atmosphere is given in Table 1. Estimates of natural emissions of windblown and volcanic dusts to the earth's atmosphere are from [12]. Previous estimates of natural lead emissions from silicate dusts [13] are excessive because the estimate of natural lead concentrations in the dust is too high by a factor of three (present-day windblown soil dusts are excessively contaminated with industrial lead), and the highest estimate for dust in air is used (it is appropriate to use the average concentration of lead in rocks that provide soils). Previous estimates for dust may be excessive because of bias by erroneously high measurements of dusts in rain and snow that were caused by failure to exclude dust contamination during collection of samples. The natural emission of windblown silicate lead in aerosols characterized by a natural Pb/(Ca + K) ratio is modified from [12]. Seaspray emissions are believed from recent preliminary investigations to contain lead enriched no more than a thousand-fold above natural concentrations in surface seawater believed to be about 0.0005 ng Pb/g during prehistoric times [14]. Lead concentrations reported in foliage forest emissions [15] are erroneously high due to excessive artifact lead contamination during collection and analysis and failure to correct for anthropogenic lead deposited by dry deposition on foliage surfaces. Lead emissions from foliage measured with ^{210}Pb tracers [16] are less than lead deposited by dry deposition [38] although the emission data are erroneous because of errors in common and radioactive lead contamination control. If an upper limit of 0.1 ppm Pb is assigned to these organic emissions, a natural lead emission can be estimated from this source. Experimental measurements of volcanic lead emissions in volcanic gases have been seriously compromised by failure to exclude artifact lead contamination during sample collection and by use of improper flux models. Recent measurements of the Pb/S ratios in fumarolic gases from high [17] and low [18] halogen emitting volcanoes suggest that the average Pb/S ratio in volcanic gas is about 2×10^{-7} g/g. Other natural sources of lead emissions to the atmosphere are insignificant in relation to those listed in Table 1. Global emissions of lead from natural sources sum to about 2×10^3 tons/yr, and with a mean residence time of ten days, the estimated natural concentration of lead in the earth's troposphere is about 0.01 ng Pb/m^3. On the basis of this and the previous estimate above, the expected natural concentration of lead in air over land areas likely to have been inhabited by humans in prehistoric times is about 0.04 ng Pb/m^3.

NATURAL LEAD CONCENTRATIONS IN MARINE WATERS

It is estimated that prehistoric natural concentrations of lead in surface waters of the North Pacific were about 0.0005 ng Pb/g water. Although it is obvious that lead effluents and atmospheric emissions added to the oceans near industrialized and urban regions have contaminated the seas on a local basis, the questions are whether the concentrations of lead in open ocean waters have been perturbed by anthropogenic inputs and whether lead concentrations in those waters have been correctly determined. No competent investigator in chemical oceanography today would claim that measurements of lead concentrations in open ocean waters made before the 1960s have any scientific significance. At that time, an unusual shape in the vertical distribution profile of common lead in the oceans had been determined by ultra-clean laboratory IDMS analytical methods [19]. The concentrations were observed to decrease with depth within the thermocline to relatively fixed concentrations in deep waters. This distribution contrasted with that for nutrients and other metals in the seas and perturbation by anthropogenic inputs of industrial lead was indicated, which on a mass inventory basis was permissible. These re-

TABLE 1   Atmospheric Lead from Natural Emissions (see text for sources of data)

Source	Total Production (10^6 t/yr)	Lead Emission Factor (g Pb/kg emission)	Lead Transfer to Atmosphere (10^3 t/yr)
Natural emissions			
Volcanic and wind-blown dust	200	1×10^{-2}	2
Sea spray	1,000	$<1 \times 10^{-7}$	<1
Forest foliage	100	$<1 \times 10^{-5}$	<0.1
Volcanic sulfur	6	2×10^{-4}	0.001
TOTAL			2

ported lead concentrations were in error because the water sample collectors were contaminated by lead effluents from research vessels. Interlaboratory calibrations concerning lead in seawater carried out in the early 1970s showed that this was true and that, in addition and without exception, all measurements of lead concentrations in open ocean waters by methods other than ultra-clean IDMS gave results that were erroneously high by very large factors. Subsequently, a seawater sampler which protects itself against effluents from ships has been used, which has allowed vertical distribution profiles of common lead in the North Pacific and North Atlantic to be determined [10]. These new profiles show that the principal source of lead in the oceans today is atmospheric deposition in a manner very similar to that for ^{210}Pb, whose radioactive precursor is emitted from continental soils as a gas [20]. There are few reliable data other than these available today relating to the concentration of lead in open ocean waters. Although great improvements have been made in analytical techniques for lead in some chemical oceanographic laboratories during the past six years, so that they can now properly collect and analyse surface samples of nearshore seawaters which contain relatively high concentrations of lead originating from local effluents, the extreme difficulty of controlling lead contamination has prevented investigators in many of those laboratories from reliably collecting and analysing seawaters from open ocean locations. Determination of present-day atmospheric input fluxes of common lead to the open oceans, when compared with the output of lead from the oceans to sediments during the ancient past, indicates about an order of magnitude more lead is entering the oceans of the Northern Hemisphere today than has done so in the past. Reliable and accurate lead concentration profiles have not yet been determined in the oceans of the Southern Hemisphere, where atmospheric input fluxes of industrial lead are certain to be less. Therefore, natural concentrations of lead in ocean waters must for the moment be estimated from past output fluxes to the sediments and residence times in surface waters. Using a mean residence time of two years and a past output flux of 2 ng nonsilicate Pb/cm^2-yr in the North Pacific, it is estimated that prehistoric natural concentrations of lead in the surface waters of the North Pacific were about 0.0005 ng Pb/g water [10].

NATURAL LEAD CONCENTRATIONS IN FRESH WATERS

It is estimated that the natural concentrations of lead in clear streams during prehistoric times was less than 0.02 ng Pb/g water. It is commonly believed that natural concentrations of lead in remote rivers and lakes range from 1–10 ng Pb/g water [21]. This estimate is based on beliefs that anthropogenic perturbations of lead concentrations in fresh waters are buffered to insignificant levels by soil chelation, together with the belief that most reported concentrations of lead in remote fresh waters are acceptable because they seem so low. The first belief may be correct in that the buffering effect of soils probably confines anthropogenic perturbations to less than order of magnitude elevations of lead concentrations in stream waters. The second belief is wrong in that, although fresh waters from urban areas may contain high concentrations of industrial lead, this is not the case for rivers and streams in remote areas. Further, most analytical methods for lead in remote waters are too insensitive for such measurements and contamination controls during sampling and analysis have been inadequate. Reliable measurements have been made of lead concentrations in streams in remote areas by means of ultra-clean IDMS laboratory methods, and observed values ranged from 6 to 50 ng Pb/kg water [22]. This magnitude of analytical error and naivete of analysts reporting erroneously high values is identical to the situation which prevailed with respect to lead in seawater. In the latter case, the matter was resolved during the following fifteen years by demonstrating that the lower values were correct. It is pointless to believe that most presently reported lead concentrations in fresh waters in remote regions determined by ordinary analytical methods have any significance.

Much of the industrial lead in precipitation is sorbed in soils, which greatly complicates relationships between lead in stream waters and precipitation in remote regions. ^{210}Pb studies, which are applicable because both ^{210}Pb common lead have atmospheric source functions in this case, show that lead in atmospheric precipitation is strongly sorbed by soils [23]. Furthermore, snow in a remote North American region contains about 0.7 ng industrial Pb/g and rain contains about 5 ng industrial Pb/g, yet local streams that drain off this precipitation contain only about 0.015 ng Pb/g water [24]. Reported mass balance studies of common lead leaving remote watershed systems via streams, which used analytical methods other than the ultra-clean IDMS technique, probably involve high positive errors in lead concentration measurements. Sufficient knowledge is not yet available to indicate the relative proportions of natural and anthropogenic leads in the total lead in streams draining remote watersheds. At present, the best estimate for a natural level of lead in fresh stream waters must originate from the few ultra-clean IDMS laboratory values that are available, and an assumption that anthropogenic contributions elevate those values by no more than two-fold. Although total lead concentrations in turbid waters of principal rivers may have been considerably higher than 0.02 ng Pb/g water, this probably was the approximate upper limit for the natural concentration of lead in clear streams during prehistoric times.

NATURAL LEAD CONCENTRATIONS IN SOIL HUMUS AND IN SOIL MOISTURE FILMS

The natural concentration of lead in soil humus may be equal to or less than several ppm, and soil moisture films in contact with such humus may have contained natural lead concentrations that were substantially less than 2 ng Pb/g water. As will be shown below, very large increases in concentrations of lead in soil humus at a remote location caused by atmospheric inputs of industrial lead occurring at concentrations of 10 ng Pb/m^3 have been indicated by observations of lead concentrations in pond sediments at that location. This means that natural concentrations of lead in humus certainly cannot be found in soils located near any populated regions, including farming areas. Most natural soils were derived from geologically old, consolidated sedimentary rocks and the constituents of most of those rocks in turn were derived from igneous sources. The occurrence of lead among minerals in igneous rocks and within various igneous rock types is reasonably well known. Although the whole-rock concentration of lead among different igneous rock types varies systematically from about 5 to 20 ppm, the proportions of these types which exist at the surface of the earth's crust are reasonably well known, so that an average value of 12 ppm Pb in igneous rocks at the earth's surface has been derived [9]. The occurrence of lead in igneous rocks is better known and understood than in sedimentary rock strata. There are great disparities among the concentrations of lead in different components of these strata. Sandstones rich in quartz contain low concentrations of lead compared to shales, while limestones contain intermediate concentrations of lead. Although soils derived for the most part from only one of these sedimentary rock types do show characteristic chemical features that are related to such associations, most soils are derived from fairly representative mixtures of types. The crucial feature in soils that is significant in determining the concentration of lead in plants, as will be shown later in this section, is not the weight fraction of lead in the soil, but the Pb/Ca ratio in soil moisture film. This ratio in the latter is apparently determined by lead and calcium concentrations in minor phases of soils such as humus and mixed phosphates and carbonates of major cations.

Lead in igneous, clay, and other mineral particles is largely chemically inactive in soil and, except for a small fraction on surfaces of these particles, is relatively unavailable for biological assimilation. Since this mineral fraction constitutes the major reservoir of lead in most soils, variations in lead concentrations in this reservoir in soils may or may not be significant in determining the concentration of biologically available lead in soils, because some minerals which account for major portions of mineral lead, such as potash feldspars, are highly intractable to weathering. Although there are many theories dealing with the transfer of lead from soil to plants, there are no trustworthy lead measurements available for natural soil-to-plant transfers of lead in remote, undisturbed systems. In spite of this lack, it is highly probable that one of the major pathways of lead transfer from soil to plant roots is via soil moisture films. It is probable that lead in this medium is derived mainly from soil humus because the reactive surface of humus is equal to or greater than that of any mineral component in soil, and it is highly reactive on a volume basis compared to minerals. Very few trustworthy measurements have been made of the concentrations of lead in soil humus from remote regions. Ultra-clean IDMS measurements of lead in humus contained in the upper 10 centimeters of remote, uncultivated soils show values of 5 to 10 ppm Pb in the humus on a dry weight basis [25]. In such soils the humus comprises about 10% on a dry weight basis and the total lead content of the soils is about 10 ppm.

Although experimental studies have been made in laboratories of effects on plant roots by lead solutions which contained unnaturally excessive concentrations of soluble lead compounds and some studies have been made of lead concentrations in artificial "soil solutions" prepared in laboratories [26], few reliable measurements have been made of lead concentrations in natural soil moisture films sampled *in situ* from remote undisturbed soils [26]. Data obtained by ultra-clean IDMS methods show that lead concentrations are about 2 ng Pb/g water in soil moisture films obtained in the field by placing ultra-clean blotters on remote uncultivated soils. It must be emphasized that this lead is not equivalent to lead in phreatic or "ground" waters which, in the above case, are observed to contain 0.05 ng Pb/g water, nor to lead in streams draining such soil which contain 0.015 ng Pb/g water.

These few data are all that are both available and pertinent to the natural concentration of biologically available lead in soils. Because of this, it is fruitless at this time to consider the range of total leads that have been measured and reported in those soils not taken from cultivated or ore-mineralized or urbanized locations as though it were significant with respect to natural levels of biologically available lead in soils. Virtually all soils have been affected by anthropogenic inputs of lead. Although some studies in urban regions suggest that insoluble, anthropogenic, inorganic precipitates in soils, such as sulfates or carbonates, may account for large fractions of soil leads in those regions [26], it is believed that soil humus, rather than inorganic minerals [26], is the major sink for anthropogenic lead in remote, uncultivated soils [28]. Anthropogenic additions of lead to such remote soils might be minor relative to the total amount of lead in the soil, but when concentrated in the small humus fraction, they can exert a major effect on the concentration of lead in that humus fraction. These anthropogenic additions are then reflected as increased concentrations of lead in soil moisture film.

It should be emphasized that possible variations in the occurrences of natural lead concentrations in plants caused by high concentrations of lead in soils developed from mineralized lead ore deposits played an insignificant role in the general occurrence of natural lead in the biosphere, because natural surface exposures of such ore deposits were only about 10^{-6} of total soil exposures in prehistoric times [29].

There is strong evidence suggesting that the concentration of lead in higher animals during prehistoric times was relatively uniform. Such evidence originates from observations of the skeletal Ba/Ca ratio in humans. There are variations in the geological occurrences of barium among ores, rocks, minerals, and soils in the same manner as for lead, yet there is a remarkable uniformity in the skeletal Ba/Ca ratio in humans who lived at different times on different continents: atomic Ba/Ca = 1×10^{-6} in an ancient Egyptian; 2×10^{-6} in ancient Peruvians; 3×10^{-6} in present-day Americans; and 7×10^{-6} in present-day British [30]. This indicates that regional variations in the barium content of human diets are small and do not fluctuate widely as a consequence of either regional variations in the barium content of soils or differences in the biopurification of calcium with respect to barium (a process which is explained later in this section). Since barium and lead are covariant within organisms and consequently in natural human foods, it is highly unlikely that the natural lead content of human diets in prehistoric times varied over a wide range because of regional variations in lead concentrations in soils and differences in biopurification.

The 2 ng Pb/g water concentration level that has been determined in a few samples of soil moisture film in soils taken from a remote location probably has been elevated by additions of anthropogenic lead through rain, snow, and dry deposition. Numerous observations which relate to increases in concentrations of lead with time in recent sediments of lakes and coastal waters near urban regions are relevant to the subject of the natural occurrence of lead in soil moisture film only where lead concentrations have been reliably determined in the ancient humus fraction of those sediments, and this has not yet been done [31]. Concentrations of lead in air, precipitation and dry deposition have been measured at remote locations [32], but many of these cannot be used to estimate reliable atmospheric input fluxes of lead to remote watersheds, because of errors due to contamination during collection and/or analysis of the samples or to the collection of types of samples that are irrelevant to the determination of the input flux or both. Excluding large contamination errors associated with lead analyses, a common error is to leave buckets unattended in the field for the collecting of samples of combined dry deposition and precipitation. The interception areas of such buckets are not representative of those of foliage in watersheds, and further such buckets usually collect large amounts of re-entrained dusts and fragments of foliage whose contributions of lead cannot be properly accounted for.

Ultra-clean IDMS analytical techniques and aerodynamically significant collection procedures show total atmospheric lead inputs of about 400 ng Pb/cm^2 yr at the remote North American watershed where atmospheric lead concentrations are about 10 ng Pb/m^3 [25]. It has been shown that this input flux of atmospheric lead has elevated the concentration of lead four-fold in the humus fraction of the upper centimeter of pond sediments in that watershed. It was measurable back to 1900 at a depth of about 8 cm, but in earlier times the perturbation was less. Lead concentrations were observed to be 3 ppm in the oldest sediment layers dated at A.D. 1700 [8]. Similar measurements have not yet been made for soils in this watershed. However, it has been estimated on the basis of mass inventories of input fluxes of lead that the contamination effect in the pond sediments is probably about 1/4th of that expected in the humus fraction in top layers of soils in the watershed of the pond. It is therefore expected that a ten-fold elevation of lead concentrations above natural levels has been caused in the humus fraction of the upper 5 cm of soil in the watershed. Since analyses of lead concentrations in humus composites from these surface soils show an average concentration of about 10 ppm

Pb, it would appear that the natural concentration of lead in soil humus at this location was about 1 ppm. Soils in this watershed are known to have been derived recently from a single type of igneous rock whose total lead concentration is twice that in average surface crustal rocks. Therefore, this estimated natural concentration of lead in humus should be regarded as an upper limit.

It has been proposed that the excess total lead observed in the upper strata of soils exposed to unmeasured and unrecognized intense atmospheric inputs of locally derived industrial lead in or near urban regions is the result of natural processes such as vertical transport by plants [33]. This transport theory is probably incorrect for soils, because another version of it is demonstrably wrong in the case of water laid sediments, where it has been shown, in both urban regions and in a remote area, by means of stable lead isotopic tracers and by chronological associations with anthropogenic activities, that recent increases of lead concentrations in the upper strata of these sediments are clearly and definitely not the result of natural vertical transport of lead in pore fluids, but are additions of industrial lead [31]. Since it is rather certain that the observed lead concentration of 10 ppm in soil humus is substantially higher than natural levels as a result of anthropogenic additions, the observed lead concentration of 2 ppb in soil moisture film in contact with that humus is probably also higher than natural levels by a similar factor.

NATURAL LEAD CONCENTRATIONS IN THE EARTH'S BIOMASS

In prehistoric times the natural concentration of lead in the main mass of the earth's biosphere was probably about 4 ng Pb/g. Trees comprise the major portion of the earth's biomass [34]. As mentioned in Section 3, all reported analyses of lead in old stemwood of trees are erroneously high by a factor of one thousand. Published estimates of the amount of lead in the earth's biomass (reviewed in [35]) are therefore wrong because erroneous data were considered and the extent of industrial pollution of the biosphere was not understood. In prehistoric times the natural concentration of lead in the main mass of the earth's biosphere probably was about 4 ng Pb/g, because century-old portions of softwood stems of trees are found to contain only about 3 ng Pb/g, while hardwood stems contain less [36], and trees comprise the major fraction of the biomass. Foliage, comprising a small fraction of tree mass, probably contained slightly higher concentrations of lead because pine needles today in North America are believed to contain about 10 ng internal Pb/g fresh weight, of which about half is anthropogenic [36]. In prehistoric times, lead in the biomass of the Northern Hemisphere probably amounted to about 3000 tons, with the annual turnover in the growth cycle amounting to only about 300 tons Pb/yr.

NATURAL LEAD CONCENTRATIONS IN HUMAN DIETS

The average natural concentration of lead in the total prehistoric human diet was less than 2 ng Pb/g wet weight. Most investigators who have either studied occurrences of lead in plants and animals from remote regions at random or who have studied the occurrences of lead in related components of ecosystems in remote regions have used analytical methods for lead which were seriously compromised by contamination effects and they failed to adapt their studies to an important principle which governs the occurrence of lead in related components of ecosystems. This principle is that lead is not processed by organisms in ecosystems as an individual entity. Instead it tends to follow calcium in its nutrient pathways as a toxic trace constituent of calcium such that Pb/Ca ratios are altered by various acceptance-exclusion processes during nutrient uptake, internal distribution, and excretion within organisms [37]. Natural occurrences of lead should be evaluated in the form of Pb/Ca ratios in various organisms connected by common nutritive calcium pathways, because it is by this means that true contamination effects can be properly ascertained. Until now such studies have been carried out in only one remote ecosystem. Nevertheless the data appear to be valid and useful because they fit into a self-consistent pattern determined by both prediction and confirmation from separate lines of investigation.

At present only the broadest aspects of the biopurification of calcium with respect to lead and barium in nutrient pathways are apparent from preliminary studies, while complications and restrictions of applicability of this concept to specific problems remain to be worked out by further investigations. A potentially significant increment of lead contamination to furred animals probably originates from grooming, and this remains to be evaluated. The inhalation of air excessively enriched with reentrained soil surface lead by animals also remains to be evaluated. Neither of these factors were accounted for in the corrections for lead contamination discussed below and illustrated in Figure 4. Such corrections, if applied, would serve to strengthen the premise set forth in Figure 4 by depressing the contamination-corrected Pb/Ca curve further downward. The pathways of calcium from rock to soil moisture are not related to those of lead in simple ways. Furthermore it is clear, as is shown in Figure 5 below by comparison of Pb/Ca in tuna bone and muscle, that calcium is not biopurified of lead in all tissues of an organism, and consumers are affected by this reversal. A major example of such an effect is in the nu-

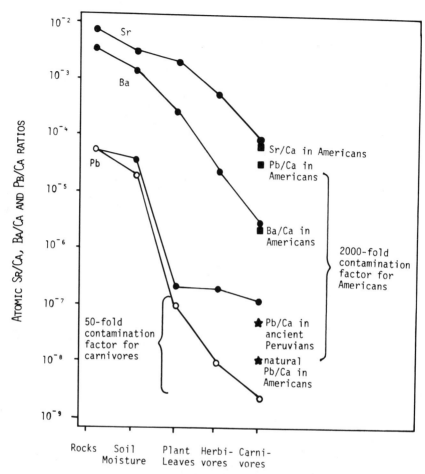

FIGURE 4 Biopurification in a remote terrestrial ecosystem and in humans. (●) indicates observed Sr/Ca, Ba/Ca and Pb/Ca atomic ratios in this ecosystem, normalized to average crustal abundances. (■) indicates observed average skeletal Sr/Ca, Ba/Ca and Pb/Ca atomic ratios in Americans. (★) indicates observed skeletal Pb/Ca atomic ratio in ancient Peruvians and natural Pb/Ca ratio predicted for Americans. In this ecosystem, the observed Pb/Ca ratios were corrected for known contaminant lead (○), showing that carnivores are contaminated 50-fold. The Sr/Ca and Ba/Ca ratios for Americans are similar to those observed in carnivores while the Pb/Ca ratios observed in Americans are 5000 times higher than for carnivores. Data from [28].

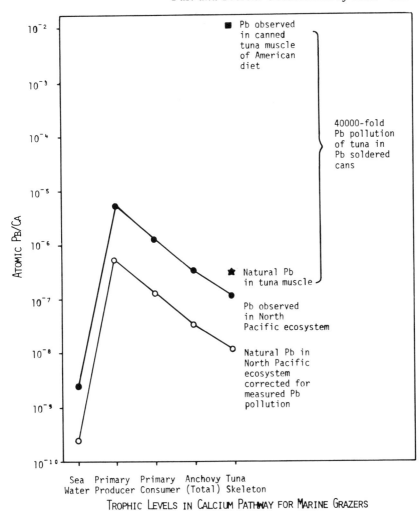

FIGURE 5 Biopurification in a Marine Ecosystem of the North Pacific. (●) indicates atomic Pb/Ca ratios observed in this ecosystem. In this ecosystem, the observed Pb/Ca ratios were corrected for known contaminant lead (○). (★) is predicted natural Pb/Ca ratio in tuna muscle based on observed muscle-skeletal relationships of lead and corrected for known contaminant lead. (■) indicates the observed Pb/Ca ratio in Pb soldered canned tuna muscle. Data from reference [39].

TABLE 2   Natural Skeletal Atomic Ratios (see text for sources of data)

Source	Sr/Ca	Ba/Ca	Pb/Ca
Martens	1×10^{-4}	4×10^{-6}	3×10^{-9}
Americans	9×10^{-5}	3×10^{-6}	2×10^{-8}
Tuna	2×10^{-3}	3×10^{-6}	1×10^{-8}

tritive calcium pathway through soil litter, insects, and insectivores, where the increase of lead in deciduous litter, accumulating biochemically and by direct atmospheric input, counteracts biopurification [28]. In addition, the nutritive pathways of calcium are not linear, but webbed, so that successive biopurification effects cannot be inferred in a simple manner. Nevertheless, the pragmatic determination of overall biopurification factors for calcium with respect to lead, barium, and strontium in going from rock to organisms at different, approximately determined trophic levels is remarkably useful, in that these overall factors appear to be similar for quite different species of animals which feed at similar trophic levels. This is shown by the remarkably close juxtapositions of natural values for Sr/Ca, Ba/Ca, and Pb/Ca ratios in martens, humans, and tuna fish, shown in Table 2 despite the enormous magnitude of the overall biopurification effects that are involved.

Studies of lead in a remote subalpine ecosystem based on soil derived from local igneous rock in California show that centuries ago the input of lead from the atmosphere to that ecosystem was only about 1/5th of the lead input from rock weathering [38]. Today the atmospheric input of lead to this same ecosystem has been elevated by anthropogenic lead-rich aerosols to about twenty times the input of lead by rock weathering. It has been found that virtually none of this recently introduced lead leaves the ecosystem by stream runoff. Although this excess industrial lead collects in soil humus, and by root uptake elevates lead in plants and consumers, new and more predominant entry routes for lead into food chains have been established by industrial lead accumulated in the form of dry deposition on foliage and fur surfaces. These new anthropogenically created reservoirs of surficial deposits of industrial lead in terrestrial ecosystems, although short-lived and of relatively small mass, elevate lead levels in consumers in great disproportion compared to the effects caused by larger masses of industrial lead collected in soil humus. These new surface deposition reservoirs of industrial lead bypass and circumvent natural so-called "biopurification" processes which formerly diminished lead levels in higher organisms under natural conditions. They exert a much greater contamination effect on organisms high up in food chains that under former natural conditions were protected by precursors. This is illustrated in Figure 4 by the much greater contamination of carnivores relative to plant leaves. As a result of these new circumstances, concentrations of lead are elevated from about 20 ng Pb/g wet weight to 300 ng Pb/g wet weight in plant leaves and from about 20 ng Pb/g wet weight to about 900 ng Pb/g wet weight in carnivore bones by lead inputs of about 270 ng Pb/cm^2 yr (projected map area of ecosystem) by dry deposition and about 130 ng Pb/cm^2 yr by precipitation in the remote ecosystem where atmospheric lead concentrations are about 10 ng Pb/m^3 [25].

Unlike its associations with other metals within igneous and inorganic systems, lead, when it occurs in organisms, belongs to the calcium, strontium, barium family of metals with respect to uptake, internal distribution, and excretion. Lead and barium are apparently processed inadvertently along with calcium by virtually all organisms, being stored in major reservoirs of calcium. Biochemical mechanisms seem to directly regulate calcium, but operate passively as a consequence of trace occurrences and less efficiently as a consequence of small differences in chemical properties on lead and barium. In this manner calcium is purified of these trace metals during plant and animal ingestion of calcium because less lead and barium are absorbed compared to calcium. Major reservoirs of calcium in most organisms generally reflect this purification process in terms of reduced Pb/Ca and Ba/Ca ratios compared to those in nutrient media. This process is called biopurification of calcium with respect to lead and barium in nutrient pathways. In food chains stepwise five-fold to twenty-fold biopurifications of calcium with respect to lead and barium are multiplicative through successive consumer stages, so that organisms at the highest ends of food chains possess calcium reservoirs with extremely low Pb/Ca and Ba/Ca ratios compared to initial rock values. This means that carnivores become contaminated by much greater factors than plants from the same quantities of industrial lead pollution. Proteins in some tissues in organisms possess such great affinities for lead relative to calcium that Pb/Ca ratios in these tissues are sometimes greater than those in nutrient media. However, the masses of lead in these tissues are such small fractions of the total masses of lead in organisms that biopurification of calcium with respect to lead holds for entire plants and animals. Biopurification factors are numbers that remain relatively fixed, independent of increases of trace lead concentrations in nutrient media due to contamination. Thus, higher levels of lead in nutrients result in elevated lead concentrations in consumers.

In North America the average atomic Ba/Ca ratio in crustal rocks is

3000×10^{-6}, whereas this ratio in the skeletons of typical Americans, British and ancient Peruvians is only 2 to 7×10^{-6} [30]. The thousand-fold difference is the result of consecutive biopurifications of calcium with respect to barium within precursors of humans in their food chains. As shown in Figure 4, field measurements in a remote ecosystem show that the initial Ba/Ca ratio of rocks is reduced at four successive trophic levels in a stepwise manner by an overall factor of one thousand in a food chain leading from rock to soil moisture, to plant, to herbivore, and to carnivore [28]. Initial rock atomic ratios in this remote ecosystem were Sr/Ca = 2.0×10^{-2}, Ba/Ca = 2.7×10^{-2}, and Pb/Ca = 3.5×10^{-4}, which are different from average crustal abundances, so observed biopurification factors for each trace metal at each stage in the food chain were applied to initial average crustal rock abundances to yield the values shown in Figure 4 which are generally applicable on a continent-wide basis. Contamination by industrial barium in remote ecosystems and in human foods is relatively minor even though the world industrial production of barium is nearly the same as that for lead (most of the barium is used in drilling muds, although some is used in paints, sugar refining, and smoke depressants). For example, it has been observed that there is an enormous contrast between the small contamination effects for industrial barium and the large contamination effects for industrial lead in tuna [12].

As shown in Figure 4, when corrections are applied for measured industrial lead contamination deposits in soil humus, on surfaces of plant leaves and animal fur, and within contaminated precursors in this North American ecosystem, the Pb/Ca ratio is observed to be reduced about fifteen thousand-fold by means of biopurification in going from rock to carnivore, which is an order of magnitude greater reduction than that for barium. The biopurification factor for short-lived carnivores should be reduced to correct for lead accumulation in longer-lived humans. A tentative correction which can be used now reduces the biopurification factor for humans to about three thousand. When this factor is applied to the atomic Pb/Ca ratio in crustal rocks of 6400×10^{-8}, a natural skeletal Pb/Ca ratio of about 2×10^{-8} is predicted. This value compares favorably with a value of 6×10^{-8} in bones of adult Peruvians who lived sixteen hundred years ago in an unpolluted environment, which indicates that the biopurification concept for lead is valid.

Figure 5 shows that biopurification factors for calcium with respect to lead in marine food chains leading from seawater to albacore are different from those in terrestrial food chains because the Pb/Ca ratio in algae at the first trophic level is about a thousand-fold greater than that in seawater due to preferential passive sorption of lead relative to calcium on surfaces of algae in oceans. Pb/Ca ratios are subsequently diminished through biopurification at successive stages in marine food chains so that tuna have approximately the same estimated natural Pb/Ca ratios as do terrestrial carnivores after corrections are applied in both of them for industrial lead contamination.

Lead concentrations in natural human foods can be estimated from the above quantitative knowledge about lead and calcium relationships in components of natural ecosystems. During prehistoric times the atomic Pb/Ca ratio in rocks was reduced by means of biopurification from about 6400×10^{-8} to about 1.3×10^{-8} in a mixture of herbivore and carnivore food animals within natural ecosystems (a mean of the natural herbivore and carnivore values shown in Figure 4). Lead concentrations in bone are about one hundred-fold higher than those in muscle, a ratio that is rather constant for a large range of skeletal lead concentrations among different species of relatively long-lived animals [40]. By assigning 17% calcium to wet bone, the average lead concentration in a mixture of terrestrial herbivore and carnivore flesh during prehistoric times is estimated to have been about 0.1 ng Pb/g wet weight (0.0001 ppm Pb). Concentrations of lead in marine animal flesh during prehistoric times can be estimated more directly from reliable observations which show that lead is 0.3 ng Pb/g wet weight in tuna muscle [12] and 6 ng Pb/g wet weight in abalone muscle [39]. These values must be reduced ten-fold to correct for a reasonably firm open ocean pollution factor [41]. The herbivorous shellfish is contaminated by an additional less quantitatively known amount (two to ten-fold) of lead originating from more intense pollution near shore. These corrections for lead contamination indicate that a mixture of marine herbivore and carnivore flesh probably contained about 0.1 ng Pb/g wet weight during prehistoric times. Data are unavailable to permit similar estimates of lead contents in edible portions of plants. The total biopurification of calcium with respect to lead observed for plants in the remote ecosystem was less than that observed for animals, which suggests that lead concentrations in vegetables probably were about fifty-fold higher than in meat. The average concentration of lead in a mixture of these two constituents in the total diet may have been approximately 2 ng Pb/g wet weight during prehistoric times.

This estimate is probably an upper limit and actual natural concentrations of lead in human diets were less than this value. Assuming that the calcium content of human diets has not changed with time, the upper limit for the atomic Pb/Ca ratio in natural diets is about 8×10^{-7}. Direct measurements of very low lead concentrations in old stemwood of trees show that the atomic Pb/Ca ratio in the main mass of the earth's biosphere (~ 1000 ppm Ca [12]) was $\sim 8 \times 10^{-7}$. It is highly unlikely that natural human foods would have had higher Pb/Ca ratios in comparison with the rest of the biosphere. On the contrary, the main mass composed of trees, is near the beginning of food chains where Pb/Ca ratios should be higher than in many substances in human diets that are nearer the ends of food chains. The most forceful confirmation of low lead concentrations in prehistoric human diets comes from the direct measurement of an exceedingly low concentration of lead in fresh tuna muscle of 0.3 ng Pb/g [12]. The natural concentration of lead in this tissue is certainly less than this value because the seas are known to be contaminated about ten-fold with industrial lead.

NATURAL LEAD CONCENTRATIONS IN HUMAN BONES

The natural skeletal atomic Pb/Ca ratio in adult humans is about 6 × 10^{-8}. The measurement of lead concentrations in bones of ancient humans is a pragmatic attempt to obtain a direct answer in the matter of natural lead levels in humans by circumventing the more difficult acquisition, through scholarly research, of knowledge concerning natural relationships among the occurrences of lead and other metals in humans and components of their environment. It has turned out that the pragmatic approach is actually not a shortcut, and much of the older data that have been obtained regarding this matter must be set aside because of failures of such studies to properly fulfill requirements of the paradigm that were either unknown or misunderstood. Reliable measurements that have been made recently of lead in ancient human bones suggest that the natural concentrations are on the order of 40 ng Pb/g dry bone [30]. This means that lead analyses of such samples are not a trivial matter that can be addressed using conventional analytical techniques which involve serious positive errors due to lack of contamination control, especially since the bone fragments are usually encrusted with and intercalated by soil in which lead concentrations are a hundred-fold higher. Furthermore, as shown in Section 2, humans have been exposed to excessive amounts of industrial lead for many thousands of years so that considerable care must be exercised in choosing only those bone specimens which originate from cultures that did not use lead. This in itself is not a trivial archaeological exercise, for it involves not just the choosing of bones associated with certain cultures, but it also requires a background of knowledge relating to metallurgical developments to guide the proper selection of cultures to be sampled. Finally, the extremely low natural concentrations of lead in bones of ancient humans who were not exposed to industrial lead are easily elevated by additions of soil moisture lead during thousands of years of burial, and this is a very complex matter which must be solved before results can be interpreted.

Some studies of lead in ancient human bones have delineated in an informative manner increases in the lead contamination of humans over the broad span of time by the mining, smelting, and dispersal of leaded products in human environments. People who received virtually no exposure to industrial lead and who lived six hundred years ago in North America are reported to have contained less than 1 ppm Pb in their bones [42]. Lead concentrations of about 1 ppm in teeth and bones of people who lived in the Old World five thousand years ago are elevated, presumably by increased additions of industrial lead to the environment, to concentrations of 3 to 10 ppm Pb in human teeth and bones at the same location about one hundred years later [43]. Lead in human bones increased to high levels during Roman and medieval times [44]. Levels of lead in teeth of contemporary primitive people isolated from some of the major sources of industrial lead are found to be far below existing lead levels in teeth of people in the United States and England [45].

In a recent study of lead in ancient human bones, the three main factors of lead contamination from soil, from cultural uses, and from ground water were carefully dealt with. Ultra-clean IDMS methods for lead were used to deal with the problem of soil and laboratory contamination. Bones were chosen from an eighteen hundred-year-old culture known on the basis of metallurgical development to use lead only in minor ways which did not introduce appreciable amounts into the diet. The problem of lead contamination from ground water during burial was solved by comparing Pb and Ba concentrations in various specimens of tooth enamel with those in various specimens of bone.

Results of these comparisons are shown in Figure 6. Data on contemporary skeletal Ba/Ca ratios indicate that there is little variation with differences in geographic area, and that the values are confined to the extreme left side of the graph. On this basis only those ratios on the extreme left of Figure 6 can be considered natural. Sorption of Ba from soil moisture causes higher values. High Pb/Ca ratios associated with high Ba/Ca ratios are also due to sorption of Pb from soil moisture. This effect is expected from observations in the relative stabilities of Pb, Ba and Ca chelates [39]. Tooth enamel can be expected to sorb less Ba and Pb than bone because apatite crystals in the former are larger, have smaller surface exposures, and are enclosed by smaller quantities of organic membrane. If lead were to be leached from bony material rather than added, the leaching of lead from tooth enamel would be expected to be less than that for bone, and bone should have less lead if this leaching process were operative, but such is not the case. Selection of tooth and bony material on the basis of minimal effects from ground water yields an observed natural skeletal atomic Pb/Ca ratio of 3×10^{-8} and a natural

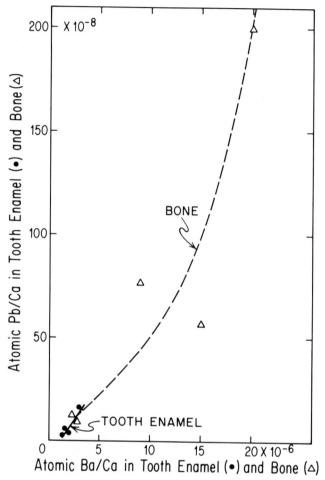

FIGURE 6   Relations between ratios of atomic barium to atomic calcium and of atomic lead to atomic calcium in tooth enamel and bone in ancient Peruvians, demonstrating differential passive sorption of lead from soil moisture.

concentration of lead in dry bone of 0.04 ppm Pb in young adults. These values convert to 6×10^{-8} and 0.08 respectively for 45-year-old ancient humans.

A natural skeletal atomic Pb/Ca ratio of 2×10^{-8} was predicted from studies of the biopurification of Ca with respect to Pb, Ba and Sr in nutrient pathways of Ca in a remote ecosystem, as shown in Figure 4 above. This prediction, which is based on an understanding on an average global

TABLE 3   Global Lead Emissions from Anthropogenic Sources [13]

Source	Production (10^9 kg/yr)	Emission Factor (g Pb/kg emission)	Lead Emission (10^3 kg/yr)
Anthropogenic emissions			
Lead alkyls	0.4	(70%)	280×10^3
Iron smelting	780	0.06	47×10^3
Lead smelting	4	6.0	24×10^3
Zinc and copper smelting	15	2.8	42×10^3
Coal burning	3,300	4.5×10^{-3}	15×10^3
TOTAL			400×10^3

scale of how natural lead in humans originates from their surroundings, conforms with the pragmatic determination of natural lead concentrations in ancient human bones at this particular site, and indicates general applicability of this natural value. The small range in values observed in skeletal Ba/Ca ratios in humans with respect to differences in time and place, discussed previously in the part of this section dealing with natural lead in soil humus and soil moisture, is strong evidence that the ranges in skeletal Pb/Ca ratios in humans were also quite small in prehistoric times because lead and barium have been shown to be covariant within organisms (see Figure 4). It is therefore probable that the few observations of natural lead concentrations that have been made in ancient human skeletons are generally applicable, with very little deviation, to all humans with respect to time and place.

COMPARISON OF NATURAL AND CONTEMPORARY LEAD EXPOSURES IN THE NORTHERN HEMISPHERE

About half of the total of anthropogenic lead emissions listed in Table 3 can be assigned to long-lived aerosols with diameters of <5 μm and residence times in the atmosphere of about ten days. Waters in the oceans, polar ice cap, and precipitation in the Northern Hemisphere are demonstrably polluted with large excesses of industrial lead which originate from the 200,000 tons of long-lived industrial lead aerosols emitted annually to the atmosphere. The quantity of natural lead originating from fluvial sources in the upper 50 meters of the world's oceans in the Northern Hemisphere in prehistoric times is estimated to have been about 4000 tons, while some 80,000 tons of industrial lead originating from atmospheric inputs are estimated to reside in these waters today [10]. The amount of natural lead in the upper 10 meters of the Greenland ice cap is estimated to have been about 10 tons in prehistoric times, while to-day the top 10 meters of ice are observed to contain about 4000 tons of industrial lead derived from atmospheric inputs [4]. It is estimated from natural dust contents that in prehistoric times the annual precipitation of rain and snow which fell on all lands in the world's Northern Hemi-sphere contained about 300 tons of lead, but today this annual precipita-tion is believed to contain about 40,000 tons of lead [25]. Contamination of trees by the emission of about 200,000 tons per year of long-lived in-dustrial lead aerosols to the Northern Hemisphere is confined mostly to bark surfaces. This is a large flux compared to the annual turnover of about 300 tons of natural lead per year in the growth cycle which took place in prehistoric times. Years of accumulation of industrial contami-nation lead, on bark and on leaf surfaces, has elevated the present average total lead content of trees about ten-fold above natural lead levels in the biomass of North America [25]. In the Southern Hemisphere today lead pollution effects in remote nondomesticated regions are estimated to be about one tenth those in the Northern Hemisphere. By far the largest proportion of industrial lead aerosols is emitted to the Northern tropo-sphere, and since the residence time of lead aerosols in the atmosphere (~ 10 days) is short compared to the half life of interhemispheric ex-change ($\sim 1–2$ years), the average concentration of lead in the atmosphere of the Northern Hemisphere is probably much larger than in the South-ern Hemisphere. This does not mean that contamination effects are nonexistent in remote regions of the Southern Hemisphere because indus-trial lead concentrations are two orders of magnitude above natural levels in aerosols in the Northern Hemisphere and it is expected that industrial lead concentrations are an order of magnitude above natural levels in the Southern Hemisphere. Average folial lead concentrations may therefore be expected to be two-fold above natural levels in remote locations.

Comparison of natural prehistoric lead concentrations in various sub-stances in North America with contemporary lead concentrations, given in Table 4, show that maximum permissible levels of lead that have been set by regulatory agencies are greatly influenced by contemporary lead concentration levels and are enormously excessive in comparison with natural levels of lead. Such excessive permissible over-exposures to lead above natural levels would seem, on a cellular biochemical basis, to invite biochemical perturbations that could prove deleterious.

A comparison of total daily lead absorptions listed in Table 5 shows that 210 ng Pb/day were absorbed into systemic blood of prehistoric hu-mans and 29,000 ng Pb/day into blood of typical American adults. It is assumed that the fraction of ingested lead absorbed by humans in prehis-toric times is similar to that for humans today despite a large difference in lead concentration in the two diets. Tracer studies indicate that substantial amounts of lead are cycled through the human portal blood–liver–bile system [46], but the fraction of lead in food that enters the systemic blood does not include this lead, so that the overall human biopurification factor for calcium with respect to lead in going from their diets to their skeletons is approximately 0.5 Ca absorption/0.07 Pb absorption, or seven-fold. An internal consistency can be demonstrated in relationships among Pb/Ca ratios in diets, biopurification factors, and skeletal Pb/Ca ratios. The estimated atomic Pb/Ca ratio of $\sim 8 \times 10^{-7}$ in natural diets was probably reduced seven-fold through biopurification to a predicted value of about 10×10^{-8} in human skeletons, which agrees well with the skeletal value of 6×10^{-8} found in ancient adult Peruvians. The observed Pb/Ca ratio in present-day American diets of 8×10^{-5}, when reduced through biopurification, yields a predicted skeletal Pb/Ca ratio of 10×10^{-6}, which compares favorably with the observed skeletal ratio of 35×10^{-6} in adult Americans (contributions from inhaled and other nondietary sources of industrial lead are included in the latter value). This internal consistency constitutes strong evidence that the fraction of ingested lead absorbed by humans from their prehistoric diets did not differ appreciably from the situation today.

On the basis of these absorptions it would appear, as shown in Table 5, that prehistoric people absorbed into their systemic blood less than 1/100th of the lead absorbed into the blood of contemporary Americans. The ten thousand-fold contamination by industrial lead of canned tuna, shown in Figure 5, documents the existence of the extremely large lead contamination effects in the American diet that are required to account for the difference in lead absorptions shown in Table 5. It is very difficult to establish such documentation, for it cannot be done in the usual manner practiced by surveillance laboratories until now, but requires comprehensive studies within different fields of basic research. Knowledge of biopurification factors indicates that more documentation of this extensive lead contamination of foods should be forthcoming from other careful tracings of natural ecological lineages of lead and calcium in other contemporary dietary items from their original natural sources to the prepared state in foods.

BIOCHEMICAL PERTURBATIONS CAUSED BY EXCESSIVE LEAD EXPOSURES

Interests of regulatory agencies regarding lead pollution, their support of research aims in this field, and the analytical capabilities of their surveillance laboratories for lead are directed exclusively to deleterious effects in a small fraction of the population caused by lead intakes which exceed the norm for the main population. During the past fifteen years a consid-

TABLE 4 Comparison of Lead Concentrations in North America

Source	Natural Prehistoric [this report]	Contemporary Remote [this report]	Contemporary Urban [47]	Maximum Permissible Levels [47]
Air (ng Pb/m^3)	~0.04	8 to 10	1,000 to 20,000	1,500
Fresh water (ng Pb/g)	<0.02	0.005 to 0.05	<1 to >50	50
Trees (ng Pb/g)	~4	~40	~200	none
Human food (ng Pb/g)	<2	~200	~200	300
Human skeletons (atomic Pb/Ca)	~6 × 10^{-8}	~3,500 × 10^{-8}	~3,500 × 10^{-8}	none

TABLE 5   Inventory of Estimated Average Daily Pb Absorbed into Blood in Adult Humans (ng Pb/day) (see text for sources)

Source	Prehistoric Natural	Contemporary Urban American
Air	0.3	6,400
Water	<2.0	1,500
Food	<210.0	21,000
TOTAL	<210.0	29,000

Natural

$$\text{Air} = 0.04 \text{ ng Pb/m}^3 \times 20.0 \text{ m}^3/\text{day} \times 0.4 = 0.3 \text{ ng Pb/day}$$
$$\text{Water} = <20.0 \text{ ng Pb/kg} \times 1.0 \text{ kg/day} \times 0.1 = <2.0 \text{ ng Pb/day}$$
$$\text{Food} = <2.0 \text{ ng Pb/g} \times 1.5 \text{ kg/day} \times 0.07 = <210.0 \text{ ng Pb/day}$$
$$\text{TOTAL} = <210.0 \text{ ng Pb/day}$$

Contemporary

$$\text{Air} = 800 \text{ ng Pb/m}^3 \times 20.0 \text{ m}^3/\text{day} \times 0.4 = 6,400 \text{ ng Pb/day}$$
$$\text{Water} = 15,000 \text{ ng Pb/kg} \times 1.0 \text{ kg/day} \times 0.1 = 1,500 \text{ ng Pb/day}$$
$$\text{Food} = 200 \text{ ng Pb/g} \times 1.5 \text{ kg/day} \times 0.07 = 21,000 \text{ ng Pb/day}$$
$$\text{TOTAL} = 29,000 \text{ ng Pb/day}$$

erable portion of this interest was shifted to possible subtle, subclinical, and asymptomatic deleterious effects caused by so-called "low levels" of lead exposures which are restricted to those ranging above the norm of the main population to those which cause easily recognized clinical symptoms of harm. This "low level" range of exposures appeared to be an important region of concern to investigators who questioned the existence of a threshold for harmful lead exposures after the basis for this concept had been undermined in 1965. The term "low level" originates from the widespread medical attitude that present "normal" lead intakes are satisfactory, because it is not generally understood that these intakes, which are typical instead of normal, are displaced from natural intakes by an enormous factor which is very much larger than the small factor which separates typical intakes from those presently recognized as poisonous.

Sometime ago it was suggested that since biochemical systems within cells could not be absolutely pure, noise levels must exist for various trace constituents within cells which biochemical processes had evolved to ignore [48]. Although the noise level suggested at that time for lead in biochemical systems was excessively high, and true natural noise levels of lead in biochemical systems of higher organisms such as mammals are extremely low, the question still remains: "To what degree must levels of lead be elevated in various biochemical systems within cells to perturb them?" Contemporary levels of lead in biochemical systems within cells of average Americans are so excessive compared to natural levels that it is highly probable that perturbations are being caused in them. Since divalent lead masquerades as calcium, biochemical reactions involving calcium are most likely to be perturbed. These effects can only be ascertained through experimental studies at cellular levels. It is virtually certain that no one has yet studied natural interactions of lead in living cells or determined how present excessive lead exposure have actually perturbed natural processes in the so-called normal control cells that have been used. Since all reagents, nutrients, and controls used so far in biochemical laboratories have been excessively contaminated with industrial lead [12], such studies will require innovative approaches to grow living organisms at natural lead levels. Nutrient media must be highly purified of lead, and growth must be carried out in a manner that will certainly challenge the abilities of the very best of investigators.

In this matter the problem arises of distinguishing between biochemical adaptations that may be relatively harmless on the one hand and biochemical dysfunctions which probably cause harm on the other. In the past, industrial toxicologists have tended to favor the former type of biochemical perturbation to justify the point of view that the existence of various clinical effects resulting from increased lead exposures below their so-called thresholds (now refuted) does not warrant undue concern. Continued growth of new knowledge has gradually supplanted the older forms of these views with recognition that undesirable dysfunctions are probably related to some of the observed clinical effects that had previously been regarded more or less as adaptive. This progressive shift from the adaptation to the dysfunction point of view for clinical effects has occurred gradually over a period of more than a decade. It has concerned only the range of lead exposures above the norm but below those causing obvious poisonings.

It is likely that this same scenario will be followed with respect to new discoveries of biochemical perturbations within cells caused by typical lead exposures. The perturbations of the haemopoietic system by lead are an example of the direction and slowness in shift of viewpoint. At present majority medical opinion leans to the biochemical adaptation point of view in this matter. Another example is the occurrence of lead in bones. Since most of the lead contained in mammals is located in their skeletons, majority medical opinion leans to adaptation and holds that the major fraction of the body lead in mammals is of no biochemical consequence. It is not generally recognized that most of the nutrient calcium and trace toxic barium in the blood is contained in plasma and not in red blood cells, and that it is expected that this should hold also for lead because of the strong covariance observed to hold between lead and barium in their distribution within organisms in the biosphere. This is not the case for the observed distribution of lead in the blood of highly contaminated mammals which are the only types that have been examined so far. It would be highly anomalous if this observed distribution in mammalian blood were to be natural. It appears that haemopoietic systems existing within mammals exposed to typical inputs of industrial lead and regarded as "normal" have been so badly perturbed by typical lead exposures that most of what is probably an overwhelming excess of lead in the blood has been transferred to red blood cells as a result of overloading and breakdown of natural biochemical processes. Such perturbations originate not just from inputs of lead to the systemic blood from the liver and lungs but also from the bone reservoir. The latter reenters the soft tissue system from the skeleton in accompaniment with inputs of skeletal calcium. There are indications that lead concentrations in blood of mammals were extremely low under natural conditions in prehistoric times, and could follow the Ba and Ca distribution pattern between plasma and cells within it. These indications come from observations that the ratio of the concentration of lead in muscle to that in bone of a given animal (about 0.01) remains relatively fixed in the face of a greater than a hundred-fold change in the absolute concentration of skeletal lead, and lead concentrations in tuna muscle of 0.3 ng/g have been observed.

In still another case, the formation of lead-rich intranuclear inclusion bodies within cells upon exposure to great excesses of lead above typical levels [49] is regarded as a protective adaptive mechanism [50], when these bodies are, instead, the probable protein debris of catastrophic biochemical dysfunctions.

It is probable that decades of basic research concerning the interaction of lead with biochemical systems will be required before medical opinion shifts from an adaptive to a dysfunction point of view with respect to just these few instances of biochemical perturbations caused by lead exposures above the norm. Future discoveries of new biochemical perturbations caused by normative lead exposures seem destined to be accorded a similar fate on a much more extended time scale.

REFERENCES

1. Chester, R., S.R. Aston, J.H. Stoner and D. Bruty (1974) Trace metals in soil-sized particles from the lower troposphere over the world ocean, *Journal de Recherches Atmospherique*, Vol. 8, 777–789. Duce, R.A., G.L. Hoffman and W.H. Zoller (1975) Atmo-

spheric trace metals at remote northern and southern hemisphere sites: pollution or natural? *Science 187*, 59–61.

2. Herron, M., C. Langway, N. Weiss and J. Cragin (1977) Atmospheric trace metals and sulfate in the Greenland ice sheet. *Geochimica et Cosmochimica Acta 41*, 915–920. Boutron, C. (1979) Past and present day tropospheric fallout fluxes of Pb, Cd, Cu, Zn and Ag in Antarctica and Greenland. *Geophysical Research Letters 6*, 159-162.

3. Duce, R.A., G.L. Hoffman, B.J. Ray, I.S. Fletcher, G.T. Wallace, J.L. Fasching, S.R. Piotrowicz, P.R. Walsh, E.J. Hoffman, J.M. Miller and J.L. Hefter (1976) Trace metals in the marine environment. Pages 40–77 *Marine Pollutant Transfer* edited by H.L. Windom and R.A. Duce. Lexington, Mass.: Heath. Chow, T.J., J.L. Earl and C.B. Snyder (1972) Lead concentrations in air, White Mountain, California. *Science 178*, 401–402. Murozumi, M., T.J. Chow and C.C. Patterson (1969) Chemical concentrations of pollutant lead aerosols, terrestrial dusts, and sea salt in Greenland and Antarctic snow strata. *Geochimica et Cosmochimica Acta 33*, 1247–1294. Hirao, Y. and C.C. Patterson (1974) Lead aerosol pollution in the High Sierra overrides natural mechanisms which exclude lead from a food chain, *Science 184*, 989–992. Elias, R., Y. Hirao, C. Davidson and C.C. Patterson (1979) The input, output, and distribution among biomass reservoirs of lead and six other metals in Thompson Canyon. *Manuscript in preparation*.

4. Murozumi, M., T.J. Chow and C.C. Patterson (1969) in Reference [3].

5. Herron, M., C. Langway, N. Weiss and J. Cragin (1977) in Reference [2].

6. Boutron, C. (1979) in Reference [2].

7. Boutron, C. (1978) Influence des aerosols naturels et anthropogeniques sur la geochimie des neiges polaires. Ph.D. Thesis. Publication #254 du Laboratoire de Glaciologie du Centre National de la Recherche Scientifique.

8. Shirahata, H., R. Elias and C.C. Patterson (1979) Chronological variations in concentrations and isotopic compositions of anthropogenic atmospheric lead in sediments of a remote subalpine pond. Accepted for publication in *Geochimica et Cosmochimica Acta*.

9. Chow, T.J. and C.C. Patterson (1962) The occurrence and significance of lead isotopes in pelagic sediments. *Geochimica et Cosmochimica Acta 26*, 263–308.

10. Schaule, B. and C.C. Patterson (1979, in press) The occurrence of lead in the Northeast Pacific and effects of anthropogenic inputs. *Proceedings of an International Experts Discussion on Lead: Occurrence, Fate, and Pollution in the Marine Environment*, edited by M. Branica. Oxford: Pergamon Press. Schaule, B. and C.C. Patterson, Lead concentrations in the Northeast Pacific Ocean: evidence for global anthropogenic perturbations (unpublished manuscript).

11. National Academy of Sciences–National Research Council (1972) *Airborne Lead in Perspective*. Washington, D.C.: National Academy of Sciences.

12. Settle, D.M. and C.C. Patterson (1979) Lead in albacore: guide to lead pollution in Americans. Accepted for publication in *Science*.

13. Nriagu, J.O. (1978) Lead in the atmosphere. Pages 137–184, *The Biogeochemistry of Lead in the Environment, Part A*, edited by J. Nriagu. New York: Elsevier.

14. Piotrowicz, S.R., R.A. Duce, J.L. Fasching, and C.P. Weisel (1979) Abstract, *EOS 60*, 276. Schaule, B. and C.C. Patterson (1979, in press) in Reference [10]. Schaule, B. and C.C. Patterson (unpublished manuscript) in Reference [10].

15. Curtin, G.C., H.D. King and E.L. Mosier (1974) Lead concentrations reported in foliage forest emissions. *Journal Chemical Exp. 3*, 245.

16. Beauford, W., J. Barker, and A.R. Barringer (1977) Lead emissions from foliage measured with ^{210}Pb traces. *Science 195*, 571.

17. Buat-Menard, P. and M. Arnold (1978) Pb/S ratios in fumarolic gases from Mount Etna. *Geophysical Research Letters 5*, 245.

18. Unni, C.K., W. Fitzgerald, D. Settle, G. Gill, B. Ray, R.A. Duce, and C.C. Patterson (1978) Abstract. Section of Volcanology, Geochemistry and Petrology, AGU Annual Meeting, San Francisco.

19. Tatsumoto, M. and C.C. Patterson (1963) The concentration of common lead in seawater. Pages 74–89, *Earth Science and Meteoritics* edited by Geiss and Goldberg. Amsterdam: North Holland. Tatsumoto, M. and C.C. Patterson (1963) Concentrations of common lead in some Atlantic and Mediterranean waters and in snow. *Nature 199*, 350–352. Chow, T.J., and C.C. Patterson (1966) Concentration profiles of barium and lead in Atlantic waters off Bermuda. *Earth and Planetary Science Letters 1*, 397–400.

20. Nozaki, Y., J. Thompson and K.K. Turekian (1976) The distribution of ^{210}Pb and [210]Po in the surface waters of the Pacific Ocean, *Earth and Planetary Science Letters 32*, 304–312.

21. Chow, T.J. (1978) Lead in natural waters. Pages 185–218, *The Biogeochemistry of Lead in the Environment, Part A*, edited by J.O. Nriagu. New York: Elsevier. U.S. Environmental Protection Agency (1976) *Quality Criteria for Water, Lead*, p. 82.

22. Kolbasuk, G. and C.C. Patterson, Total lead concentrations in samples from 3 rivers, unpublished work. Hirao, Y. and C.C. Patterson (1974) in Reference [3].

23. Lewis, D.M. (1977) The use of ^{210}Pb as a heavy metal tracer in the Susquehanna River. *Geochimica et Cosmochimica Acta 41*, 1557–1564. Nozaki, Y., D.J. DeMaster, D.M. Lewis and K.K. Turekian (1978) Atmospheric ^{210}Pb fluxes determined from soil profiles, *Journal of Geophysical Research 83*, 4047–4051.

24. Hirao, Y., and C.C. Patterson (1974) in Reference [3].

25. Elias, R., Y. Hirao, C. Davidson, and C.C. Patterson (1979) in Reference [3].

26. Zimdahl, R.L. and J.J. Hassett (1977) Lead in soil. *Lead in the Environment* edited by W. Boggess. NSF-RA-770214. Washington, D.C.: U.S. Government Printing Office.

27. Hinkley, T. (1979) Concentrations of metals in very small volumes of soil solution. *Nature 277*, 444–446. Hirao, Y., and C.C. Patterson (1974) in Reference [3]. Hirao, Y., R.W. Elias, L. Hewbern, and C.C. Patterson. Anthropogenic lead aerosols circumvent the biopurification of calcium in natural subalpine nutrient pathways. Manuscript in preparation.

28. Hirao, Y., and C.C. Patterson (1974) in Reference [3]. Hirao, Y., R.W. Elias, L. Newbern, and C.C. Patterson (manuscript in preparation) in Reference [27].

29. Patterson, Clair C. (1971) Native copper, silver, and gold accessible to early metallurgists. *American Antiquity 36*, 286–321.

30. Ericson, J.E., H. Shirahata, and C.C. Patterson (1979) Skeletal concentrations of lead in ancient Peruvians. *New England Journal of Medicine 300*, 946–951.

31. Published work and summary of new work given in Reference [8].

32. Lindbergh, S.E. (1979) Mechanisms and rates of atmospheric deposition of selected trace elements and sulfate to a deciduous forest watershed. Ph.D. Dissertation, Florida State University. Publication No. 129, Environmental Sciences Division. Oak Ridge: ORNC. Reiners, W.A., R.H. Marks and P.M. Vitonsek (1975) Heavy metals in subalpine and alpine soils of New Hampshire, *OIKOS 26*, 264–275. Cawse, P.A. (1974) A survey of atmospheric trace elements in the U.K. (1972–73). AERE Report No. R-7669, H.M.S.O., London, 84 pages. Getz, L.L., A.W. Hancy, R.W. Larimore, J.W. McNurney, H.V. Leland, P.W. Price, G.L. Rolfe, R.L. Wortman, J.L. Hudson, R.L. Solomon, and K.A. Reinbold (1977) Transport and distribution in a watershed ecosystem. Pages 105–134, *Lead in the Environment*, edited by W. Boggess. NSF-RA-770214. Washington, D.C.: U.S. Government Printing Office. Siccama, T.G. and W.H. Smith (1978) Lead accumulation in a northern hardwood forest. *Environmental Science and Technology 12*, 593–594.

33. Jenkins, D.A., and R.I. Davies (1966) *Nature 210*, 1296.
34. Bowen, H.J.M. (1965) Page 48, *Trace Elements in Biochemistry*, London: Academic Press. Rodin, L.E., N.I. Bazilevich, and N.N. Rozov (1975). Page 13, *Productivity of World Ecosystems*, Proceedings, Edited by D. Reichle, J. Franklin and D. Goodall. Washington, D.C.: National Academy of Sciences.
35. Nriagu, J.O. (1978) Properties and the biogeochemical cycle of lead. Pages 1–14, *The Biogeochemistry of Lead in the Environment*, edited by J.O. Nriagu. New York: Elsevier.
36. Published work and summary of new work given in Reference [12].
37. Elias, R.W. and C.C. Patterson (1979) The biopurification of calcium in natural ecosystems. Manuscript in preparation.
38. Elias, R., Y. Hirao, C. Davidson and C.C. Patterson (1979) in Reference [3]. Hinkley, T.K. (1975) Weathering mechanisms and mass balance in a High Sierra Nevada watershed—distribution of alkali and alkaline earth metals in components of parent rocks and soil, snow, soil moisture, and stream outflow. Ph.D. Thesis, Division of Geological and Planetary Sciences, California Institute of Technology, Pasadena, California.
39. Burnett, M., A. Ng, D. Settle and C.C. Patterson (1979, in press) Impact of man on coastal marine ecosystems. In *Proceedings of an International Experts Discussion on Lead: Occurrence, Fate, and Pollution in the Marine Environment*, edited by M. Branica. Oxford: Pergamon Press. Burnett, M. (1979) Occurrences and Distribution of Ca, Sr, Ba, and Pb in Marine Food Chains. Ph.D. Thesis, Division of Geological and Planetary Sciences, California Institute of Technology, Pasadena, California.
40. Burnett, M., A. Ng, D. Settle and C.C. Patterson (1979, in press) in Reference [39]. Burnett, M. (1979) in Reference [39]. Hirao, Y., R.W. Elias, L. Newbern, and C.C. Patterson (manuscript in preparation) in Reference [27].
41. Patterson, C.C., D. Settle and B. Glover (1976) Analysis of lead in polluted coastal seawater. *Marine Chemistry 4*, 305–319.
42. Becker, R.O., J.A. Spadaro and E.W. Berg (1968) The trace elements of human bone. *Journal of Bone Joint Surgery 50* (AM), 326–334.
43. Grandjean, P., O.V. Nielson, and I.M. Shapiro (1979) Lead retention in ancient Nubian and contemporary populations. *Journal of Environmental Pathology and Toxicology 2*, 781–787.
44. Gilfillan, S.C. *Rome's Ruin by Lead Poison*. Book to be published. Gilfillan, S.C. (1965) Lead poisoning and the fall of Rome. *Journal of Occupational Medicine 7*, 53–60. Mackie, A., A. Townsend and H.A. Waldren (1975) Lead concentrations in bones from Roman York. *Journal of the Archaeological Society 2*, 235–237. Jawarowski, Z. (1968) Stable lead in fossil ice and bones. *Nature 217*, 152–153.
45. Shapiro, I.M., G. Mitchell, I. Davidson, and S.H. Katz (1975) The lead content of teeth: evidence establishing new minimal levels of exposure in a living preindustrialized human population. *Archives of Environmental Health 30*, 483–486.
46. Chamberlin, A.C., M.J. Heard, P. Little, D. Newton, A.C. Wells, and R.D. Wiffen (1978) *Investigation into Lead from Motor Vehicles*. AERE-R9198. Harwell, U.K. Atomic Energy Authority.
47. *Air Quality Criteria for Lead* (1977) EPA-600/8-77-017, Washington, D.C.: U.S. Environmental Protection Agency.
48. Hutchinson, G.E. (1964) The influence of the environment. *Proceedings of the National Academy of Sciences U.S.A. 51*, 930–934.

49. Goyer, R.A., P. May, M.M. Cater and M.R. Krigman (1970) Lead and protein content of isolated intranuclear inclusion bodies from kidneys of lead-poisoned rats. *Laboratory Investigations 22*, 245–251.

50. Goyer, R.A. (1971) Lead toxicity: A problem in environmental pathology. *American Journal of Pathology 64*, 167–182.

Recommendations

It is intrinsically wrong to mine and smelt a highly toxic substance such as lead on a scale of millions of tons per year and then disperse it within human environments. The majority of this Committee on Lead in the Human Environment fails to explicitly acknowledge this obvious truth. The analysis presented here indicates why the majority of the Committee responded to the challenge of the lead pollution situation as they did in their report. They propose tedious investigations to see whether various poisoning problems caused by lead technology exist, and then to use applied engineering solutions which supposedly, on the basis of cost/benefit analysis, would involve control of the dispersal of lead products. This type of approach has always failed in the past and has generally led to a worsening of the situation.

The question is, what is to be done? Increasing concern and pressure from the public will almost certainly curtail and probably halt the mining and smelting of lead sometime in the future. This can and undoubtedly will be done because there are nontoxic substitutes for most uses of lead today. The economic costs of producing these nonleaded alternatives are in many cases demonstrably less than are the costs of producing leaded materials. Lead alkyls, for example, cost more in terms of manufacturing and engine deterioration alone than does the cost of refining nonleaded gasolines with equivalent anti-knock characteristics. This excludes the enormous costs that result from poisoning effects associated with the use of leaded gasolines. Setting aside the incalculable costs of darkening the lives of entire populations by lead poisoning, the costs of mining and smelting lead are enormously outweighed by the later costs of cleaning up the dispersed lead residues in a manner that renders them nonhazardous.

Important steps have already been taken to reduce lead intakes within the general population. Lead alkyl production has been reduced significantly during the past four years. Leaded closures in food and drink cans have been replaced on a significant scale by the use of aluminum cans, die-punched steel cans, and plastic seals in crimped steel seams. Plastic or aluminum foil covers are being substituted for lead foil covers over cork on wine bottles. Nonleaded paints and putties are available in increasing quantities. Nonleaded glazes are being used on dinnerware.

On the other hand, pressure by the lead industry continues to erode these accomplishments. The American Petroleum Institute, in responding to the energy crisis has declared a need to "dispense with the limitations on the use of lead and aromatic additions in gasoline production." In April 1979 President Carter, under pressure from the petroleum related industries "directed the Enviromental Protection Agency to defer for one year the further phase-down of (lead anti-knock compounds)." The Food and Drug Administration is under pressure from the canning industry to rule that the use of lead soldered cans should receive "prior sanctioning," since approval for this process may have been given before 1958. It is clear from these reports that lead industries will continue to resist efforts by the government to reduce environmental lead pollution, even after governmental decisions have been made and regulatory policies have been established. *Therefore it is recommended that regulatory actions be promoted by means of stronger restrictions and controls with the aim of total phasing out, in as short a time as feasible, the manufacture and use of leaded products in the categories listed above.* Home and municipal water systems in some localized zones probably contribute a much larger portion to the total lead in the diet than is indicated by the average figures for dietary intakes given in Section 4. Intakes of lead from these sources are difficult to estimate because studies have shown that lead concentrations in potable waters are related, not just to the types of leaded pipes used to carry the water, but also to the length of time the waters are exposed to the pipes before the water is drained out of them. Other studies indicate that commercial drying and milling of food substances may introduce excessive amounts of lead into some processed foods. *A new uniform code regulating the construction of new potable water distribution systems in cities and homes so as to require that they be lead-free is needed to halt the proliferation of this source of lead in people. The extent of lead contamination introduced during various drying and milling processes of foods should be investigated immediately, and such studies should have high priority.*

It is not necessary to engage in lengthy studies before acting on behalf of inner-city babies. The HUD study showing positive correlations between lead in infant blood and rates of use of leaded gasolines indicates that reduction of the use of leaded gasolines within cities would probably significantly reduce lead exposures to infants within cities. Other sources of lead exposures to infants within cities are more intractable to prophylaxis. Nevertheless, the creation of small lead-free zones within cities where infants and small children spend a great deal of their time should help reduce lead exposures to them. Temporary lead-free coatings of playgrounds, nurseries, and schools, together with educational programs that would enable parents to reduce lead exposures to children in their homes through improved environmental hygiene, should reduce lead intakes in many infants and children within cities. The costs of such programs are not large compared to the much larger value of the lives that probably would be saved from destruction by neurological damage. *The burning of lead alkyls within cities should be halted within the shortest possible time. Priority should be given to provide lead-free coatings for inner-city playgrounds, nurseries, and schools and to provide educational programs that will enable parents to reduce lead exposures to their children in their homes by means of environmental hygiene.*

The probable existence of unrecognized forms of lead poisoning among most Americans indicates that *investigations into biochemical perturbations within cells caused by lead exposures ranging down from typical to 1/1000th of typical, as well as investigations which trace the biogeochemical lineages of lead from natural sources to processed components in human diets, should be supported.* The nature of this work renders it unsuitable for mission oriented agencies to carry out. The reason for this is that the manner in which lead is analyzed must be enormously improved before such investigations can be properly undertaken, and it is doubtful that such improvements will take place in mission oriented laboratories. It is probable that this change will be slow and difficult and it is unlikely that it can be accelerated by such prosaic remedies as widely distributing suitable standards for lead that would challenge most analysts and cause them to improve their analytical techniques for lead. Investigators in the pure sciences who produce accurate and reliable new scientific knowledge have no other recourse but to solve their technical problems with certainty before acquiring the new knowledge they seek. They sharpen their techniques against what is known until they are convinced they can modify and extend what is known. By the time investigators in such laboratories are capable of correctly handling standards, they usually don't need them. This manner of resolving technical problems during the process of acquiring basic knowledge usually evolves through attempts among different investigators in the pure sciences to modify, disprove, or extend each other's findings in an atmosphere of mutual interaction in a common field of study. Mission oriented agencies seldom allow, and in fact generally prohibit, such freedom because they exert strong pressures on investigators to generate data in accordance with narrowly defined goals. They seldom allow individuals the freedom to pursue challenges presented by the scientific aspects of problems.

The basic research activities mentioned above are important and require support but they should be considered to be entirely academic pursuits. They should not serve either as alternatives to actions that would alleviate lead poisoning among Americans, or primarily as attempts to obtain information which might accelerate the phasing out of the mining and smelting of lead. These research activities should instead be supported with the aim that they should provide knowledge which would serve as a longstanding source from which additional knowledge of the biogeochemistry of metals could grow in the future.

Funding for this kind of research may properly be taken from the budgets of mission oriented government agencies already involved in studies of lead pollution by means of interagency transfers of funds to the National Science Foundation. The past use of outmoded applied chemical techniques to acquire large amounts of erroneous lead data has been so wasteful it would be wise to divert a small portion of these funds to useful purposes. It is suggested that this transfer be formalized by requiring that applicable government agencies assign through interagency transfer, a mandated fraction of their annual mission oriented investigations budget to the National Science Foundation. These agencies would have no control over the disbursement of these transferred funds. They could only recommend categorically general areas of interest to the National Science Foundation. The NSF would be in complete control of proposal evaluations, peer reviews, and disbursal of funds. These additional increments of monies administered by the National Science Foundation would not be designated as belonging to the NSF budget, but would appear as items in the budgets of the other agencies concerned.

The ability of the National Science Foundation to fund basic scientific studies which extend knowledge in unexplored areas and directions is being seriously eroded by legislative actions that require funding of mission oriented investigations to enlarge knowledge in defined areas along conventional lines using applied science and engineering. This is occurring in two ways. First, legislative mandates are made directly to the National Science Foundation to fund investigations related to social problems believed to have high priority. Second, mission oriented agencies, such as the Department of Energy and the Environmental Protection Agency, have, through reorganizations associated with redefinitions of goals and missions in recent years, taken over the disbursement of some funds which used to flow to universities to support nonmission oriented, basic scientific research and have diverted these funds to mission oriented applied science and engineering studies. This second process has shunted substantial numbers of scientists in nonmission oriented, basic research to the funding responsibility of the National Science Foundation, which has placed such excessive demands on the National Science Foundation that it has seriously diminished its ability to fund young, unestablished scientists and to upgrade the physical qualities of instrumentation.

The need for support of nonmission oriented basic research related to social problems has been demonstrated in the case where knowledge about lead pollution has been made available through ultra-clean IDMS research. In that instance the investigative techniques were far too expensive and the research aims were much too foreign compared to accepted views for that research to have received support from industry or mission oriented government agencies. Without the National Science Foundation, this work would never have been carried out. This is not a singular situation, and it is urgent that the scope of NSF funding for these kinds of studies be enlarged in the fields of anthropology, ethnology, and archaeology.

It cannot be emphasized strongly enough that the history of the development of lead technology with its attendant social problems indicates that if the total cessation of mining and smelting of lead were to be brought about by applied engineering approaches devoid of humanitarian considerations, it could have disastrous consequences. Needed for such actions are new approaches that are guided by conscious humanitarian interests which draw upon the broad base of human experience in many fields and which consider the long-term future interests of humans, rather than of existing industrial enterprises.

The story of our difficulties with lead has kinship with many other present and potential social problems ranging from those in their infancy, such as atomic energy and the pollution of our environment with petrochemicals incompatible with natural biochemical processes, to older ones, such as war and overpopulation. *Strong support is recommended for substantial enlargement of research and scholarly studies in the fields of anthropology, ethnology, and archaeology, including support to greatly increase faculty and facilities within universities in these fields.* Research into the origins of *H.s.sapiens* and into factors which determined developments in both engineering technology and esthetic culture will probably provide insight which may suggest how humanitarian principles might be used to guide future developments of engineering technology, something which has never occurred before in human history. A holistic appraisal of the story of lead suggests that these fields of study are truly of paramount importance to the future well-being of *H.s.sapiens*. The presence or absence of certain vital kinds of knowledge from these fields may very well turn out to be the factor which tips the scales for or against the survival of our hominid species in the face of challenges presented by impending developments in genetic engineering.

Appendixes to the
Main Report

A Guide to Major Recent Reviews and Assessments of the Literature on Lead in the Environment

INTRODUCTION

The purpose of this appendix is to provide the reader with a guide to the "first layer" of recent literature on lead, i.e., major survey and assessment documents. The documents abstracted here were selected from the literature that the Committee has become familiar with over the course of this study; no systematic search of the literature was conducted. However, a substantial effort was made to assemble all of the current review and assessment documents available.

The documents selected can direct the reader to the primary literature and to detailed information on issues that this report does not treat extensively. In fact, the Committee chose to present this guide instead of repeating detailed information and assessments that are available elsewhere in the literature. Gaps in the data or in the assessment of issues are identified and discussed elsewhere in this report (see Chapter 2).

A large number of documents reviewing and assessing scientific knowledge of lead in the environment has become available in recent years. Most of these documents focus on human exposures and effects. Some have been highly comprehensive, covering the distribution and effects of lead in ecosystems as well; others have been concerned mainly with the effects of lead on people; and still others focus on health effects from a single source of exposure. Reviews of lead biogeochemistry and techniques or strategies for controlling lead emissions are fewer in number. Most of the reports abstracted here were prepared or sponsored by regulatory agencies, to support standard-setting activities.

Of the 16 documents included in this appendix, all but one appeared since 1976. Eight provide thorough assessments of major exposure routes and effects on humans (Drill et al. 1979; Ewing et al. 1979; Jaworski 1979; NRC 1972; Nriagu 1978; U.S. EPA 1977a, 1978; WHO 1977); five deal with effects from a single source of exposure (Bridbord 1977, motor vehicle emissions; NIOSH 1978, workplace environments; NRC 1976, paint; NRC 1977, drinking water; U.S. DOL 1978, workplace environments); three deal thoroughly with biogeochemistry (Lovering 1976, Nriagu 1978, U.S. EPA 1977a), and several others review the topic more briefly; and several reports deal with limited aspects of control for specific sources or pathways (Bridbord 1977; Drill et al. 1979; Ewing et al. 1979; Jaworski 1979; NIOSH 1978; NRC 1976, 1977; U.S. DOL 1978), but only one does an extensive assessment of control techniques and attendant costs (U.S. EPA 1977b, air emissions).

The purpose of the following material is not to summarize the conclusions of or to evaluate the various reports, but rather to indicate the topics and issues that each document covers. Each abstract provides information on the depth of treatment of given topics, the extent and currency of the literature surveyed, the primary purpose and focus of the report, and any special or unique characteristics of the document. No evaluation of the scientific quality of these documents has been attempted in the abstracts; if any documents are especially strong or weak on some points, this may be reflected in evaluative comments in the body of this report.

Finally, this Committee does not endorse the interpretations made and conclusions drawn in the various documents; those are the responsibility of the reports' authors. In fact, readers are encouraged to go to original (primary) literature to check the accuracy of the citations and interpretations in the review documents.

ABSTRACTS
(in alphabetical order)

1. Bridbord, K. (1977) *Human Exposure to Lead from Motor Vehicle Emissions.* Office of Extramural Coordination and Special Projects, National Institute for Occupational Safety and Health. DHEW (NIOSH) Publication No. 77-145. Washington, D.C.: U.S. Department of Health, Education, and Welfare; 757–141/6767. Washington, D.C.: U.S. Government Printing Office (1978). 94 pages.

The primary purpose of this study is to review and assess what is currently known about the effect of exposure to lead emissions from motor vehicles upon absorption of lead into the bodies of children and adults. The difficulties involved in determining the contribution from a single route of exposure, given the multimedia nature of lead exposure, are addressed. The advantages and disadvantages of the various approaches taken to studying the contribution from motor vehicle emissions to lead absorption are discussed, and some conclusions are drawn from an evaluation of the results of all the approaches combined.

The literature reviewed (approximately 85 references) is all more recent than 1970 and covers the following types of information: (a) epidemiological studies correlating concentrations of lead in the ambient air with levels of lead in the blood; (b) studies of occupational groups exposed to motor vehicle emissions; (c) studies of populations residing near roadways; (d) clinical studies; (e) studies correlating blood lead levels in children with exposure to lead in dirt and dust; (f) sources of lead in dirt and dust; (g) impacts of reducing lead in gasoline upon emissions of other potentially harmful materials; and (h) health benefits of reducing lead emissions from motor vehicles.

2. Drill, S., J. Konz, H. Mahar, and M. Morse (1979) *The Environmental Lead Problem: An Assessment of Lead in Drinking Water from a Multi-Media Perspective.* Office of Drinking Water. EPA-570/9-79-003. Washington, D.C.: U.S. Environmental Protection Agency. 149 pages.

This report was requested by the Criteria and Standards Division of EPA's Office of Drinking Water to assist in their evaluation of the adequacy of the current interim primary drinking water standard for lead. The approach taken is multimedia: The authors estimate the degree to which each major environmental source of lead exposure contributes to an individual's total daily lead uptake (using a "source contribution model"), relate this to blood-lead values in order to assess health impacts, and then identify those areas of exposure where regulatory action will have the greatest impact on blood-lead levels. This report differs from the others in this appendix in that it makes an original contribution by developing an exposure-hazard model. Of the 225 references listed, 80 percent are more recent than 1973.

The report defines and quantifies the major environmental sources of lead exposure; identifies and characterizes sensitive populations; describes the metabolism of lead and its compounds in humans via each exposure route; briefly synopsizes human health effects, reviews the association between biological change and lead in the body, and reviews the use of various exposure indicators; estimates total daily lead uptake by humans for each exposure pathway on the basis of ambient exposure levels and absorption/retention characteristics; relates the contribution of lead from each exposure to an individual's blood-lead level; assesses the relationship between varied water-lead exposures and resultant blood-lead values for sensitive populations; and assesses the public health significance for sensitive populations of various levels of lead in drinking water, given current ambient lead contamination in other environmental media (air, food, and dust/soil) to which these populations are exposed.

3. Ewing, R.A., M.A. Bell, and G.A. Lutz (1979) *The Health and Environmental Impacts of Lead: An Assessment of the Need for Limitations.* Office of Toxic Substances. EPA-560/2-79-001. Washington, D.C.: U.S. Environmental Protection Agency. 494 pages, 42 figures, and 105 tables.

This report was prepared for EPA's Office of Toxic Substances to assess the need for and opportunities for additional controls on human exposure to lead. The report takes a multimedia approach to analyzing potential limitations, and it considers areas (e.g., lead in foods) for which other federal agencies may have responsibility. (Under the Toxic Substances Control Act, EPA is required to determine whether other laws and other agencies may be applied to specific regulatory problems before EPA may promulgate regulations using the Act's authority.)

The primary objectives of the report are to examine systematically the uses and releases of lead and related health and safety hazards; to assess present and future needs for limitations on lead based on such an overall examination; and, if further limitations are needed, to identify the types of limitations that appear to be the most justified. The study evaluates the nature and structure of the lead industry, the myriad uses of lead and its compounds, the losses of lead to and fate of lead in the environment, the resultant health and environmental hazards, and where the most effective reduction of those hazard levels might be effected. Of the 690 references listed (disregarding possible duplication), 57 percent are from 1973 or later.

The coverage given to the lead industry and sources of lead release into the environment is quite comprehensive and detailed; this is one of the most thorough studies available on these topics. The sections on health and ecological hazards, on the other hand, are more superficial, probably because a related report (U.S. EPA 1978, reviewed elsewhere in this appendix), whose authors include the authors of this report, covers those topics in great detail.

The report assesses the relative contribution of various sources of exposure to lead to total body burden for the general adult population and contains detailed reviews of human exposure via two primary routes, i.e., air and food. The effects of existing regulations on those exposures are evaluated, and an assessment is made of the need for further control of lead and how to approach it. The health implications of reducing adventitious lead in foods are thoroughly assessed in terms of effects on blood lead levels. Finally, the report presents a detailed analysis of the technological aspects of lead in canned foods, and of methods for reducing lead in such products and the economic implications of such reduction.

4. Jaworski, J.F. (1979) *The Effects of Lead in the Canadian Environment.* Report from NRC Associate Committee on Scientific Criteria for Environmental Quality, National Research Council, Canada. Pub. No. NRC 16736 of the Environmental Secretariat. Ottawa, Canada: Publications NRC/NRC. 805 pages, 212 figures, and 187 tables.

This report was written by J.F. Jaworski for the National Research Council of Canada. It replaces an earlier, now outdated, NRC report and contains about 1,200 references, selected from more than 4,000 papers and documents that were obtained principally through computer title-search methods. The literature evaluated covers mainly the period from January 1973 to April 1978, although earlier papers are included to clarify certain points.

The primary purpose of the report is to review and evaluate the recent literature on biological effects of lead in the environment; subtle effects of low-level prolonged exposures are emphasized. This is one of the most comprehensive and thorough reports available on the topics addressed.

Chapter 2 is a summary of the document in which key information is cited according to the page, table, or figure in which it is presented. Chapters 3 and 4 evaluate lead cause–effect data concerning terrestrial vegetation and aquatic life, respectively. Chapter 5 describes lead metabolism in animals and humans (adults and children) as well as the effects of lead on the biochemistry of life forms, expeically mammals. The asssociations between biological changes and lead in the various systems of the mammalian body are discussed in detail in Chapter 6, including an evaluation of the usefulness and reliability of the various indicators of exposure to lead. Sources of environmental lead and their health implications are the subject of Chapter 7, including a detailed assessment of the contributions of automotive and industrial emissions of lead to exposures of the general population, children, people living near smelters, and workers. Sampling and analytical methods for measuring lead and body metabolites affected by lead are covered in two appendixes.

5. Lovering, T.G., ed. (1976) *Lead in the Environment.* Geological Survey Professional Paper 957, U.S. Department of the Interior. Stock number 024-001-02911-1. Washington, D.C.: U.S. Government Printing Office. 90 pages, 11 figures, and 37 tables.

This report is a collection of 11 papers, edited by T.G. Lovering. The papers follow a brief (6-page) summary by Lovering and average about 6 pages in length, with one exception at 20 pages. Of the 384 references listed, about 20 percent are more recent than 1970, 57 percent are later than 1965, and 76 percent are later than 1960.

This report is primarily a review and summary of the biogeochemistry of lead, covering in some detail the occurrence of lead in all media, "natural" levels and the anthropogenic contribution, cycling, chemistry, and analytical methods. Health effects and control techniques were mainly outside the scope of this report, although the summary does briefly relate the report contents to the significance of lead to human health, and the paper on lead in the atmosphere considers human exposures from all sources and reviews health effects.

Specific paper topics include: inorganic chemistry of lead in water (J.D. Hem); organic chemistry of lead in natural water systems (R.L. Wershaw); principal lead deposits in the continental United States (A.V. Heyl); oxidation and weathering of lead deposits (L.C. Huff); lead content of igneous, metamorphic, and sedimentary rocks, sediments, fossil fuels, and water (M. Fleischer, T.G. Lovering, M.J. Fishman, and J.D. Hem); occurrence and movement of lead in soils (R.R. Tidball); vegetation (H.L. Cannon); and the atmosphere (H.L. Cannon); and analytical methods (F.N. Ward and M.J. Fishman).

6. National Institute for Occupational Safety and Health (1978) *Criteria for a Recommended Standard . . . Occupational Exposure to Inorganic Lead, Revised Criteria—1978.* HEW (NIOSH) Publication No. 78-158. Washington, D.C.: U.S. Department of Health, Education, and Welfare. 757-141/1801. Washington, D.C.: U.S. Government Printing Office. 199 pages.

The NIOSH Office of Research and Standards Development had primary responsibility for this report, which is a revision of the 1973 criteria document for *Occupational Exposure to Inorganic Lead.* The literature review and evaluation on which the revised criteria are based were conducted by J. Santodonato and S. Lane of Syracuse Research Corporation and are included as an 84-page appendix; over 85 percent of the 185 references in the appendix are from 1973 or later. The body (53 pages) of the document is supported by 87 references, the most recent of which (20 percent) range from 1970 to 1972.

The primary purpose of the report is to support recommended changes in the standard for permissible workplace air exposure levels (from 150 to 100 $\mu g/m^3$, 8-hour time-weighted average). The permissible maximum blood lead level in workers is also lowered (from 80 to 60 $\mu g/100$ ml), and improved respiratory protection measures, work practices, and sanitation are recommended. The specific population reviewed is adults with occupational exposure and the only transport pathway considered is air; other populations and pathways are outside the scope of the report. The recommended standards are based on data correlating airborne concentrations of lead with blood lead levels that have been associated with adverse health effects and symptoms, with an emphasis on epidemiological studies.

Topics addressed include: the extent of occupational exposures; the association between clinical and subclinical biological change and lead in the body; the use of blood lead versus other measures as indicators of occupational hazard; the "acceptable" biological change in workers and the associated "acceptable" level of lead in workplace air; and sampling and analytical methods.

7. National Research Council (1972) *Lead: Airborne Lead in Perspective.* Committee on Biologic Effects of Atmospheric Pollutants, Division of Medical Sciences. Washington, D.C.: National Academy of Sciences. 330 pages.

This report was written by an ad hoc panel consisting of P. Hammond (Chairman), A. Aronson, J. Chisolm, J. Falk, R. Keenan, H. Sandstead, and B. Dinman (Associate Editor), together with 39 acknowledged consultants and contributors. The body of the report (220 pages) gives thorough coverage to the topics addressed and is accompanied by 50 pages of technical appendixes. The references listed are not intended to comprise a comprehensive bibliography but rather are (in the panel's judgment) the most important primary literature sources on lead up to early 1971. Of the 600 references, approximately half are from 1965 or later.

The primary goals of this report are to assess the likelihood that humans, animals, and plants would be brought into the range of harmful exposure to lead then (1971) or in the near future, and to identify the circumstances that might make that likely. The report reviews and evaluates the scientific knowledge of the biological effects, and points out areas where data are lacking. It is an attempt to place in perspective the role of airborne lead in the biosphere; to gain this perspective the report considers the biologic effects of lead from a wide range of sources and levels of exposure.

Topics addressed include: natural and anthropogenic sources of lead to the environment; the magnitude, distribution, and cycling of lead in the biosphere (air, precipitation, soils, and biota); sources and effects in plants, domestic animals, and wildlife; general population (adult and child) exposures from natural and human-made contributions in food, water, and air; occupationally exposed adults and young children as special cases with high exposure; the association between lead in the human body and biological change (high-dose, metabolic, and behavioral effects); the association between biological change and lead in the environment; "acceptable" biological change; the occurrence and effects of lead alkyl vapors in air; nonbiological effects (e.g., textile fibers, glass, and atmospheric visibility—treated briefly); and research recommendations.

8. National Research Council (1977) *Drinking Water and Health*. Safe Drinking Water Committee, Advisory Center on Toxicology, Assembly of Life Sciences. Washington, D.C.: National Academy of Sciences. 939 pages.

The primary purpose of this report was to assess the significance of the adverse effects that the constituents of drinking water may have on public health. The economic or technological feasibility of controlling the concentration of these constituents was outside the scope of the study. In addition to identities, concentrations, and toxicities of the various water constituents, other questions were considered in the review, namely:

a. What reason is there for concern about the material? What risks are associated with its presence in water?

b. How does the material get into water?

c. What sources are there other than water?

d. What contaminants need to be controlled?

e. Are there special places or persons at higher-than-average risk?

f. Are there essential nutritional requirements for this material?

g. In view of the data at hand, can one say that this is a material that causes temporary ill effects? Permanent ill effects? Reversible effects?

h. In view of these effects—and their reversibility (or lack of it)—is it possible to set "no-observed-adverse-health-effects" levels?

i. For materials with special health benefits, what concentrations will maximize these benefits, while keeping the health risks associated with them at an acceptably low level?

j. What additional information is required to resolve the outstanding problems?

One chapter (112 pages) deals with trace metals; of that, 26 pages are devoted to overview discussion of all the metals with 10 additional pages on lead specifically. There are 63 references in the passages that deal with only lead; 76 percent are more recent than 1970 and 44 percent are from 1975 or later. The authors of the trace metal sections were C. Kruse, J. Chisolm, Jr., T. J. Chow, R. Engelbrecht, F. Gartrell, J. McKee, and J. Pierce.

Topics addressed for lead were necessarily brief and the assessments presented succinct. These included "natural" lake and river concentrations; a review of the occurrence of lead in drinking water (raw and finished water supplies, distribution system, and tap); sources to drinking water; chemical characteristics of lead in water; estimates of average adult and child lead intake from all routes of exposure; identification of the fetus and children under 3 as populations at special risk; discussion of factors influencing their susceptibility; the association between biological change and lead in the body; "acceptable" levels of lead in drinking water; a brief review of water treatment methods to remove lead and a semiquantification of removal efficiencies; a brief description of analytical methods and problems with reference to publications where details are available; and a list of research needs.

9. National Research Council (1976) *Recommendations for the Prevention of Lead Poisoning in Children.* Committee on Toxicology, Assembly of Life Sciences. Washington, D.C.: National Academy of Sciences. NTIS No. PB-257-645. Springfield, Va.: National Technical Information Service. 65 pages.

This report was written for the Consumer Product Safety Commission by an ad hoc committee consisting of J. Chisolm, Jr. (Chairman), E. Bingham, R. Goyer, P. Hammond, V. Newill, P. Rosser, and J. Wilson. It is a succinct (11-page) response to the primary question the committee was asked to answer, supported by 40 pages of referenced appendixes. The report is based on an evaluation of data from over 200 studies; of the 140 references listed, 80 percent are more recent than 1970.

The primary question addressed by this report is: "Given the fact that some children eat paint, what is a safe level of lead in paint?" The committee notes that, although the total amount of lead assimilated may be derived from a variety of environmental sources, the scope of this report is basically confined to a consideration of lead absorption from one source—paint—by one specific population—preschool-age children.

In order to answer the primary question, three preliminary questions are discussed first, namely: (1) What are the adverse effects of lead? (2) What dose of lead is sufficient to produce adverse effects? and (3) What is the estimated daily intake of lead in a child with pica for paint? Following this is a discussion of the lead content of paints available on the current retail market and a discussion of future research needs. Committee recommendations appear at the end of the report. Detailed appendixes were prepared by the committee in support of the report.

Topics addressed include: the occurrence of lead in paint, children with pica as the exposed population, factors influencing susceptibility, the association between biological change and lead in the body, and the association between biological change and the resulting "acceptable" levels of lead in paint.

10. Nriagu, J.O., ed. (1978) *The Biogeochemistry of Lead in the Environment.* Part A, Ecological Cycles (Chapters 1–10); Part B, Biological Effects (Chapters 11–19). Topics in Environmental Health Volume 1. New York: Elsevier/North Holland Biomedical Press. Part A: 422 pages, 96 tables, and 81 figures. Part B: 379 pages, 58 tables, and 11 figures.

The purpose of the two-part volume is to provide a holistic framework for looking at the vast recent literature on the chemical behavior and biological effects of lead in the geosphere, hydrosphere, atmosphere and biosphere. It contains the most in-depth treatment of lead biogeochemistry that the Committee has found. It is composed of 19 chapters written by experts in the various scientific disciplines, and was edited by J. Nriagu. The chapters in the two parts vary from 12 to 84 pages and include more than 2,500 references (disregarding possible duplication), with approximately 50 percent more recent than 1972.

Both parts provide a comprehensive review, assessment, and guide to the literature, covering almost every topic of interest, on their respective subjects, i.e., ecological cycles (Part A) and biological effects (Part B) of lead. Topics addressed include: sources (natural and anthropogenic) and levels of lead in soils, sediments, major rock types, the hydrosphere, and atmosphere (Chapters 2, 6, and 7); global and regional distribution and cycling of lead (Chapters 1, 2, and 5 through 8), with a case study of Missouri's New Lead Belt; use of equilibrium models to study the behavior of lead in the aqueous environment (Chapter 8); biogeochemical prospecting for lead (Chapter 10); uses of radioisotopes of lead in geochemistry and medicine (Chapters 9 and 12); mining, uses, and lead as a factor in the world economy (Chapters 3, 4, and 5); strategies to control atmospheric pollution and a summary of recommended "safe" levels of lead in air (Chapter 6); environmental exposures of humans and other biota (Chapters 11 and 16 through 19); the distribution, metabolism, and storage of lead in humans (Chapters 12 through 14); clinical and subclinical effects on organs and body systems in adults and children (Chapters 14 and 15); the value of various indices of subclinical effects (Chapter 15); and occurrence and effects of lead in other biota (Chapters 16 through 19).

11. U.S. Department of Labor (1978) *Final Environmental Impact Statement, Inorganic Lead.* Office of Environmental and Economic Impact, Occupational Safety and Health Administration, Washington, D.C. NTIS No. PB-284-746. Springfield, Va.: National Technical Information Service. 98 pages.

This document was prepared by OSHA's Office of Environmental and Economic Impact to assess the impact of a proposed standard for occupational exposure to lead on both the workplace and external environments. Beneficial impacts on worker health are projected; expected impacts on external air quality, water quality, and solid waste generation are examined; and economic impacts (compliance costs, employment/ productivity impacts, energy, inflation, and medical removal protection impacts) are evaluated. Emphasis is given to summarizing the major studies and information concerning the types and severity of health effects that have been associated with occupational exposure to lead.

The proposed standard (8-hour time-weighted average, 100 μg/m^3 of workplace air) relies heavily on the NIOSH *Criteria for a Recommended Standard . . . Occupational Exposure to Inorganic Lead* (1973) and the National Research Council's report *Airborne Lead in Perspective* (1972). The impact statement also draws upon approximately 50 recent references, oral and written submissions to OSHA through public hearings, comments on the draft statement, and reports by D.B. Associates, Inc., and the Center for Policy Alternatives at M.I.T. on economic and technological feasibility and costs of a medical removal requirement.

In addition to stating and describing the proposed regulatory action in detail and its relationship to other federal actions, topics addressed in support of the impact assessment include: sources and levels of lead in the environment (natural and anthropogenic); transport pathways; physical and chemical properties of lead relevant to human exposure; exposure of the general population via food, water, and air; high exposure of adults in occupational settings (reviewed with great care); children as a special population; the association between biological change and lead in the body; the "acceptable" biological change in occupationally exposed people, and the associated "acceptable" level of lead in the workplace; air monitoring of workplace and biological surveillance of workers; methods to reduce worker exposure; and the economic impacts of implementing the proposed standard.

12. U.S. Environmental Protection Agency (1977a) *Air Quality Criteria for Lead.* Office of Research and Development. EPA-600/8-77-017. Washington, D.C.: U.S. Government Printing Office. 273 pages, 69 figures, and 114 tables.

This document was prepared by EPA's Office of Research and Development, with major contributions and reviews by other branches of EPA, other government agencies, numerous independent experts, and EPA's independent Science Advisory Board. The document provides the scientific assessment of health and welfare criteria upon which EPA's Administrator based his promulgation of a national ambient air quality standard for lead. It emphasizes the potential hazards of general exposure to lead, and because of the very public way it was reviewed and revised, it attempted to produce a consensus statement on this topic.

The criteria formulated here are based on an extensive review of current scientific knowledge of sources, occurrence, exposure to and effects of lead. Control techniques and the assessment of alternative control strategies are addressed in a separate EPA document (U.S. EPA 1977b). The scientific literature through March 1977 is reviewed; of the 1,186 references listed (disregarding possible duplication), 62 percent are from 1972 or later.

Although *Air Quality Criteria for Lead* deals primarily with airborne lead, it also examines other environmental routes of exposure and evaluates the relative contribution from inhalation and ingestion of atmospheric lead to the total body burden. The first portion of the document (Chapters 3 through 7, 67 pages) is devoted to lead in the environment: its physical and chemical properties; monitoring and measurement for lead in the various environmental media; environmental sources, emissions and concentrations of lead; and the transport and chemical and physical reactions of lead in the environment.

Chapters 8 through 13 (178 pages) examine effects of lead on ecosystems and, most importantly, on human health. Topics addressed include: exposure of the general population and populations at special risk; routes and mechanisms by which lead enters the body; metabolism of lead in adults and children; dose–effect and dose–response relationships; the advantages and disadvantages of use of blood lead levels as an indicator of exposure; quantitative relationships between blood lead levels and air and soil/dust lead levels; and the magnitude of the risk from airborne lead in terms of the number of persons exposed in various subgroups of the population.

13. U.S. Environmental Protection Agency (1977b) *Control Techniques for Lead Air Emissions*. Office of Air Quality Planning and Standards. EPA-450/2-77-012. 2 Vols. Research Triangle Park, N.C.: U.S. Environmental Protection Agency. Vol. I, 212 pages. Vol. II, 370 pages, 94 tables, and 89 figures.

This document was prepared by PEDCo Environmental, Inc., for EPA's Office of Air Quality Planning and Standards. Its primary purpose is to assess the methods of controlling atmospheric emissions of lead and its compounds from various sources, and to estimate approximate costs for implementing these control methods; control of lead in food and water are outside its scope. It is one of relatively few in-depth evaluations of the topics addressed. A companion document, *Air Quality Criteria for Lead*, evaluates the effects of lead on health and welfare (U.S. EPA 1977a, summarized immediately preceding). Of the 310 references listed for this document (disregarding possible duplication), approximately 69 percent are from 1972 or later.

A background chapter characterizes lead emissions; documents and estimates stationary and mobile source emissions; discusses emission factors, trends, and projections; describes major control devices (electrostatic precipitators, wet scrubbers, and fabric filters); explains how estimates of control costs for 11 categories of industrial sources are derived; and summarizes anticipated impacts from specific control devices for those 11 industries. The remainder of the report is devoted to an in-depth review and evaluation of the major sources: combustion of gasoline, coal, oil, waste oil, and solid wastes; production of lead alkyls, storage batteries, primary and secondary nonferrous metals, ferrous metals and alloys, and lead oxide; and lead-handling operations and miscellaneous sources. For each of these sources, the specific process involving lead and the resulting emissions are described, and feasible control techniques and related control costs and impacts are assessed.

14. U.S. Environmental Protection Agency (1978) *Review of the Environmental Effects of Pollutants*. VII. Lead. Draft Report from Battelle Memorial Institute. Health Effects Research Laboratory, Office of Research and Development. EPA-600/1-78-029. Cincinnati, Ohio: U.S. Environmental Protection Agency. 472 pages, 50 figures, and 101 tables. (NOTE: The final draft is expected to be available in late 1979 from Health Effects Research Laboratory, U.S. Environmental Protection Agency, Cincinnati.)

This report was prepared for EPA's Health Effects Research Laboratory as one in an ongoing series of reports (REEPs) on selected pollutants. The purpose of these reports is to provide the scientific and technical background for developing criteria documents to be used in regulatory decision making. The lead REEP is an extensive survey of relevant research and an up-to-date compendium of data on the environmental effects of lead. Of the 933 references listed (disregarding possible duplication), approximately half are from 1973 or later.

This extensive review of the literature is preceded by an assessment chapter, written by P. Hammond. This chapter summarizes and interprets the large volume of factual information presented in the subsequent chapters, and presents an overall evaluation of the potential hazards resulting from present concentrations of lead in the environment. A related report (Ewing et al. 1979, reviewed elsewhere in this appendix), which assesses the need for further limitations on human exposure to lead, is based in large part on the information and assessment presented in this report.

A major portion of this report (40 percent) reviews human metabolism and health effects of lead, including: effects on cell and organ systems; the various indicators of human exposure to lead; lead toxicity in children; epidemiological studies; dose–response relationships; and a separate treatment of organic lead. Other topics addressed are: sampling and analytical methods; effects on microorganisms, plants, and animals; the sources, distribution, and transformation of lead in air, water, and soil; and the movement of lead within ecosystems. The occurrence of lead in food is reviewed in detail and the relative contribution to general population exposure from food and air is assessed. Research needs are identified.

15. U.S. Environmental Protection Agency (1979) *Lead: Ambient Water Quality Criteria, Criterion Document.* Office of Water Planning and Standards. Washington, D.C.: U.S. Environmental Protection Agency. Springfield, Va.: National Technical Information Service. 151 pages.

This report is one of 65 criteria documents recently developed for use by EPA's Office of Water Planning and Standards in establishing water quality criteria for toxic pollutants. The primary purpose of the report is to summarize and evaluate literature that is most relevant to the question of what is an "acceptable" level of human and aquatic life exposure to lead via water. From this literature evaluation water quality criteria are developed that specify the maximum recommended concentrations of lead in water consistent with the protection of aquatic life and human health. Of the 237 references listed, approximately 64 percent are from 1973 or later.

In concept, the criteria and supporting criterion document are scientific entities, based solely on data and scientific judgment. The criteria are not enforceable, although they can be used in developing standards. The report contains no economic or technological feasibility considerations.

The criterion document is divided into sections on aquatic life toxicology (28 pages) and mammalian toxicology and human health effects (80 pages). The aquatic life section reviews the scant literature on acute and chronic toxicity to fresh and saltwater fish, invertebrates, and plants. The approach used to develop criteria involves fitting an exponential equation that describes the relationship of toxicity to water hardness for each species. The resulting criteria are in terms of hardness.

The human health section is divided into subsections on exposure, pharmacokinetics, effects, and criteria formulation. The approach taken to assessing the impact of lead in water on human health is basically the same as that taken by EPA for lead in air (U.S. EPA 1977a, reviewed elsewhere in this appendix). First, the critical target organ or system is identified (the hematological system), and the value of the various indices of exposure to lead is assessed. Then the highest internal dose of lead that can be tolerated without injury to the target organ is specified. Finally, the impact of lead in water on the maximum tolerated internal dose and the likely consequences of specific reductions in the maximum allowable concentration of lead in water are estimated.

In applying the above approach, the report considers all major routes of exposure to the general population and to children with special exposures; briefly reviews what is known about lead metabolism and the factors influencing absorption; assesses the relative contributions to blood lead levels from diet (food and water) versus air; presents a fairly thorough review of the relative effects on blood lead of different levels of lead in water; and summarizes what is known about dose–effect and dose–response relationships for the general population and children, with emphasis on hematological, neurological, behavioral, and carcinogenic effects.

16. World Health Organization (1977) Environmental Health Criteria 3. Lead. Geneva: World Health Organization. (Available in U.S.A. from Q Corporation, Albany, N.Y.) 160 pages.

The first and second drafts of this document were prepared by P. Hammond with the collaboration of national institutions, international organizations, WHO collaborating centers, and individual experts. A WHO Task Group then reviewed and revised the second draft in May 1975, and made its own evaluation of the health risks from exposure to lead and its compounds. The document is based primarily on original publications, although several recent broad review documents and comprehensive symposia proceedings were cited as well. Of the 573 references listed, over 55 percent are from 1970 or later; 19 percent are from 1974 or later.

The primary purpose of this report is to evaluate human health risks from exposure to lead and its compounds. Conclusions are based on a consideration of: (a) the significance of different natural and anthropogenic environmental sources of lead and pathways of exposure; (b) the probability of occurrence of biological effects at different levels and rates of lead intake; (c) the significance for human health of the various known biological effects of lead; and (d) the validity and limitations of various indicators of lead exposure and of resultant effects.

Three populations are identified: the general population exposed through ingestion of food and water and by inhalation; infants and children exposed by eating nonfood items (soil, dust, paint); and occupationally exposed adults. Exposure levels and blood lead levels are reviewed for each population identified. The current state of knowledge about the absorption, distribution, retention, and elimination of inorganic and organic lead compounds is evaluated. Studies on the effects of lead and factors influencing susceptibilty are thoroughly reviewed under three categories: experimental, epidemiological, and clinical. For the epidemiological and clinical studies, where doses are more likely to approximate what can occur in environmental or occupational exposure, an attempt is made to establish, as far as possible, dose–effect relationships and the frequency of such effects.

Other topics addressed include: sampling and analytical problems; blood lead levels, hematological effects, and other measures as an indication of exposure; dose–effect relationships for specific organs and body systems; and research needs.

Federal Research on Lead in the Environment

SUMMARY

This appendix surveys research on lead in the environment sponsored by the U.S. federal government in fiscal years 1977 through 1979. It describes studies on various topics related to lead that were conducted or supported by different federal agencies, and presents an integrated, topic-by-topic assessment of the total government research effort. The lead research programs of each agency involved are briefly described and related to the various missions of the agencies. The survey was made to provide a context for the recommendations in Chapter 5 about research needs and an appropriate role for this study's sponsor, the Department of Housing and Urban Development, in federal research on lead hazards.

Throughout the appendix, abbreviations are used instead of lengthy names of agencies (Table B.1).

KINDS OF RESEARCH

The individual projects that make up the research programs described here can be divided into two broad categories. The first consists of studies that are primarily concerned with lead, its behavior in the environment, or its biological effects. The second category consists of studies concerned with broader topics, such as the geochemical cycling of trace elements or the effects of heavy metals in sludges on soil organisms, which include lead among the group of elements examined. In the 3

368

TABLE B.1   Abbreviations Used in This Report

Abbreviation	Agency
ADAMHA	Alcohol, Drug Abuse and Mental Health Administration, PHS, HEW
BM	Bureau of Mines, Department of the Interior
CDC	Center for Disease Control, PHS, HEW
CPSC	Consumer Product Safety Commission
CRS	Congressional Research Service, Library of Congress
DOE	Department of Energy
DOI	Department of the Interior
DRR	Division of Research Resources, NIH, HEW
EPA	Environmental Protection Agency
FDA	Food and Drug Administration, HEW
FWS	Fish and Wildlife Service, Department of the Interior
HEW	Department of Health, Education, and Welfare
HUD	Department of Housing and Urban Development
ILZRO	International Lead Zinc Research Organization, Inc.
IRLG	Interagency Regulatory Liaison Group
NBS	National Bureau of Standards, Department of Commerce
NCI	National Cancer Institute, NIH, HEW
NHLBI	National Heart, Lung and Blood Institute, NIH, HEW
NICHD	National Institute of Child Health and Human Development, NIH, HEW
NIEHS	National Institute of Environmental Health Sciences, NIH, HEW
NIH	National Institutes of Health, HEW
NIMH	National Institute of Mental Health, HEW
NINCDS	National Institute of Neurological and Communicative Disorders and Stroke, NIH, HEW
NIOSH	National Institute for Occupational Safety and Health, CDC, PHS, HEW
NMFS	National Marine Fisheries Service, NOAA, Department of Commerce
NOAA	National Oceanic and Atmospheric Administration, Department of Commerce
NRC	National Research Council
NSF	National Science Foundation
OMB	Office of Management and Budget
ORD	Office of Research and Development, EPA
OSHA	Occupational Safety and Health Administration, Department of Labor
OWRT	Office of Water Research and Technology, Department of the Interior
PHS	Public Health Service, HEW
USDA	Department of Agriculture
USGS	Geological Survey, Department of the Interior
WHO	World Health Organization

years covered by this survey, the government supported $18 million worth of research on lead per se, and $63 million worth of multi-element studies that included lead. Since the fraction of the latter sum that was actually devoted to the study of lead cannot be precisely determined, consideration of the two kinds of research has been kept separate in this survey. Generally, the term "lead research" is used to refer only to studies that focused primarily on lead. Those that were only partially or peripherally concerned with lead are called "multi-element studies" or, occasionally, "lead-related research."

RESEARCH ON SPECIFIC TOPICS

Table B.2 lists 18 research topics, grouped under 7 major headings, and shows the level of effort of the federal government as a whole on each topic for the last 3 years. If the fraction of total funds spent on a topic is taken as an index of the aggregate level of importance the various agencies assigned to the topic, some obvious conclusions can be drawn about the government's priorities.

Lead Research

In the category of research concerned primarily with lead, topics under the heading of biological effects were overwhelmingly the top priority, receiving 67.4 percent of total expenditures. Two topics related to estimating human exposures—measurement of levels of lead in foods and studies of the contributions of specific sources to total exposure to lead—drew another 12.8 percent of the funds, and studies of the absorption and pharmacodynamics of lead received 6.2 percent. In all, the topics that constitute research on potential hazards of lead to human health accounted for 86.4 percent of the federal government's expenditures for lead research in the last 3 years.

The only other subject area that was emphasized in studies concerned primarily with lead was pollution control and hazard abatement, which received 10.1 percent of the expenditures. However, these statistics reflect primarily the activities of one agency (HUD), and less than a quarter of the funds were spent on development of improved methods for managing lead hazards (see detailed discussions on each topic).

Seven other topics, including several that have been stressed throughout this report as critical for making decisions about lead in the environment, received a combined total of only 3.5 percent of the funds that the government spent for lead research over the last 3 years. However, this does not necessarily reflect low priority; it might mean instead that the needed information can be more readily or logically obtained through multi-element studies.

Multi-element Research

Within multi-element research that includes lead, the most heavily studied topic was levels of trace elements in environmental media, and the four topics under the heading Sources and Environmental Pathways received 53.3 percent of the total outlay for multi-element studies. However, this sum includes the extensive environmental sampling programs of USGS, which are only marginally relevant to an assessment of lead in the human environment. The value of the research for decision making is therefore probably less than the fraction of funds allocated to the topics would otherwise suggest.

The remainder of funds for multi-element studies was divided chiefly among analytical and measurement methodology (18.5 percent), biological effects (12.5 percent) and pollution control (9.8 percent). For two of those topics, the amounts spent were also inflated by a single agency's efforts on projects that were only peripherally concerned with lead: the USGS was most active in developing analytical methods to support its sampling programs; and the BM spent $5.2 million for studies on controls of trace contaminants from mineral and metals industrial operations.

Areas Not Studied

A few topics were either noticeably absent from both the lead and the multi-element categories or received little attention. None of the agencies appears to have sponsored any research in the social or behavioral sciences, either to estimate the value of lead-related risks, to explore social approaches to hazard management, or to project costs and benefits of policy alternatives. Studies of ecological effects, beyond data gathering on the accumulation of toxic elements by organisms, received very little support. Research on humans concentrated heavily on a few populations known to be at high risk; very few studies were conducted to assess the magnitude and distribution of risks among the general population. The general problem of integrated assessment of the contributions by critical sources to multiple-pathway exposures drew little attention from agencies other than HUD, and no agency except HUD undertook research to assess the effectiveness of current programs to manage lead hazards.

TABLE B.2 Levels of Effort in Research on Topics Related to Lead in the Environment Supported by the Federal Government in FY 1977-1979 (in thousands of dollars)

Topic	Studies Concerned Primarily With Lead					Multielement Studies That Include Lead [d]				
	1977	1978 [a]	1979 [b]	Total [c]	%	1977	1978 [a]	1979 [b]	Total [c]	%
Sources and Environmental Pathways										
Character of sources and emissions	—	—	—	—	0.0	1,641	1,777	1,539	4,957	7.9
Transport, fate, geochemical cycling	41	164	25	230	1.3	2,998	3,006	3,208	9,212	14.6
Levels in environmental media	—	—	—	—	0.0	4,565	5,259	6,050	15,884	25.2
Levels in biota, foods, housewares	605	597	413	1,615	9.0	924	1,359	1,325	3,608	5.7
Populations with Exposures										
Assessment of exposures	—	—	—	—	0.0	65	60	60	185	0.3
Contributions of specific sources	176	67	446	689	3.8	13	13	—	26	<0.1
Absorption and Pharmacodynamics	519	324	282	1,125	6.2	334	268	304	906	1.4
Biological Effects										
Clinical studies	683	453	244	1,380	7.7	61	68	20	149	0.2
Epidemiology	1,238	342	312	1,892	10.5	340	274	210	824	1.3
Toxicology	3,027	2,288	2,284	7,599	42.1	2,281	1,583	1,670	5,534	8.8
Ecological effects	3	16	—	19	0.1	624	247	348	1,219	1.9
Interactions with other substances	452	449	364	1,265	7.0	123	57	41	221	0.3

Pollution Control/Hazard Abatement									
Development of technological methods	133	166	100	399	2.2	2,386	1,389	2,268	6,043	9.6
Non-technological approaches	309	235	135	679	3.8	74	18	18	110	0.2
Evaluation of current programs	—	633	100	733	4.1	—	—	—	—	0.0
Analytical and Measurement Methodology									
Chemical analysis of samples	108	41	40	189	1.0	2,929	3,435	3,731	10,095	16.0
Sampling and monitoring methods	141	26	27	194	1.1	1,004	300	300	1,604	2.5
Miscellaneous	21	—	—	21	0.1	476	1,016	1,071	2,563	4.1
TOTALS	7,456	5,801	4,772	18,029	100	20,838	20,129	22,173	63,140	100

[a] EPA and USDA did not report expenditures for FY 1978. Government totals shown for the year are therefore lower than actual expenditures, by an undetermined amount.

[b] EPA, USDA, and OWRT did not report expenditures for FY 1979. Estimated government totals shown for the year are therefore lower than actual expenditures, by an undetermined amount.

[c] Some interagency contracts may have been reported by both the sponsoring agency and the performing agency. There may therefore be a small amount of double-counting in some of the totals.

[d] For some agencies (OWRT, NBS, USDA, and NSF), information was provided on an element-by-element breakdown, and total costs of multielement studies could not be determined. (Such studies are therefore reported as amounts spent primarily on lead.) Most other agencies did not specify all elements included in most multielement studies; it was therefore not possible to identify all projects that might have included lead. Both of these considerations make the levels of effort shown in the table for multielement studies that include lead likely to be underestimates. The fraction of such expenditures that may properly be allocated to work on lead varies from topic to topic, and may range from a few percent to one-fourth or one-third of the amounts shown for particular items.

AGENCIES INVOLVED IN LEAD RESEARCH

The survey identified research on lead or relevant multi-element studies in the research programs of 21 federal agencies. It is possible that isolated projects in other agencies were overlooked, but it is apparent that a handful of agencies dominates the field in each category of research. Table B.3 displays the amounts spent by each of the agencies in the last 3 fiscal years.

Lead Research

Six agencies supported 86 percent of the research on lead that was funded in the 3-year period. The biggest source of funds, NIEHS, accounted for 30.5 percent of the expenditures, almost all of which was devoted to study of the biological effects and pharmacodynamics of lead. DOE (18.2 percent) spent all of its $3.3 million on toxicological studies. FDA (14 percent) surveyed lead levels in foods and supported biological studies of toxic effects and interactions. HUD, ranked fourth in support of lead research (12.6 percent), divided its efforts among studies of the sources of lead in children, development of improved techniques to abate lead paint hazards, technical support for local projects, and evaluation of current programs. NIOSH (6 percent) conducted epidemiological studies of workers in lead industries; and EPA (4.6 percent) supported a variety of studies, chiefly on biological effects. (EPA reported data only for 1977; its activities over the 3-year period therefore have been substantially underestimated.)

Six of the other 15 agencies supported no research that was primarily concerned with lead. Most of the nine remaining agencies were specialized units of HEW that contributed one or two studies within their primary research areas. NBS carried out several studies to improve methods for chemical analysis for lead, and provided technical support for projects supported by other agencies.

Multi-element Research

Six agencies also dominated the multi-element category; in this case, the leaders spent 93 percent of the total. USGS alone accounted for 47.1 percent, spending $29.7 million for geochemical surveys and related development of analytical techniques. DOE (14.7 percent) spent about $9 million to assess trace element pollution associated with a variety of energy sources, and the BM (13.2 percent) supported a comparable effort to assess and develop controls for such pollution from mining and mineral operations. NIEHS, which supported primarily toxicological studies of effects of heavy metals, was fourth in this category, with 7.9 percent of expenditures. EPA (on the basis of 1 year of funding) was fifth, with 6 percent. EPA's studies were balanced among biological effects, analytical and monitoring methods, control technology, and sources and environmental pathways. FDA spent 4.1 percent of the total, almost all of it for the development of analytical methods to measure trace contaminants in foods.

Nine other agencies made some contribution to this multi-element research, each in its own specialized area. Seven divisions of HEW collectively sponsored 3 percent of the research, almost all of it in the area of biological effects of trace contaminants. NOAA spent $1.5 million (2.3 percent) on a survey of trace elements in ocean fish; and FWS contributed 1.6 percent of the research through its studies of the effects of heavy metals on wildlife and its program to monitor pollutant levels in freshwater fish. Unfortunately, the information available on the support of multi-element studies by OWRT, NBS, USDA, and NSF was not sufficient to permit an estimate of their contributions to this category.

RECENT TRENDS IN LEAD RESEARCH

The total reported government outlay for lead research (studies primarily concerned with lead) was $7.5 million in fiscal year 1977, and only $4.7 million in fiscal year 1979. Disregarding inflation, this represents a decline of about 36 percent in the level of support. However, three agencies (EPA, USDA, and OWRT) did not provide data for 1979. If those 3 are excluded from the total for 1977 as well, expenditures by the other 12 agencies that supported research on lead declined 25 percent over the 2-year span (again making no adjustment for inflation).

Table B.2 shows that this decline in effort was distributed fairly uniformly over the range of topics investigated. Table B.3, on the other hand, shows that the drop in support was more dramatic in some agencies than in others. NIOSH and NICHD completed major studies, and have apparently turned their attention to other priorities. NIEHS, the leading source of support, reduced its reported funding on lead by 33 percent. DOE and FDA, however, showed only 11 and 19 percent decreases, and HUD and a few others showed net increases from fiscal year 1977 to fiscal year 1979.

The 3-year period covered by this survey is too brief to provide insight into the long-term strength of support for lead research, but certain obvious influences may explain the short-term trends. In 1977 (and in 1976, when fiscal year 1977 research funding decisions were made), EPA, FDA, CPSC, and OSHA were preparing to set criteria or standards for lead in ambient air, drinking water, industrial effluents, foods, paints, and occupa-

TABLE B.3 Levels of Support by Various Federal Agencies for Research on All Topics Related to Lead in the Environment for FY 1977-1979 (in thousands of dollars)

Agency	Studies Concerned Primarily With Lead					Multielement Studies That Include Lead[c]				
	1977	1978[a]	1979[b]	Total	%	1977	1978[a]	1979[b]	Total	%
HUD	510	1,028	725	2,263	12.6	—	—	—	—	0.0
EPA	822	n.a.	n.a.	822[d]	4.6	3,762	n.a.	n.a.	3,762[d]	6.0
HEW										
FDA	904	895	728	2,527	14.0	819	805	978	2,602	4.1
NIEHS	2,183	1,841	1,468	5,492	30.5	1,605	1,700	1,685	4,990	7.9
NINCDS	62	135	147	344	1.9	91	215	230	536	0.8
NICHD	388	114	—	502	2.8	112	171	111	394	0.6
NHLBI	9	17	9	35	0.2	54	54	22	130	0.2
NCI	—	—	—	—	0.0	59	170	5	234	0.4
NIH-DRR	129	102	105	336	1.9	110	116	119	345	0.5
NIOSH	719	193	251	1,163	6.4	60	38	155	253	0.4
CDC	117	102	105	324	1.8	—	—	—	—	0.0
ADAMHA	—	—	—	—	0.0	91	—	—	91	0.1
DOE	1,191	1,026	1,059	3,276	18.2	2,881	3,262	3,112	9,255	14.7
Interior										
BM	—	—	—	—	0.0	2,233	2,602	3,515	8,350	13.2
USGS	—	—	—	—	0.0	8,200	10,100	11,420	29,720	47.1

FWS	—	—	—	—	0.0	304	345	361	1,010	1.6
OWRT	47	158	n.a.	205[d]	1.1	n.a.	n.a.	n.a.	n.a.[c]	—
Commerce										
NBS	50	90	65	205	1.1	n.a.	n.a.	n.a.	n.a.[c]	—
NOAA	—	—	—	—	0.0	457	551	460	1,468	2.3
USDA	221	n.a.	n.a.	221[d]	1.2	n.a.	n.a.	n.a.	n.a.[c]	—
NSF	104	100	110	314	1.7	n.a.	n.a.	n.a.	n.a.[c]	—
TOTALS[e]	7,456	5,801[a]	4,772[b]	18,029	100	20,838	20,129[a]	22,173[b]	63,140	100

[a] EPA and USDA did not report expenditures for FY 1978. Government totals shown for the year are therefore lower than actual expenditures, by an undetermined amount.

[b] EPA, USDA, and OWRT did not report expenditures for FY 1979. Estimated government totals shown for the year are therefore lower than actual expenditures, by an undetermined amount.

[c] For some agencies (OWRT, da, and NSF), information was provided on an element-by-element breakdown, and total costs of multielement studies could not be determined. (Such studies are therefore reported as amounts spent primarily on lead.) Most other agencies did not specify all elements included in most multielement studies; it was therefore not possible to identify all projects that might have included lead. Both of these considerations make the levels of effort shown in the table for multielement studies that include lead likely to be underestimates. The fraction of such expenditures that may properly be allocated to work on lead varies from topic to topic, and may range from a few percent to one-fourth or one-third of the amounts shown for particular items.

[d] EPA and USDA reported expenditures only for FY 1977, and OWRT reported expenditures only for FY 1977 and 1978. Each agency's total effort is undoubtedly greater than the amount shown in the table, but the correct totals cannot be determined from information available.

[e] Some interagency contracts may have been reported by both the sponsoring agency and the performing agency. There may therefore be a small amount of double-counting in some of the totals.

tional environments. Several of those actions were completed in 1978, and some are still pending (see Appendix C). Three of the six top agencies in terms of funding for lead research (NIOSH, FDA, and EPA) are conducting such studies primarily to support regulatory decisions, and the priorities of NIEHS also respond, albeit less dramatically, to urgent, decision-related information needs. It therefore seems likely that the trend observed here does not reflect a dramatic decrease of interest in a formerly strong research field, but rather a return from an aberrant peak of activity to a more nearly normal level.

In the multi-element category of research, total funding appeared to increase by about 6 percent over the 3 years. This is a slower rate of growth than government support of R & D in general has shown (17 percent from fiscal year 1977 to fiscal year 1979 [Greenberg 1978]). If EPA is excluded as before, however, the level of effort of the other 14 agencies in this category actually increased by nearly 30 percent. Table B.3 shows that this trend affected most agencies and was most pronounced in USGS and BM. Table B.2 (adjusted to exclude EPA) suggests that work increased primarily on monitoring for trace elements in the environment and in the food chain, on analytical methods, and on miscellaneous research (chiefly metallurgical studies by BM). The level of effort in biological research apparently dropped by 31 percent, but if EPA's contributions in 1977 are subtracted, the net change was a 7 percent *increase* in work by other agencies on these topics.

Since it appears that support for trace element studies in general has experienced healthy growth in the last 3 years, the strong trend in the opposite direction in research on lead seems almost certain to be the descending phase of a short-term pulse of activity in support of recent regulatory decision making.

INTERAGENCY COORDINATION

The large number of agencies involved in lead research and the apparent overlapping areas of interest of many of them suggest a need for effective coordination of research programs, both to avoid wasteful duplication and to help ensure that most of the important topics are being studied. There are both some areas of duplication and some significant gaps in activity in the federal program on lead research, but there is little to indicate that improved interagency coordination would do away with these problems. Furthermore, two factors make it likely that recent research on lead has been as well coordinated as can be expected. First, the flurry of regulatory activity on lead in recent years has stimulated interest in some of the same issues in several agencies, and motivated both research managers and regulators in each agency to be aware of what their colleagues in the other agencies are doing. Second, the predominant subject matter of lead research—biological effects (and especially toxicology)—is an area in which strong, formal interagency coordinating mechanisms are already operating effectively.

The multi-element research surveyed here, however, is dominated by nonregulatory agencies with diverse missions and information needs. There appears to be an opportunity worth exploring for valuable interaction between the regulators and such agencies as DOE, USGS, BM, FWS, or USDA, whose large data-gathering efforts might be modified to generate some information needed by decision makers without weakening the basic nature of the research.

INTRODUCTION

APPROACH AND METHOD

The purpose of this survey was to provide an overview of federal research activities related to lead in the environment. No attempt was made to evaluate the scientific quality of the research. Also, no judgments were made about the appropriateness of the agencies' programs, except in the case of HUD, which specifically asked for such advice. Recommendations for HUD's lead-based paint research program are presented in Chapter 5.

The primary sources of information for the survey were materials compiled by the agencies in late 1978 for the Subcommittee on Science, Research and Technology of the U.S. House of Representatives. Congress, through the Congressional Research Service of the Library of Congress, was conducting a survey of research by federal agencies on trace elements (CRS 1979); the staff of the CRS generously made the information they collected available for this study. Also, in October 1978 the Committee on Lead in the Human Environment met with representatives of 10 federal agencies that support lead research, to discuss their programs, priorities, interagency coordination, and the relationships between lead research and the missions of the agencies. The Committee's staff subsequently obtained additional information from numerous individuals in the various agencies. A list of those who supplied information appears in Appendix E.

ACTIVITIES ENCOMPASSED BY "RESEARCH"

The federal expenditures reported here include support of virtually all lead-related research and development projects, and some testing and monitoring activities. However, it is likely that some of the government's information-gathering activities have been omitted from this survey. For instance, regulatory agencies collect extensive information on the nature of problems, including data they obtain from the regulated industries, and support some environmental monitoring programs to identify hazardous conditions or to determine compliance with regulations. Such agencies also make substantial efforts to obtain, review, and interpret previously published information, in order to develop criteria and standards. Although these are all primarily scientific activities, they are frequently supported as part of regulatory programs, rather than out of appropriations for research, and therefore may not have appeared in the agencies' summaries of their research programs (NRC 1977).

LEAD RESEARCH IN PERSPECTIVE

The survey identified $18 million worth of research on lead and $63 million worth of related multi-element studies that the federal government sponsored in fiscal years 1977 through 1979. In the same period, total federal obligations for research and development averaged $26 billion per year (Greenberg 1978), and federal expenditures for environmental research averaged about $2 billion per year (U.S. OMB 1979). NSF surveyed government research, development, testing, and monitoring activities on toxic substances for fiscal year 1977 and reported a total outlay of $644 million for that year (Myers et al. 1978). According to another study, 13 federal agencies spent an average of $548 million per year for support of environmental health research in fiscal years 1977 through 1979 (U.S. NIEHS 1978). The recent survey by the CRS put total federal spending for research on trace elements at $100 million per year over the same period (CRS 1979). Finally, a recent survey of current (1977–1978) research in 7 federal agencies, carried out by the Interagency Regulatory Liaison Group, identified $15.7 million worth of studies on toxic metals supported by the agencies (Williams et al. 1978). Against this background, studies on lead appear to have accounted for between 1 and 6 percent of federal spending on environmental pollutants and their effects.

RESEARCH IN SUBJECT AREAS

Government research on each of the 6 major topics and 18 subtopics shown in Table B.2 is described in the sections that follow, in terms of the specific subjects investigated and the agencies that sponsored the research. The brief discussions summarize detailed information that is presented in tabular form in Supplement 1 of this appendix.

SOURCES AND ENVIRONMENTAL PATHWAYS

Research in this category, which includes four subtopics, consists almost entirely of studies classed as multi-element research. Among the six major topics, this one received the greatest support, accounting for 53 percent of expenditures for multi-element studies and 10 percent of the funding for studies focused on lead.

Character of Sources and Emissions

Three agencies spent a total of $5 million in the period surveyed for research on the potential impacts on air and water quality of a variety of mobile, stationary, and nonpoint sources of pollutants (Table B.7). Most of the studies were only peripherally concerned with lead. The most active agency in this area, DOE (84 percent of expenditures on the topic), conducted assessments of the environmental impacts of fossil fuel and refuse combustion, coal gasification, and geothermal energy sources. The BM (11 percent) supported studies of fugitive emissions and dusts from the mining, mineral processing, and metals industries, and examined the mobility of trace elements in surface mining areas. EPA, which reported only for 1977, conducted four studies of automobile emissions and one of trace metal emissions from nonferrous smelters.

Between 1971 and 1976, HUD spent $887,000 on research into the nature and extent of lead paint hazards; and FDA is likely to need to examine sources of lead in foods in the near future. However, neither of these efforts appears in the fiscal years 1977 through 1979 research programs of the agencies.

Transport, Fate, and Geochemical Cycling

The government spent more than $9 million on studies in this category during fiscal years 1977 through 1979, almost all of it for multi-element research (Table B.8). Of 10 agencies involved in this field, the USGS is most active (65 percent of expenditures), supporting basic research on the geochemistry of elements and applied studies of human impacts on elemental cycles, for example, in surface mining areas. DOE (27 percent) supports broad studies of the environmental behavior of energy-related pollutants, including several projects on the fate of trace metals in fresh-water, coastal, and marine systems. EPA is more involved in this field than its 1-year total suggests, and has conducted a wide array of studies of the transport and fate of pollutants in the air, water, and soil.

Table B.8 shows a slight increase in the government's level of effort on this topic from 1977 to 1979, due almost entirely to expansion of the USGS program.

Levels in Environmental Media

The government spent nearly $16 million in the period surveyed to gather data on the occurrence of multiple elements in the environment (Table B.9), making this topic the most heavily supported of the 18 on the list. Virtually all of that work was conducted by the USGS, which collects and analyzes geochemical samples of rocks, soils, waters, and vegetation. In fiscal year 1978, USGS laboratories made an estimated 5 million elemental determinations on 300,000 environmental samples. Lead is one of about 50 elements for which analyses are commonly made.

Other projects in this category in the period surveyed include studies by EPA of air quality in the Four Corners region and of rural water quality, and a study by NIEHS of airborne contaminants in New York City.

Many agencies, especially at the state and local levels, support extensive monitoring programs to determine the levels of contaminants in the environment, including lead. However, such activities by the federal government are usually not considered research and are not included in this survey.

Levels in Biota, Foods, and Housewares

In the period surveyed, five federal agencies spent $1.6 million on research to determine levels of lead in human food items and housewares, and another $3.6 million on studies of trace elements in general in the human food chain (Table B.10). FDA has conducted recent major surveys of lead levels in fish, raw agricultural products, canned foods, typical diets of adults and children, and ceramic and hollowware products. DOE supports a large program to measure levels of trace metals in biological samples, with emphasis on pathways to humans. NOAA surveys the trace element content of edible ocean fishes, and the FWS monitors pollutant levels in freshwater fish. USDA conducts studies of trace element levels in crops and animal products, primarily from the standpoint of assessing their nutritional value.

POPULATIONS WITH EXPOSURES

This category received the lowest level of funding among the six major topics during the period surveyed; however, some research in other categories (e.g., epidemiology) also includes some assessment of exposures. Only three studies were of a general sort that might serve to identify populations at risk; the studies included an appraisal of environmental exposure to heavy metals, sponsored by NIEHS, and two assessments of the exposure of the general population to trace metals, supported by NHLBI. Most of the effort in this category has been devoted to research on the contributions of specific environmental sources of lead to lead absorbed by specific populations, notably children.

Five agencies have supported work on this topic in the last 3 years (Table B.11). HUD heads the list. Since an earlier study showed a strong correlation between a decline in sales of leaded gasoline and blood lead levels in children in New York City, HUD has stepped up its effort in this area in an attempt to clarify the relative contributions of atmospheric lead, soil and dust, and lead-based paint to children's total exposure. EPA sponsored one study to assess the importance of automobile traffic and other sources in contributing to elevated blood lead levels in children. NIEHS supported two studies of the home environments of children with high blood lead, and FDA examined dietary patterns of the same group. NSF spent $6,000 in 1977 for a pilot study on the feasibility of an intensive investigation to determine where individual children get the lead they absorb; however, the project apparently has not been pursued further.

Table B.11 does not include one important study, sponsored by EPA in 1978, that reviewed all earlier studies and attempted to develop a simple model to project the contributions of specific sources of lead to lead hazards for different populations under a variety of conditions. The report of that study (by Drill et al.) is summarized in Appendix A.

ABSORPTION AND PHARMACODYNAMICS

Four agencies sponsored $1.1 million worth of studies in the period surveyed that looked at the absorption, distribution, storage, mobilization, and excretion of lead in humans or in experimental animals (Table B.12). NIEHS spent more than three-fourths of the total on projects that studied lead metabolism in bone, renal handling of lead, distribution of lead in the central nervous sytem, and effects of chelating agents on the distribution and excretion of lead. FDA studied mechanisms of absorption of lead from the gastrointestinal tract, and NIH–DRR supported a study of the metabolism of lead-210 in infant monkeys.

Nearly a million dollars also went to support similar studies concerned with multiple substances. NIEHS sponsored 6 studies, including 2 devoted to the development of a compartment model for body burdens of heavy metals. DOE investigated the role of plasma lipoproteins in the transport of environmental pollutants, and EPA explored the relationship between body burdens of pollutants and their appearance in saliva. NIOSH recently undertook a study of the bioavailability of constituents of inhaled dust.

Federal support for studies on the pharmacodynamics of lead has declined over the 3 years surveyed. NIEHS, the primary source of funds, supported 11 studies on this topic in fiscal year 1977, but only 6 in fiscal year 1979.

BIOLOGICAL EFFECTS

More than two-thirds of the amount the government has spent for research primarily concerned with lead in the last 3 years has gone to support studies of the biological effects of the metal. In addition, nearly $8 million more has been spent to study toxic effects of heavy metals or other groups of elements. At least 17 federal agencies have supported some research in this category during the period surveyed. Among the five research areas that make up the category, toxicological studies have received almost twice as much funding as the other four topics combined.

Clinical Studies

Three of the NIH institutes have sponsored about $1.5 million worth of studies of effects of lead in humans with known conditions of lead intoxication (Table B.13). NICHD supported a major investigation, concluded in 1978, of the developmental effects of exposure to lead in childhood. NIEHS funded five studies, including three concerned with neuropsychological and behavioral effects of lead intoxication, and two that examined metabolic effects. The DRR supported a study of lead in fetal erythrocytes, an investigation of the role of lead in childhood hyperkinesis, and a study of dose–effect relationships for lead intoxication in young children. NICHD also sponsored a project to study interactions among lead and certain essential elements in pediatric development.

Epidemiology

Six federal agencies have spent $1.9 million in the last 3 years for studies of the mortality, morbidity, and lead body burdens of populations with various levels of exposure to lead (Table B.14). Eight agencies have supported an additional $800,000 worth of epidemiological research concerned with effects of metals in general. The largest effort was carried out by NIOSH, which conducted extensive surveys of the health, reproductive histories, and mortality of workers in lead industries and is pursuing work now on early signs of neurological, hematological, or renal effects of occupational exposure to lead. EPA (which reported only its fiscal year 1977 projects) studied the relationships between lead in the water supply of Boston and blood lead levels and hypertension in residents, and supported an investigation of biochemical, nutritional, and growth indicators in children with varying body burdens of lead. EPA also funded a study of the behavior and school performance of children in relation to lead levels in their teeth, and is providing some support to an anthropological expedition to Nepal in hopes that it may bring back some blood lead data typical of populations that are remote from any sources of lead pollution. EPA and NCI collaborated on a study of the incidence of cancer in communities with nonferrous smelters, and FDA and CDC joined in an effort to determine the range of typical blood lead levels in the general population of the United States. NIEHS and NHLBI provided smaller amounts of funds for several studies, including investigations of the effects of subclinical lead intoxication in preschool years on subsequent school performance, of mortality of gravure pressmen, of exposure to and effects of lead in the air in police firing ranges, and of relationships between public drinking water and urban mortality.

The aggregate level of effort in lead-related epidemiology has declined substantially in the 3 years surveyed. NIOSH and EPA completed major regulations on lead in 1978 (see Appendix C); epidemiological research in support of those actions is continuing in both agencies, but at much lower levels than those of 2 years ago.

Toxicology

Within the research programs primarily concerned with lead, toxicological studies of the effects and mechanisms of effects of lead on cells, tissues, and animals received far more support (42 percent of the total) than any other of the 18 topics considered. The nine agencies that sponsored such research spent $7.6 million on toxicology in the period surveyed, and a different combination of agencies spent another $5.5 million on multi-element toxicological tests (Table B.15).

NIEHS led the government's effort in toxicology, supporting 28 studies on lead per se and 20 related multicontaminant studies. Half (24) of the studies were concerned with effects on the developing nervous system or behavior; the remainder examined effects on the kidney, reproduction and fetal development, the immune system, several other target organs, and the functions of cells (see Table B.27, in Supplement 2 of this appendix). Over the 3-year period, the level of support NIEHS gave to toxicological studies on lead declined by one-third, while the agency's efforts in multisubstance toxicology increased about 13 percent.

DOE spent about $1 million per year in 1977 through 1979 on studies of the effects of lead and lead compounds on hematopoiesis, development and differentiation of the nervous system, hormone biosynthesis and metabolism, and behavior of animals. DOE has also investigated effects of lead on the replication of genetic material, and is sponsoring one study of mutagenic and carcinogenic effects of lead.

EPA sponsored studies of effects of lead on the developing nervous system, behavior, and the immune system in 1977, and (although it is not reported in Table B.15) work on these topics is continuing. EPA also is studying the relationships between atherosclerotic disease and trace constituents of "hard" and "soft" waters; lead is one of the factors being examined.

Other agencies supporting toxicological studies on lead include NINCDS, which has conducted neurochemical studies of effects of lead on cerebral metabolism; FDA, which sponsored a histochemical and histopathological study of effects on the central nervous system; and NIOSH, which is sponsoring a study of effects on the offspring of female rats exposed to lead. NIOSH also has begun a study of the teratogenic potential of lead and copper, and is sponsoring two studies of the carcinogenic potential of smelter dusts, conducted by NCI. NICHD has supported studies of the role of trace metals in mental retardation and congenital malformations, and NIH–DRR provided small amounts of funds for 17 studies of toxic effects of lead, primarily on the nervous system and behavior.

In summary, the strongest emphasis in government-sponsored toxicological studies on lead is clearly on effects of early exposure on the central nervous system and behavior. The several agencies that are significantly involved are using a variety of neurochemical, histological, physiological, and behavioral tests to assess toxic effects in the subclinical range. Although the level of effort in toxicology has declined from 1977, its position relative to other topics has improved. In fiscal year 1979, this category received 48 percent of federal research funds spent on lead.

Ecological Effects

In contrast to the amount spent to predict effects of lead on human health, federal expenditures to study potential hazards of lead to domestic and wild animals and ecosystems were miniscule during the last 3 years. Virtually all of the research in this category was in the multi-element class, where it accounted for less than 2 percent of the total effort. The fraction of that support that was devoted to lead probably amounted to no more than $300,000 over the period surveyed.

Table B.16 summarizes the efforts of five agencies that supported studies of ecological effects of lead. The FWS studied the accumulation of lead in bats and rodents near a highway, and assessed hazards to organisms that feed on worms and other invertebrates that have absorbed heavy metals from contaminated soils. EPA, which reported only its 1977 studies, supported investigations of the impact of air pollutants on soil systems and of the effects of geothermal effluents on aquatic fauna. NIEHS sponsored one study of the environmental distribution and biological effects of heavy metals and one on effects of nongaseous air pollutants on plants, over the 3 years surveyed.

Interactions With Other Substances

About 10 percent of the experimental research on biological effects of lead has examined the effects of other substances or conditions, especially nutritional factors, on the toxicity of lead. (Some clinical studies, discussed above, also have been concerned with this subject.) Table B.17 shows that NIEHS provided about two-thirds of the support for studies on this topic during the period surveyed. Studies funded by NIEHS explored interactions of lead with zinc, iron, general nutrition, and cadmium. FDA supported a study of interactions between lead and dietary constituents, particularly vitamin D, over the last 3 years. Projects sponsored by other agencies were either only peripherally related to lead or received very small amounts of funds.

POLLUTION CONTROL AND HAZARD ABATEMENT

This category was third among the six major topics in terms of the fraction it comprised of the research directed at lead, and it received about 10 percent of the total funds expended for both lead studies and multi-element studies over the period surveyed. The majority of studies were concerned with developing technological methods for preventing pollution; almost all of this research was the multi-element variety. Work on lead per se was concentrated in two other categories, nontechnical approaches to hazard abatement and evaluation of the effectiveness of current programs.

Development of Technological Controls

Although federal agencies spent more than $6 million on this topic in fiscal years 1977 through 1979, most of it was devoted to research by the BM on controls of emissions and runoff of trace elements from mining, smelting, and metal processing sites (Table B.18). Many of the 16 studies BM conducted were directed toward developing economic methods for the recovery of minerals from wastes and geothermal brines. This research may help preserve environmental quality, but it has very little effect on the exposure of the typical urban child to lead. EPA devoted most of its efforts in this field to studies of the treatment of industrial waste waters and sludges to remove metals. One of EPA's studies was concerned with corrosion control in water distribution systems, and another examined methods for removing metals and other pollutants from drinking water.

The only significant research program concerned primarily with the abatement of lead hazards was HUD's continuing effort to develop improved methods for removing lead paint or rendering it inaccessible to ingestion by children. HUD spent $389,000 on this research over the last 3 years, and has devoted $5.5 million to development of methods of detecting and removing lead paint hazards since 1971 (see section on HUD, below).

Nontechnological Approaches to Control

Table B.19 summarizes federal efforts in hazard abatement that did not involve development of new technology. Only three agencies were involved, and each program was quite different. HUD has spent $590,000 over the last 3 years on technical support for lead poisoning control programs, to assist local officials in choosing the most appropriate combination of currently available techniques for removing lead paint hazards. The effort is not research, but it involves the effective transfer of the results of HUD's earlier research to potential users, and is an integral part of HUD's total program. CDC also provides technical support to local governments; its expenditures in this category were for quality-control evaluations of laboratories that do blood lead analyses for lead poisoning screening programs. NIEHS sponsored three studies to test new chelating agents for use in cases of heavy metal poisoning.

There appear to be many potentially effective nontechnical forms of intervention to reduce hazards of lead poisoning (such as education of parents or provision of day care for toddlers). However, except for one project supported by HUD, the agencies included in this survey have not sponsored significant amounts of research to examine the potential effectiveness of social approaches to the control of lead hazards during the last 3 years. On the other hand, most lead poisoning control projects are sponsoring outreach and awareness programs; they are operational programs, not research activities. There would appear to be an opportunity for research to examine existing programs in order to learn which elements have had the most beneficial impacts.

Evaluation of Current Programs

The only agency that has sponsored research in this category is HUD (Table B.20); however, other agencies (such as CDC) have allocated a portion of program funds to program evaluation. Ordinarily, such activities would not be considered research, and although evaluations of programs may be going on in several agencies, they would not have been reported in the information collected for this survey.

One of HUD's projects was the study that produced this report. The others have examined blood lead data, information on lead paint hazard removal efforts, measurements of atmospheric lead levels, and other data to determine whether the number of children with seriously elevated blood lead is decreasing, and if so, what other variables may be correlated with any improvements that have been registered.

ANALYTICAL AND MEASUREMENT METHODOLOGY

Only 2 percent of the funds spent on research primarily on lead fell into this category, but about $11.7 million of the amount expended for multi-element studies went into the development of improved analytical, sampling, and monitoring methods. The amount was 18.5 percent of the total funding for multi-element studies in the 3 years studied, and placed this topic second out of the 6 categories in level of effort within that class.

Chemical Analysis of Samples

Ten agencies spent $10.3 million over the period surveyed to develop improved analytical methods (Table B.21). Only one, NBS, spent more than $100,000 on methods for lead per se. NBS has worked on improving the methods for analysis of lead in blood and other biological and environmental samples, and on developing standard reference materials for lead in particulate air pollutants, river sediments, leaded fuels, tomato leaves, oyster tissues, and bovine liver. CDC also supported one study to develop an improved method for measuring lead in blood.

The multi-element category on analytical methods is dominated by

USGS, whose program supports the vast network of geochemical sampling stations that the agency maintains (see discussion in earlier section on the topic, Levels in Environmental Media). USGS has spent $7.3 million on some 27 different projects in analytical methodology during the period covered by this survey.

FDA has spent $2.3 million in the same period; three-fourths of that amount went to support research on methods for multi-element analysis of food samples. FDA also spent substantial amounts on developing methods for analyzing laboratory animal chows and shellfish for their heavy metal and trace element contents. The FWS supported $240,000 worth of studies to improve methods for detecting heavy metal residues in fish, and to develop techniques for multi-element analysis of fish and other biological samples.

Sampling and Monitoring Methods

Research to develop improved sampling or monitoring instruments for lead or to design strategies for gathering environmental samples or establishing monitoring systems received $1.8 million in federal funds during the past 3 years (Table B.22). Of that total, $1.6 million was spent on multi-element research by two agencies. The USGS supported the largest portion of this research, in conjunction with its geochemical data gathering program. EPA supported several studies on sampling methods for aerosols, and two studies on biological monitoring (e.g., using accumulation of heavy metals by mussels to indicate pollution levels). EPA also supported a study to develop an integrated monitoring system for a multipathway pollutant, using lead as the model pollutant. NIEHS sponsored one project on the effectiveness of air filters in capturing lead particles, and the USDA spent a small amount on a study of techniques of sample preparation and storage for analyses of lead in foods.

MISCELLANEOUS LEAD RESEARCH

Only a few projects reported by the agencies, totaling about 4 percent of expenditures on the multi-element side, would not fit into one of the previous categories (Table B.23). The BM spent almost $2 million on research on the physical chemistry and thermodynamics of metallurgical processes, some of which applied to lead. BM spent $331,000 for two studies by the NRC on environmental and geochemical issues related to the development of mineral lands, and another $305,000 over the 3 years collecting and analyzing mineral commodities data. Finally, the USDA declined to indicate a subject area for $21,000 it reported that it spent on lead research.

LEAD RESEARCH PROGRAMS OF FEDERAL AGENCIES

Table B.3 compares the levels of effort of 21 federal agencies that were found to support some research on lead in the environment during fiscal years 1977 through 1979. In the sections that follow, the lead-related research program of HUD is examined in some detail, and the roles of each of the other agencies are summarized briefly. Tables B.24 through B.40, which make up Supplement 2 of this appendix, present details of the expenditures of each agency according to the topics investigated. The discussions here assess the relative magnitude of effort and general subject areas studied by each agency in the last 3 years, and place the lead research programs in the context of each agency's basic missions and its overall research program. Important specific studies supported by different agencies were mentioned earlier in summaries of research on each topic; that information is not repeated here.

U.S. DEPARTMENT OF HOUSING AND URBAN DEVELOPMENT

During the last 3 fiscal years, HUD supported $2.3 million worth of studies primarily concerned with lead, or 12.6 percent of the total federal program in lead research. Although three other agencies ranked ahead of HUD in total spending for lead research, HUD was the leading source of support in each of the four topics on which it supported studies. Those topics, and HUD's fraction of the federal research effort in each case, were: contributions of specific sources to exposures (80 percent), technological methods for abatement of lead hazards (98 percent), nontechnological approaches to control (87 percent), and evaluation of the effectiveness of current programs (100 percent).

HUD's lead research program grows out of its mission as the focal agency in the government's effort to eliminate the problem of childhood lead poisoning from leaded paints in old housing units (see Appendix C). In order to assess the appropriateness of the research for meeting that goal, it is necessary to examine the research program HUD has conducted since the agency began lead research in 1971.

Evolution of HUD's Lead Research Program

The Lead-Based Paint Poisoning Prevention Act of 1971 (PL 91-695) and subsequent amendments to it gave HUD a broad mandate to conduct research and demonstrations related to lead paint hazards. In the past 9 years, HUD has spent nearly $9 million on lead research, in three temporal phases; the objectives of the program have changed with each transition to a new phase, as shown in Table B.4. The initial phase

TABLE B.4   Research Priorities of HUD'S Lead-Based Paint Poisoning Prevention Research Program, 1971-1978.

Phase I: Spring 1971 to Fall 1973
  1. Determine Nature and Extent of Problem
  2. Evaluate Current Methods and Techniques for Hazard Detection and Removal
  3. Support Development of Innovative Methods and Techniques for Hazard Detection and Removal if Required
  4. Demonstration of Selected Lead Hazard Removal Programs in Cities
  5. Provide Cities with Technical Backup
  6. Provide a Report to the Congress
Phase II: Fall 1973 to Winter 1976
  1. Define Lead-Based Paint Hazard on Surfaces
  2. Determine Extent of Lead-Based Paint Problem in Housing
  3. Determine Extent of Lead Poisoning Problem in Children
  4. Improve Lead Detection Methods
  5. Improve Hazard Elimination Methods
  6. Improvement of Local Programs and Resource Identification
  7. Disseminate and Utilize Research Products
Phase III: Winter 1976 to Spring 1978
  1. Field Testing and Evaluation of New Hazard Abatement Technology
  2. Demonstration and Increasing Utilization of New or Innovative Hazard Abatement Technology
  3. Continuing Identification and Development of New or Innovative Hazard Abatement Technology
  4. Improvement of Local Program Capabilities
  5. Evaluation of the Effectiveness of Lead-Based Paint Hazard Abatement in Controlling Elevated Lead Levels in Children
  6. Monitoring of the Extent of Lead Poisoning in Urban Children

(1971–1973) was concerned chiefly with defining the dimensions of the lead paint problem and assessing the state-of-the-art for detecting and removing lead paint hazards, as part of a required report to the Congress. Phase I also identified major research needs in these areas. In Phase II (1973–1976), the evaluation of existing hazards and abatement techniques continued, and greater emphasis was put on developing new methods of detecting and removing lead paint, in order to improve the cost-effectiveness of local lead poisoning control projects. Phase III (1976–1978) was concerned primarily with further development of improved paint hazard abatement methods, with transfer of results to potential users, and with evaluating the progress that has been made toward reduction of children's blood lead levels since the 1971 legislation was enacted.

Table B.5 summarizes the funding allocated to eight research goals during HUD's 9-year program. By far the greatest share of the funds

($5.5 million) has been spent on evaluating or developing technological methods to detect and remove lead paint hazards (research objectives 3 through 7 in the table). About one-fourth of the research ($2 million) has been devoted to efforts to determine the nature and extent of the lead paint hazard, and the relative role of paint as a source of lead in the bodies of urban children (objectives 1 and 2 in the table).

Present Status of the Research Program

The report on HUD's in-house evaluation of its lead research (Billick and Gray 1978) concludes that many of the goals of the program have been achieved: (a) the report to Congress was delivered; (b) new, improved lead-detecting instruments and calibration standards have been developed and tested, and are now commercially available; (c) the effectiveness and costs of myriad methods for removing paint have been systematically evaluated; (d) nearly $2 million has been spent on development of new and improved hazard abatement methods (with limited success); and (e) extensive data have been gathered that document the occurrence of lead paint hazards in housing, the occurrence of lead in children's blood, and the relationship between these two variables.

At present, HUD's lead research has entered a new (fourth) phase. Few new contracts have been let for hazard abatement research since 1976; instead, efforts have been concentrated on providing technical assistance to help local lead control officials choose up-to-date and appropriate methods to meet their specific needs. Further research to improve abatement methods is being deferred for three reasons: (1) in HUD's judgment, significant progress in identifying and developing methods of choice and evaluating their cost-effectiveness has been made; (2) research managers at HUD are highly skeptical that a "technical fix" to the lead paint hazard can be achieved at any reasonable cost; and (3) results of HUD's recent epidemiological studies have caused HUD to question the long-held assumption (fundamental to the 1971 legislation) that removal of lead paint would eliminate lead poisoning in children. (See Chapter 2 for more discussion of the substance of these issues.) In the current fiscal year, most of the $725,000 HUD will spend on lead research is supporting environmental and epidemiological studies to improve knowledge of the relative contribution of different environmental sources to total lead exposure.

HUD is now looking to this Committee for recommendations on the level of effort it should devote to technical aspects of paint hazard abatement; on the relative importance of research on abatement and of research to quantify sources of lead exposure; and on whether work on the latter topic, if important, should be done by HUD or by other agencies.

TABLE B.5 Lead Research Contracts Supported by HUD in Various Subject Areas, 1971-1979[a]

Topic	1971-1976		FY 1977		FY 1978		FY 1979[b]	
	No.	$1,000's	No.	$1,000's	No.	$1,000's	No.	$1,000's
1. Nature and extent of lead paint hazard	4	887	—	—	—	—	—	—
2. Nature, sources, and extent of lead poisoning	5	515	3	100	2	26	4	425
3. Existing methods of detection/analysis	1	337	—	—	—	—	—	—
4. Improved methods of detection/analysis	6	545	—	—	—	—	—	—
5. Existing methods of hazard abatement	6	1,797	—	—	—	—	—	—
6. New/improved methods of hazard abatement	18	1,663	3	128	5	161	1	100
7. Technical assistance to local programs	1	185	1	282	2	208	1	100
8. Evaluate effectiveness of efforts to date	2	629	—	—	3	379	1	100
9. Miscellaneous contracts[c]	10+	94	—	—	1	254	—	—
TOTALS	53+	6,652	7	510	13	1,028	7	725

[a] Information from Appendix C of Billick and Gray (1978), and from personal communications from I. H. Billick and V. E. Gray, Lead Based Paint Poisoning Prevention Research Program, HUD, 1979.

[b] Estimates.

[c] Includes several small contracts (less than $10,000) prior to 1977, and the contract with the National Academy of Sciences in FY 1978.

U.S. ENVIRONMENTAL PROTECTION AGENCY

EPA is a regulatory agency, and six separate laws give EPA authority to set standards for lead (see Appendix C). The primary purpose of research in EPA is to support the agency's regulatory activities. EPA's appropriation for research and development is $328 million for fiscal year 1979; about one-third of that will be spent on in-house research and the remainder will support contracts, interagency agreements or grants to individual scientists (U.S. EPA 1977). The CRS (1979) reports that EPA spent about $20 million in fiscal year 1977 for research on trace contaminants.

Table B.24 summarizes EPA's lead research in fiscal year 1977 (no data are available for 1978 and 1979). In 1977, EPA supported $822,000 worth of research that was primarily concerned with lead, and an additional $3.7 million worth of multipollutant studies that included lead. These amounts were 12 and 18 percent, respectively, of total federal spending in each category in fiscal year 1977. For that year, EPA ranked third in support of lead research and second among the agencies in expenditures for multi-element studies.

From EPA's perspective, health protection is the chief reason for its regulations, and toxicology and epidemiology are its top research priorities, accounting for 75 percent of the funds spent for studies primarily concerned with lead in fiscal year 1977. Assessments of human exposures and uptake accounted for 13 percent, and a study to develop an integrated monitoring system drew 11 percent of the funding. EPA's multi-element studies were more evenly divided among biological effects (34 percent), control techniques (22 percent), analytical methods (22 percent), and sources and environmental pathways (21 percent). In virtually every subject area in which it was active, EPA ranked second or third among the agencies in level of effort for fiscal year 1977, yielding first place to agencies with more specialized missions in each case while maintaining a broad, balanced program of its own.

EPA faces pending regulatory decisions on several lead issues (see Appendix C), and the agency's lead research is continuing with a varied agenda of projects. In the absence of complete data on fiscal years 1978 and 1979, trends in either the level of effort or the topics investigated cannot be assessed.

In addition to the original investigations it supports, EPA has devoted a considerable amount of its resources recently to preparing reports that compile, integrate, and assess current knowledge of lead and its effects. Six of the major reports reviewed in Appendix A were products of such efforts by EPA. Although they are not always considered "research," studies to prepare such documents have been a substantial, important fraction of EPA's recent contributions on lead.

FOOD AND DRUG ADMINISTRATION

FDA, like EPA, is a regulatory agency, and its research priorities are set largely in response to or in anticipation of regulatory needs. Under its enabling legislation, FDA has authority to set limits on contaminants in foods; and the agency's Bureau of Foods is now preparing to propose a comprehensive program to restrict lead levels in foods, especially canned foods to which young children may be exposed (see Appendix C). Research on lead therefore has a relatively high priority within the bureau at present.

In the last 3 years FDA spent about $13.1 million for research on all trace elements (CRS 1979). Of that total, the agency spent $2.5 million on lead research and another $2.6 million on multi-element studies that included lead. These amounts are 14 percent of the federal effort in lead research (placing FDA third among agencies) and 4 percent of the total in multi-element studies (sixth place). FDA's level of effort in lead research per se has declined somewhat during the last 3 years, but may increase again as the agency prepares to regulate lead content in foods. Most of this research has been done in-house; a small part has been conducted through contracts or interagency agreements.

FDA's research on lead (Table B.25) is designed to assess human exposures to lead through foods and housewares, and the possible hazards to health posed by them. The agency devoted 63 percent of its recent lead research effort to surveys of dietary exposures, and 89 percent of the expenditures for multi-element studies were spent on developing analytical methods to support those surveys. FDA spent more to determine lead levels in foods than any other agency, and ranked second in level of effort on analytical methods. Research on biological effects accounted for 30 percent of FDA's lead-focused studies in the 3 years surveyed; most of the work on this topic consisted of toxicology and studies of interactions between lead and other dietary constituents. FDA sponsored only 6 percent of the total on biological effects of lead, but this was sufficient to place the agency fourth among federal agencies in support for toxicological studies in each of the 3 years studied.

NATIONAL INSTITUTE OF ENVIRONMENTAL HEALTH SCIENCES

NIEHS, one of the National Institutes of Health, supports and conducts a broad research program in the biomedical sciences, with particular emphasis on studies of the metabolism, mechanisms of toxicity, and health effects of enviromental contaminants. NIEHS sees its mission as providing a bridge between broadly focused, basic research in biology and toxicology and the more narrow information needs of EPA, FDA, and other regulatory agencies. For fiscal year 1979, the research budget of NIEHS was $78 million; about $8.5 million of that was spent on trace element studies (CRS 1979). Most of the work the institute supports is conducted extramurally, through grants and contracts.

Tables B.26 and B.27 summarize lead-related research supported by NIEHS during the period surveyed. NIEHS spent $5.5 million for studies that were primarily concerned with lead; 99 percent of the research dealt with exposures, uptake, and biological effects. That work was 30.5 percent of the total federal effort on lead in fiscal years 1977 through 1979. For that period, NIEHS was the largest source of funds for research on lead (all topics combined), and ranked fourth in terms of support for multi-element studies. Research on multiple contaminants also emphasized exposure, absorption, and effects (90 percent of the total), but included some studies of the environmental distribution and fate of pollutants and a small program to develop new chelating agents for the treatment of metal poisoning.

Within the scope of its research on health hazards of lead, NIEHS divided its efforts among toxicology (50 percent), absorption and pharmacodynamics (16 percent), interactions (16 percent), clinical studies (13 percent), epidemiology (3 percent), and assessment of exposures (1 percent). NIEHS was the top-ranked agency in support of studies of interactions between lead and other substances, investigations of uptake and pharmacology of lead, and clinical studies of lead poisoning. The agency also spent the greatest amount on toxicological research (including lead projects and multi-element studies) of all the agencies, although DOE spent more for toxicological research on lead alone. Table B.27 shows the topics of the toxicological studies NIEHS has sponsored. More than half of the studies have examined effects on the central nervous system and behavior.

In neurobiology and in other areas, NIEHS has supported integrated multidisciplinary programs that combine epidemiological, physiological, biochemical, metabolic, morphological, and behavioral methods for assessing the biological effects of lead. Subclinical effects and the refinement of methods to measure them have been prominent concerns in many of the recent studies NIEHS has supported.

Table B.26 shows that research specifically concerned with lead has received progressively decreasing funding from NIEHS over the past 3 years, although funding for multimetal studies has increased slightly. (On the other hand, a more recent and more detailed analysis of grants and contracts supported by NIEHS in 1977, 1978, and 1979 suggests that the *total* spent for projects that include lead—both primary lead research and multi-element studies—has remained about about the same level [$3.8 million per year] since 1977 [Alan Hough, Extramural Programs, NIEHS, personal communication, April 1979]. The decline in projects focused specifically on lead may have been offset by an increased number of multi-element investigations that include lead. Also, funds on lead per se may have been awarded in excess of the estimates given to Congress in mid-1978, the chief source of our information.)

To the extent that support for studies on lead has in fact declined, the trend suggests that lead research reached its highest priority in the mid-1970s, and that the attention of NIEHS has begun to turn toward other anticipated or emerging problems where research needs are perceived to be more urgent. However, since scientific merit reviews of research proposals are the direct basis for the allocation of funds by NIEHS, the trend may also indicate changes in the interests of the biomedical research community as a whole, or in the quality of proposals received.

OTHER INSTITUTES OF THE NATIONAL INSTITUTES OF HEALTH

NIEHS sponsored nearly 80 percent of the research on lead supported by NIH in the last 3 years, but 4 other institutes of NIH and the Division of Research Resources also provided some funds for lead studies. The work included both intramural and extramural projects, but the fraction in each category was not indicated in the information available. The collective efforts of NIH are summarized in Table B.28, and broken down by institutes in Table B.29.

With the exception of NICHD, which supported a substantial share of the clinical studies of lead poisoning, none of the institutes played a large role in any aspect of research on lead and health. However, taken collectively, NIH provided $1.2 million of support for studies on lead, and $1.6 million of additional funds for relevant multi-element research. These expenditures included 9 and 16 percent, respectively, of the support for work on absorption, pharmacodynamics, and biological effects in those two classes of research.

National Institute of Child Health and Human Development

NICHD has spent $896,000 over the last 3 years for clinical investigations of developmental effects of low-level lead exposure and nutritional interactions among lead, calcium, phosphorus, magnesium, and zinc. These two studies account for 46 percent of the total federal effort in clinical studies of lead poisoning in the period surveyed. NICHD also has sponsored toxicological investigations that are partly concerned with lead, including studies of trace metals in mental retardation, trace metals and congenital malformations, neurobiology of environmental pollutants, and interactions among trace metals, which cost a total of $245,000 over the last 3 fiscal years.

National Institute of Neurological and Communicative Disorders and Stroke

NINCDS is currently supporting a study on the neurochemistry of lead poisoning and one on cerebral metabolism in newborn and young lead-poisoned animals, at a combined cost of $344,000 for the 3 years surveyed. NINCDS also supports a study of animal models of neurological disease ($536,000 over 3 years), which is concerned with the effects of lead and other toxins on the central nervous system.

National Heart, Lung, and Blood Institute

The NHLBI has given limited support to several epidemiological studies concerned with exposure of the general population to trace elements, including a study (with EPA) of exposure to lead through drinking water in Boston, investigations of exposure to trace elements in Seattle and of trace elements in human tissues in Missouri, a more general survey of exposure to trace metals through drinking water, and a study of public water supplies and urban mortality. The total funding for these 5 studies was $165,000 for the 3 years examined.

National Cancer Institute

NCI spent only $234,000 for research related to lead in the period covered by this survey, and all the work was concerned primarily with substances other than lead. NCI carried out two studies for NIOSH on the carcinogenicity of smelter dusts, and supported an epidemiological study of the incidence of lung cancer in communities with nonferrous smelters, conducted by EPA. NCI appears to be supporting no research that is concerned primarily with the possible role of lead in environmental carcinogenesis. (However, DOE has sponsored one study on this topic.)

Division of Research Resources

The DRR provides assistance in a variety of ways for some of the 13,000 extramural projects that NIH sponsors. In general, DRR provides backup resources for projects that have other support, either through one of the NIH institutes or from another source altogether. DRR supports regional primate centers and similar animal colonies; provides special-purpose grants to investigators with ongoing funding from NIH, NIMH, or the PHS;

makes high-cost equipment available to investigators who could not otherwise afford it; provides hospital facilities and ancillary support for clinical studies; and supports programs to enhance the opportunities for minority students to choose careers in the biomedical sciences.

At least 34 projects that are concerned with lead received some support from DRR during the period covered by this survey. Since DRR support is supplemental to other funds, the amount DRR spent was relatively small—only $681,000 over the 3 years. The resources were divided among the following topics (with the percentage spent on each): clinical studies (21), toxicology (16), environmental fate (14), occurrence in water (14), interactions (12), epidemiology (10), ecological effects (7), and pharmacodynamics (6). Through DRR, NIH plays a small part in supporting a much broader range of studies related to lead than those that receive their major support through any of the specialized institutes except NIEHS.

Other Institutes of NIH

Certain other studies with broad objectives that NIH supports probably include lead among the substances investigated. For instance, the National Institute on Aging is sponsoring two studies, one on trace elements and enzymatic activity in tissues, and another on effects of metals and proteins on nucleic acids and information transfer, from the perspective of assessing factors in the aging process. The National Institute of General Medical Sciences supports several studies on trace element analysis in biological samples and on the biochemical behavior and functions of metals. It is not possible to estimate the extent to which such studies involve lead, but it seems likely that not all lead-related studies supported by NIH have been included in this survey.

Summary of NIH Research

With the possible exception of NINCDS, none of these institutes has an integrated, continuing program objective in lead research. The information summarized in Table B.28 does not suggest any consistent trends in support of lead studies by NIH. The total declined sharply in fiscal year 1979 largely because of the completion of two studies supported by NICHD. Since each institute of NIH has its own objectives, and awards grants on the basis of the scientific merit of proposals, it seems likely that NIH will continue to support a variety of studies related to lead at some level, as long as they address scientifically important questions. The support should be relatively independent of the national level of interest in lead as a regulatory problem.

NATIONAL INSTITUTE FOR OCCUPATIONAL SAFETY AND HEALTH

Although it is located administratively in the Center for Disease Control of the Department of Health, Education, and Welfare, NIOSH was created chiefly to provide scientific support for the regulations and standards enacted by the Occupational Safety and Health Administration of the Department of Labor. OSHA issued a final revised standard for occupational exposure to inorganic lead in November 1978 (see Appendix C). In preparation for that action, the NIOSH criteria document on lead, first issued in 1973, was substantially revised and updated. (See Appendix A for a summary of that document.) While the revision was in progress (1976–1978), research on lead had high priority in NIOSH. During that period NIOSH spent about $2 million on in-house studies related to lead, and more than $300,000 on extramural lead-related research. In comparison, NIOSH spent a total of $39 million for research, including $3.9 million on extramural grants, in fiscal year 1978. In the 3 years covered by this survey, NIOSH devoted $1.2 million to studies of the effects of occupational exposures to lead, and another $253,000 to related multicontaminant studies. The research is summarized in Table B.30.

Most of the research NIOSH supported that was strictly concerned with lead consisted of epidemiological studies of workers in lead industries; the agency also initiated a toxicological study on effects of lead on reproduction, to pursue a suggestion of such hazards gained from studies of occupational groups. NIOSH was the leading federal agency in epidemiological research, spending 57 percent of the government's total outlays for such studies in the last 3 years. The effort represented 6 percent of the total federal program over that time, and placed NIOSH fifth among agencies in terms of total support for studies on lead.

The work that NIOSH supported under the multi-element category consists of toxicological studies of the bioavailability and carcinogenicity of components of smelter dusts. The agency also conducted one small in-house study of control techniques to minimize worker exposure to harmful agents (among them lead) in secondary nonferrous smelters. In the future, the emphasis of lead research in NIOSH will probably shift away from health and toward assessments of control techniques needed to implement the new standards that OSHA has established.

CENTER FOR DISEASE CONTROL

Title I of the Lead-Based Paint Poisoning Prevention Act of 1971 called for federally supported screening programs to identify children with elevated blood lead levels. Under subsequent amendments to the legislation and interagency agreements, the surveillance programs are carried out by local agencies, with funding and technical assistance provided primarily through the CDC (see Appendix C). The small amount of research that CDC conducts in support of its public health programs is a very modest part of the government's lead research effort (2 percent of the total). In the past 3 fiscal years, CDC has spent a total of about $400,000 on 4 projects concerned with blood lead screening programs. The research included a study to improve and validate analytical methods for blood lead and erythrocyte protoporphyrin, a toxicological study, an epidemiological study to determine the normative distribution of blood lead levels in the U.S. population, lab support for studies of lead exposure in high-risk areas (e.g., near smelters), and technical assistance to and quality assessments of 105 laboratories involved in regional childhood lead poisoning detection programs. Table B.31 shows the amounts CDC spent on each of these topics during the period surveyed.

The data gathered through CDC-sponsored local screening programs are a valuable information base for further epidemiological research, but CDC's primary mission in this area is to detect and prevent childhood lead poisoning. The use of such data for research purposes therefore will depend largely on the interests and priorities of other agencies.

U.S. DEPARTMENT OF ENERGY

DOE spent $4.6 billion on research and development in fiscal year 1979; only the Department of Defense spent more. DOE's broad research program encompasses the development and demonstration of new energy technologies; integrated assessments of the health, environmental, and social impacts of different energy systems; and basic science in support of these objectives (U.S. Energy Research and Development Administration 1976). DOE spent an estimated $537 million on environmental research in fiscal year 1979, according to the U.S. OMB (1979); $11.2 million worth of the research was concerned with environmental pollution by trace substances released in the extraction, processing, or combustion of fossil fuels, or in the development and use of nuclear, geothermal, or other forms of energy (CRS 1979). Lead is a common trace contaminant in coal and may be released in the production, use, or recycling of batteries; consequently, DOE supported about $3.3 million worth of research directed at lead during the 1977 through 1979 fiscal years, and another $9.3 million worth of related multi-element studies.

The multi-element research that DOE supports amounts to almost 15 percent of total federal spending in this category, and consists of studies of emissions, environmental transport, and biological fates of trace contaminants in general (Table B.32). DOE spent more than any other agency ($4.2 million) on research to characterize sources of trace elements, and was the second largest source of support for studies of the environmental behavior and cycling of pollutants. DOE also supported a major program to measure contaminants in human food chains.

All the research supported by DOE that was specific to lead fell into one subject area, toxicology. DOE was first among the agencies in support of toxicological studies of lead; the $3.3 million that DOE spent on this topic exceeded the combined total of NIEHS and FDA (which ranked second and third) for the period of this survey (Table B.15). DOE's expenditures were 43 percent of the government total on toxicology of lead, and 18 percent of the federal support for all research that was primarily concerned with lead.

In short, because some energy processes release lead into the environment, DOE has a substantial research interest in the environmental behavior and biological effects of this element. The studies that involve lead amount to less than 1 percent of DOE's environmental program but they represent more than one-sixth of the total federal effort in lead research.

U.S. BUREAU OF MINES

The Bureau of Mines of the Department of the Interior conducts mission-oriented research to support efficient, environmentally sound development of mineral resources. The BM spent $8.5 million on multi-element studies relevant to lead in the last 3 fiscal years, and its level of effort in this research increased by 57 percent from 1977 to 1979. The BM provided 13.5 percent of total federal funding for multi-element studies in the period surveyed, and ranked third among the agencies in that category. None of the BM's research was primarily concerned with lead, and most was only marginally relevant to the subject of this survey.

Table B.33 shows how BM spent its funds for research related to lead. More than $5 million (63 percent) was devoted to studies of methods for reducing or preventing environmental impacts of mining, mineral processing, and metal producing industries, and another 7 percent was put into closely related efforts to identify the characteristics of such sources. The BM's work on control techniques was far and away the largest effort by any agency on methods for preventing environmental pollution by trace elements (Table B.18). The BM also gave $331,000 to the NRC for independent assessments of some of these problems, and spent the remainder of its total (27 percent) on miscellaneous studies related to production of metals, but only peripherally relevant to lead in the environment.

U.S. GEOLOGICAL SURVEY

The U.S. Geological Survey, in the Department of the Interior, has broad research responsibilities for assessing national mineral, energy, and water resources. In the current (1979) fiscal year, the USGS appropriation for research and development was about $640 million. That research included the collection and analysis of geochemical samples of rocks, soils, waters, and vegetation, obtained from thousands of sites around the country. In USGS environmental surveys, samples are analyzed for up to 50 or 60 elements, including lead. The results of USGS geochemical research are published in many forms; a recent professional paper on lead is summarized in Appendix A of this report.

Few of the projects USGS has supported are concerned with single elements; all of the work related to lead falls in the multi-element category (Table B.34). In the period covered by this survey, USGS spent $29.7 million for studies of the occurrence and geochemical cycling of trace elements in the environment, and for development of related analytical methods. USGS spent more than any other agency on each of these topics, and this research accounted for nearly half of the total federal effort on multi-element studies that include lead. However, because of the great number of elements included in USGS surveys, only a small fraction of the total (perhaps $1 million over the 3 years) is likely to have been spent gathering data on lead.

U.S. FISH AND WILDLIFE SERVICE

The U.S. Fish and Wildlife Service, in the Department of the Interior, monitors the occurrence of environmental pollutants in wildlife, fish, and shellfish, and conducts research to evaluate potential physiological and ecological effects of toxic substances on fish and wildlife species. The OMB (1979) estimates that the FWS will spend about $54 million on environmental research in fiscal year 1980.

Table B.35 summarizes research that the FWS conducted on the environmental occurrence and effects of trace metals in fiscal years 1977 through 1979. None of the studies was concerned exclusively with lead. The FWS effort is a modest one; the 3-year total of $1 million is only 1.6 percent of total federal spending on multi-element studies that include lead. Nevertheless, the $700,000 that FWS spent on studies of ecological and physiological effects of heavy metals on wildlife species was 57 percent of the total spent by all agencies on that topic. The remainder of FWS research shown in the table was devoted primarily to monitoring pollutant levels in fish and developing analytical methods to support that program. Two small projects examined the influence of human activities on levels of trace metals in the environment.

During the last decade, the FWS has done additional work on specific hazards to wildlife posed by lead, especially on lead poisoning in waterfowl that eat lead shot. More recently, however, the emphasis in FWS wildlife studies has shifted toward a broader concern with the impacts on wildlife of general environmental pollution by metals. The level of effort in FWS research on lead and other metals has increased slightly over the 3-year period.

OFFICE OF WATER RESEARCH AND TECHNOLOGY

The OWRT of the Department of the Interior is responsible for a wide spectrum of research on the nature and quality of the nation's water resources. OWRT's studies on water quality include the collection of biogeochemical data on elements in aquatic ecosystems, and a limited number of investigations of biological effects of pollutants and of techniques for controlling contaminants. Most of the studies OWRT conducts are concerned with many substances; however, the information that the agency provided included an element-by-element breakdown of expenditures. Table B.36, therefore, shows amounts spent on lead alone in the context of multi-element studies. The data include only the 1977 and 1978 fiscal years. In that time, OWRT spent $205,000 on studies of lead; two-thirds of that amount was allocated to studies of the environmental geochemistry of the element. If it is assumed that only 5 to 10 percent of the cost of multi-element studies on that topic is rightfully assigned to lead, the OWRT effort seems to be at about the same level in this area as that of DOE (see Table B.8). OWRT contributions on other topics, however, were generally an insignificant fraction of the total government program.

NATIONAL BUREAU OF STANDARDS

The NBS, part of the U.S. Department of Commerce, conducts research to develop standard methods and reference materials for the chemical analysis and measurement of innumerable substances, including many environmental pollutants. NBS has spent $130,000 for work on improved analysis of lead in the period surveyed (see Table B.37). The entire budgetary appropriation for NBS for fiscal year 1979 is only $87 million; however, the Center for Analytical Chemistry of NBS provides analytical support on a contract basis for many studies sponsored by other agencies. In this manner, the role of NBS in lead research has been enlarged beyond its studies in analytical chemistry. For instance, NBS has provided technical assistance to HUD throughout the latter agency's 9 years of research on lead paint hazards, and has assisted CDC by checking the accuracy of blood lead analyses performed by the laboratories employed by local projects supported by CDC. (For a list of NBS technical publications on lead paint research, see Appendix D of the report by Billick and Gray [1978].)

NATIONAL OCEANIC AND ATMOSPHERIC ADMINISTRATION

NOAA, presently part of the U.S. Department of Commerce, conducts a broad-based program of research to map the oceans and coastal zones, to understand and predict weather and climate, and to monitor and predict changes in the environment. NOAA will spend about $474 million in fiscal year 1980 on environmental research (U.S. OMB 1979). Only one research activity of NOAA is significant in terms of lead; that is the ongoing program of the National Marine Fisheries Service measuring microconstituents in edible fish tissues, which absorbed $1.5 million over the last 3 years (Table B.38). The NMFS collects data on the occurrence of 15 or more elements (including lead) in more than 200 species of fish. The funds spent on this project represented 41 percent of the government's reported expenditures on studies of trace elements in human food chains (Table B.10); NOAA ranked second, behind DOE, on that topic.

U.S. DEPARTMENT OF AGRICULTURE

The USDA conducts research to support efficient production of crops and livestock, to improve the yield and quality of foods, and to promote the conservation and proper use of soil and forest resources. USDA will spend an estimated $664 million on research in fiscal year 1980. The CRS (1979) estimates that USDA's programs in crop and animal sciences, nutrition, and soil and environmental sciences include about $10 million worth of research on trace elements each year, and some of the research includes lead. Table B.39 summarizes the amounts spent on lead research by USDA in fiscal year 1977. USDA provided information only for that year, and broke the data down into element-by-element expenditures. Even though most of the studies involved several elements, the level of effort in multi-element studies cannot be determined from the available information.

USDA's role in lead research is small (less than 1 percent of the total federal effort), and is likely to decrease. A few years ago, scientists at the Agricultural Environmental Quality Institute in the USDA Beltsville Agricultural Research Center studied the deposition and fate of lead and other metals in soils and vegetation along highways and near smelters. That work has been completed, and the topic has been abandoned in favor of other priorities. Similarly, USDA investigated the fate of lead in sludges applied to soils, but the results suggested that lead is not readily taken up by crops, and the emphasis of the research has shifted to cadmium and other toxic hazards. Current research at USDA involving lead includes studies of the biochemical basis of interactions between lead stress and vitamin E deficiency in rats, and support of efforts by states to develop capabilities to include lead and cadmium in analyses of soil samples from urban gardens.

NATIONAL SCIENCE FOUNDATION

NSF has the fifth largest research budget among federal agencies, with an estimated research appropriation of $819 million in fiscal year 1979. Several of NSF's programs are concerned with environmental trace substances and with effects of pollutants on health and ecosystems. Earlier in this decade, NSF supported a 6-year, multimillion dollar study of environmental pollution by lead, which was completed in 1977. Since then NSF has been only minimally involved in support of research on heavy metals. Table B.40 shows that NSF sponsored only three projects on lead in fiscal years 1977 through 1979, and only one—an assessment of health and related effects of lead—is now under way. The other two studies in 1977 were the completion of the 6-year study mentioned above and a small pilot project to examine the feasibility of an attempt to trace sources of lead in children with elevated blood lead levels.

NSF also supports many multi-element projects that are concerned with the occurrence, geochemistry, and health and ecological effects of trace substances. Some of the projects in this category may include lead, but no breakdown is available of the research according to elements covered. NSF spent $2.63 million in fiscal year 1977 and $1.49 million in fiscal year 1978 on multi-element studies, and it expected to support about the same amount of work in this category when all of its fiscal year 1979 funds were awarded.

OTHER FEDERAL AGENCIES

The Alcohol, Drug Abuse, and Mental Health Administration, a unit of the Public Health Service in the Department of HEW, supported one study on the toxic effects of lead, copper, and mercury on the uptake and metabolism of substrates by brain tissue, completed in fiscal year 1977. Several other federal agencies have major environmental or health research programs, and at least one other agency (CPSC) has made a recent regulatory decision on lead. However, neither the information on trace element research that the agencies gave to Congress nor inquiries by the staff of this Committee have indicated that agencies not discussed above are currently supporting or conducting significant amounts of research on lead. This conclusion applies to the Department of Defense, Department of Transportation, the National Aeronautics and Space Administration, the Veterans Administration, the Smithsonian Institution, and the Council on Environmental Quality. Some other agencies, such as the Department of State or the Treasury Department, were not contacted because of the small likelihood that they would be involved in any research related to lead in the environment.

The Consumer Product Safety Commission enacted regulations in 1978 that limit the sale and use of lead-based paints (see Appendix C). While that action was under consideration, CPSC supported some research on lead, including a study by the NRC to determine a safe level of lead in paint. However, when the regulations had been promulgated, CPSC's research priorities shifted to other problems, and the agency currently is not supporting any studies on lead.

INTERAGENCY COORDINATION

The summary of research in subject areas identified several topics on which a large number of agencies appear to be gathering similar data. This is particularly true in the health field; 17 different agencies support toxicological studies on lead or related multi-element research. The apparent potential for overlap suggests a need for coordination among agencies to avoid excessive duplication of efforts, to speed the transfer of research results to potential users, and to help ensure an adequate breadth of coverage by the government's program as a whole.

Myers et al. (1978) examined the coordination of federal research on toxic substances and assessed the effectiveness of seven different coordinating mechanisms. The most widely used and highly rated form of coordination was informal contact among scientists and administrators of the agencies. Formal and informal multi-agency coordinating committees and joint sponsorship of projects were also rated as effective mechanisms. (Reliance on outside advisory groups, such as NAS, was ranked lowest of the mechanisms considered.)

Each of the effective mechanisms for coordination cited by Myers et al. has been used in federal lead research, at least in the last few years. The high level of regulatory activities on lead in the last 5 years (Appendix C) has prompted extensive contacts among agencies, especially the regulatory bodies, to exchange information and to attempt to coordinate research on topics of mutual interest. Representatives of the various agencies agreed, in a discussion at the Committee's October 1978 meeting, that participation in hearings and other less formal contacts among their staffs had been the most common and effective form of interaction.

Nevertheless, there is no shortage of more formal mechanisms to coordinate lead research. A number of jointly sponsored studies were noted in the summaries of federal research programs. The Interagency Regulatory Liaison Group (IRLG), which consists of the heads of EPA, FDA, OSHA, CPSC, and the Food Safety and Quality Service of USDA, was formed in 1978 to coordinate the regulatory and research efforts of the participating agencies. An IRLG task force recently completed an assessment of research on metals by EPA, FDA, CPSC, OSHA, NIOSH, NIEHS, and NCI and found no significant duplication of efforts (Williams et al. 1978). IRLG has supported several other task forces that were concerned with lead, mostly in the regulatory realm.

Another factor that has contributed to coordination of lead research is the predominant emphasis on health aspects by most of the agencies involved. Eleven agencies collectively supported 95 percent of the toxicological studies on lead in the last 3 years, and only two of them (EPA and DOE) are not divisions of HEW (see Table B.15). HEW established a formal Committee to Coordinate Toxicology and Related Programs in 1973, and in 1978 created the National Toxicology Program to coordinate and set priorities for toxicological research. An executive committee that includes the heads of OSHA, EPA, and CPSC will oversee the new program. The health-related research on lead summarized earlier in this appendix is a diversified, balanced program, suggesting that some effective coordination has taken place.

In short, there has been a considerable amount of contact among many of the agencies involved in lead research, and coordination appears to have been relatively effective. Nevertheless, a number of opportunities exist to improve coordination. HUD and CDC, which have major responsibilities for preventing childhood lead poisoning, might profitably participate in IRLG activities related to lead. Also, the regulatory agencies could benefit from expanded contacts with their more research-oriented colleagues in agencies like USGS, DOE, BM, FWS, NOAA, and USDA. Much of the research conducted by these nonregulatory agencies is similar in nature to some studies conducted by EPA and FDA; however, the programs differ in scope, purpose, and kinds of information collected, according to the diverse missions of the agencies. While the nonregulatory agencies could not be expected to change the basic thrust of their research programs, increased awareness of each other's research needs could potentially uncover some broad areas of mutual interest to those agencies and the regulatory bodies.

LEAD RESEARCH SUPPORTED BY INDUSTRY

The primary concern of this survey has been with research on lead performed or supported by agencies of the U.S. federal government. Extensive work on lead in the environment and on biological effects of lead has also been carried out in many other countries, and in this country some additional lead research has been sponsored by state or local agencies, or by nongovernmental entities. It is not intended that the contributions of research done outside the auspices of the federal government be overlooked or made to seem unimportant; however, neither the scope of this study nor the resources available for it allowed this survey to include *all* research on lead.

Nevertheless, to present a balanced picture, some research supported by the industries that produce, smelt, and refine lead and zinc throughout the world was included in the survey. Those industries have formed a nonprofit corporation, the International Lead Zinc Research Organization, Inc., to sponsor cooperative research on problems of mutual interest. While individual member companies also conduct their own proprietary studies, ILZRO supports research on all areas of the uses of lead and zinc, including a large number of environmental health studies. ILZRO also sponsors various seminars, symposia, and conferences to present the results of work it has supported; the most recent of these was an international symposium on environmental lead research, held in Cincinnati, Ohio, in December 1978. Through its contracts, ILZRO has supported studies on many of the same topics (and enlisted the services of many of the same research teams) that make up the research programs of federal agencies, described above.

Table B.6 summarizes ILZRO's research on lead through 1978. Almost half of the current projects and about one-fourth of those that have been completed have dealt with environmental health aspects of lead. In the last 3 years (1977–1979) ILZRO has spent $1.3 million for environmental studies on lead.

Specific topics investigated recently with ILZRO support include the following: assessment of the state-of-the-art in blood lead analysis; epidemiological studies of the health of workers exposed to lead, and epi-

TABLE B.6   Lead Research Sponsored by the International Lead Zinc Research Organization[a]

Topics	Number of Projects	
	Current (1978)	Completed
Chemistry of lead compounds	9	38
Metallurgical studies	2	23
Electrochemistry of lead compounds	7	17
Development of lead products	3	1
Lead and environmental health		
Character of sources and emissions	—	1
Environmental transport, fate, biogeochemistry	2	4
Sources of human exposure	3	3
Absorption and pharmacodynamics	1	3
Effects of occupational exposures	5	2
Effects of pediatric lead exposure	2	1
Toxicological studies	2	7
Effects on wildlife species	1	—
Interactions of Pb, Fe, Zn	1	—
Treatment of pediatric lead poisoning	1	—
Pollution control and hazard abatement	—	1
Sampling and analytical methods	—	4
Miscellaneous	1	1
Subtotal	19	27
TOTALS	40	106

[a] Based on information in ILZRO (1979).

demiological assessments of body burdens and biological effects of lead in populations with varying degrees of nonoccupational exposure; studies of the absorption of lead in children; investigations of the absorption of inhaled lead by rats; an assessment of the role of lead in hyperactivity in rodents; studies to improve dose–effect data for effects of lead in humans; a study on management of children with abnormal lead exposure; a study to determine whether lead is essential to any biological processes; several studies to improve the information base on the relative contributions of soil and dust, automobile exhaust, drinking water, and lead on household surfaces to the total amount of lead absorbed by humans, especially children; a study to improve air sampling methods for particulate lead; a review of the effects of heavy metals on aquatic life; and a study of the biotransformation of lead in the environment.

In summary, most of the studies ILZRO is sponsoring on lead and environmental health are on topics that were identified earlier in this report as critical information needs for making policy decisions about acceptable exposures to lead. The support that ILZRO has provided is equivalent to about 7 percent of the total spent in the last 3 years by U.S. federal agencies for studies concerned primarily with lead.

REFERENCES

Billick, I.H. and V.E. Gray (1978) Lead Based Paint Poisoning Research: Review and Evaluation, 1971-1977. Office of Policy Development and Research. Washington, D.C.: U.S. Department of Housing and Urban Development.

Congressional Research Service (1979) An Overview of Research in Biogeochemistry and Environmental Health. Report prepared for the Subcommittee on Science, Research and Technology of the Committee on Science and Technology, U.S. House of Representatives, 96th Congress, First Session, by the Congressional Research Service, Library of Congress. Washington, D.C.: U.S. Government Printing Office.

Greenberg, D.S. (1978) Carter and Science: A two-year scorecard. Science and Government Report 8(21):1–4, December 15.

International Lead Zinc Research Organization, Inc. (1979) Lead Research Digest. No. 36—1978. New York: ILZRO, Inc.

Myers, W., R. Abel, and C. Thiel (1978) Toxic Substances: A Review of Federal Research, Development, Testing and Monitoring Activities. Prepared for the Toxic Substances Strategy Committee of the Council on Environmental Quality. Washington, D.C.: National Science Foundation.

National Research Council (1977) Research and Development in the Environmental Protection Agency. Volume III, Analytical Studies for the U.S. Environmental Protection Agency. Environmental Research Assessment Committee, Environmental Studies Board, Commission on Natural Resources. Washington, D.C.: National Academy of Sciences.

U.S. Energy Research and Development Administration (1976) A National Plan for Energy Research, Development, and Demonstration: Creating Energy Choices for the Future. Volume 1: The Plan. ERDA-76-1. Washington, D.C.: U.S. Government Printing Office.

U.S. Environmental Protection Agency (1977) Research Highlights, 1977. Office of Research and Development, EPA-600/9-77-044. Washington, D.C.: U.S. Environmental Protection Agency.

U.S. National Institute for Environmental Health Sciences (1978) Federal Agency Support for Environmental Health Research. Research Triangle Park, N.C.: U.S. Department of Health, Education, and Welfare.

U.S. Office of Management and Budget (1979) Special Analysis K: Environment. Pages 273-293, The Budget for Fiscal Year 1980. Washington, D.C.: U.S. Government Printing Office.

Williams, S., J. Lee, S.D. Lee, and S. Molinas (1978) Report of the Metals Task Force to the Research Planning Work Group. Washington, D.C.: Interagency Regulatory Liaison Group.

SUPPLEMENT 1

SUMMARIES OF FEDERAL RESEARCH IN SPECIFIC SUBJECT AREAS

(Tables B.7 through B.23)

CONTENTS

TABLE B.7   Research Efforts of Federal Agencies to Characterize Sources and Emissions of Lead in the Environment for FY 1977-1979 (in thousands of dollars)

Agency	Studies Concerned Primarily With Lead					Multielement Studies That Include Lead				
	1977	1978	1979	Total	%	1977	1978	1979	Total	%
DOE	—	—	—	0	—	1,227	1,570	1,363	4,160	83.9
BM	—	—	—	0	—	185	207	176	568	11.5
EPA	0	n.a.	n.a.	0[a]	—	229	n.a.	n.a.	229[a]	4.6
TOTALS	0	0	0	0	—	1,641	1,777	1,539	4,957	100

[a] EPA totals are for 1977 only; 1978 and 1979 data not available.

TABLE B.8 Research Efforts of Federal Agencies on the Transport, Fate, Environmental Geochemistry and Cycling of Lead for FY 1977-1979 (in thousands of dollars)

Agency	Studies Concerned Primarily With Lead					Multielement Studies That Include Lead				
	1977	1978	1979	Total	%	1977	1978	1979	Total	%
USGS	—	—	—	0		1,600	2,100	2,300	6,000	65.1
DOE	—	—	—	0		923	773	759	2,455	26.7
EPA	—	n.a.	n.a.	0[a]		346	n.a.	n.a.	346[a]	3.8
NIEHS	—	—	—	0		98	100	100	298	3.2
All others[b]	41	164	25	230[c]	100	21	33	49	113[c]	1.2
TOTALS	41	164	25	230	100	2,998	3,006	3,208	9,212	100

[a] EPA totals are for 1977 only; 1978 and 1979 data not available.
[b] Includes OWRT, NBS, NIH-DRR, FWS, NSF, and USDA.
[c] Does not include 1978-1979 data for USDA or 1979 data for OWRT.

TABLE B.9 Research Efforts of Federal Agencies to Determine the Levels of Lead in Environmental Media for FY 1977-1979 (in thousands of dollars)

Agency	Studies Concerned Primarily With Lead					Multielement Studies That Include Lead				
	1977	1978	1979	Total	%	1977	1978	1979	Total	%
USGS	—	—	—	—	—	4,300	5,200	6,000	15,500	97.6
EPA	—	n.a.	n.a.	0[a]	—	209	n.a.	n.a.	209[a]	1.3
All others[b]	—	—	—	—	—	56	59	60	175	1.1
TOTALS	0	0	0	0	—	4,565	5,259	6,060	15,884	100

[a] EPA totals are for 1977 only; 1978 and 1979 data not available.
[b] Includes NIEHS and NIH-DRR.

TABLE B.10 Research Efforts of Federal Agencies to Determine the Levels of Lead in Biota, Foods, and Housewares for FY 1977-1979 (in thousands of dollars)

Agency	Studies Concerned Primarily With Lead					Multielement Studies That Include Lead				
	1977	1978	1979	Total	%	1977	1978	1979	Total	%
FDA	581	597	413	1,591	98.5	—	—	—	0	—
USDA	24	n.a.	n.a.	24 [a]	1.5	n.a.	n.a.	n.a.	n.a. [b]	57.9
DOE	—	—	—	0	—	465	783	840	2,088	40.7
NOAA	—	—	—	0	—	457	551	460	1,468	1.4
FWS	—	—	—	0	—	2	25	25	52	100
TOTALS	605	597	413	1,615	100	924	1,359	1,325	3,608	

[a] USDA totals are for 1977 only; 1978 and 1979 data not available.

[b] USDA conducts multielement surveys of trace metals in foods, but the data reported were broken down by elements, rather than by studies. Totals spent on multielement surveys are therefore not available for USDA, and the proportional efforts of other agencies are thus made to appear larger than they are in fact.

TABLE B.11   Research Efforts of Federal Agencies on Exposures of Populations to Lead and on Contributions of Specific Routes of Exposure to Total Exposure for FY 1977-1979 (in thousands of dollars)

Agency	Studies Concerned Primarily With Lead					Multielement Studies That Include Lead				
	1977	1978	1979	Total	%	1977	1978	1979	Total	%
HUD	100	26	425	551	80.0	—	—	—	0	—
NIEHS	28	21	21	70	10.2	65	60	60	185	87.7
EPA	42	n.a.	n.a.	42^a	6.1	—	n.a.	n.a.	0^a	—
NHLBI	—	—	—	0	—	13	13	—	26	12.3
FDA	—	20	—	20	2.9	—	—	—	0	—
NSF	6	—	—	6	0.8	—	—	—	0	—
TOTALS	176	67	446	689	100	78	73	60	211	100

[a] EPA totals are for 1977 only; 1978 and 1979 data not available.

TABLE B.12 Research Efforts of Federal Agencies on the Absorption of Pharmacodynamics of Lead in Animals and Humans for FY 1977-1979 (in thousands of dollars)

Agency	Studies Concerned Primarily With Lead					Multielement Studies That Include Lead				
	1977	1978	1979	Total	%	1977	1978	1979	Total	%
NIEHS	388	259	207	854	75.9	145	132	103	380	41.9
FDA	50	50	60	160	14.2	—	—	—	0	—
EPA	67	n.a.	n.a.	67[a]	6.0	53	n.a.	n.a.	53[a]	5.8
NIH-DRR	14	15	15	44	3.9	136	136	150	422	46.6
DOE	—	—	—	0	0	—	—	51	51	5.7
NIOSH	—	—	—	0	—	—	—	—	—	—
TOTALS	519	324	282	1,125	100	334	268	304	906	100

[a] EPA totals are for 1977 only; 1978 and 1979 data not available.

TABLE B.13 Research Efforts of Federal Agencies on Clinical Studies of Humans with Excessive Lead Absorption for FY 1977-1979 (in thousands of dollars)

Agency	Studies Concerned Primarily With Lead					Multielement Studies That Include Lead				
	1977	1978	1979	Total	%	1977	1978	1979	Total	%
NIEHS	228	303	207	738	53.5	—	—	—	0	—
NICHD	388	114	—	502	36.4	61	68	20	149	100
NIH-DRR	67	36	37	140	10.1	—	—	—	0	—
TOTALS	683	453	244	1,380	100	61	68	20	149	100

TABLE B.14 Research Efforts of Federal Agencies on Epidemiological Studies of Morbidity, Mortality, and Body Burdens Related to Exposure to Lead for FY 1977-1979 (in thousands of dollars)

Agency	Studies Concerned Primarily With Lead					Multielement Studies That Include Lead				
	1977	1978	1979	Total	%	1977	1978	1979	Total	%
NIOSH	719	193	176	1,088	57.5	60	28	—	88	10.7
EPA	334	n.a.	n.a.	334[a]	17.7	150	n.a.	n.a.	150[a]	18.2
NIEHS	93	37	37	167	8.8	—	—	—	0	—
CDC	62	75	70	207	10.9	67	66	144	277	33.6
FDA	20	20	20	60	3.2	41	41	22	104	12.6
NHLBI	9	17	9	35	1.8	—	116	—	116	14.1
NCI	—	—	—	0	—	22	23	24	69	8.4
NIH-DRR	—	—	—	0	—	—	—	20	20	2.4
Others[b]	1	—	—	1	<0.1	—	—	—	0	—
TOTALS	1,238	342	312	1,892	100	340	274	210	824	100

[a] EPA totals are for 1977 only; 1978 and 1979 data not available.
[b] Includes USGS and USDA.

TABLE B.15 Research Efforts of Federal Agencies on Toxicological Studies of Biological Effects of Lead for FY 1977-1979 (in thousands of dollars)

Agency	Studies Concerned Primarily With Lead					Multielement Studies That Include Lead				
	1977	1978	1979	Total	%	1977	1978	1979	Total	%
NIEHS	1,107	885	731	2,723	35.8	1,094	1,206	1,235	3,535	63.9
DOE	1,191	1,026	1,059	3,276	43.1	100	—	—	100	1.8
EPA	276	n.a.	n.a.	276[a]	3.6	790	n.a.	n.a.	790[a]	14.3
FDA	157	108	130	395	5.2	—	—	—	0	—
NINCDS	62	135	147	344	4.5	91	215	230	536	9.7
NICHD	—	—	—	0	—	51	103	91	245	4.4
NCI	—	—	—	0	—	59	54	5	118	2.1
NIH-DRR	29	31	32	92	1.2	5	5	5	15	0.3
NIOSH	—	—	75	75	1.0	—	—	104	104	1.9
ADAMHA	—	—	—	0	—	91	—	—	91	1.6
USDA	115	n.a.	n.a.	115[a]	1.5	—	n.a.	n.a.	0[a]	—
OWRT	—	3	n.a.	3[b]	<0.1	—	—	n.a.	0[b]	—
NSF	90	100	110	300	3.9	—	—	—	0	—
TOTALS	3,027	2,288	2,284	7,599	100	2,281	1,583	1,670	5,534	100

[a] EPA and USDA totals are for 1977 only; 1978 and 1979 data not available.
[b] Totals for OWRT are for 1977 + 1978; data for 1979 not available.

TABLE B.16 Research Efforts of Federal Agencies on Physiological and Ecological Effects of Lead on Wildlife Species for FY 1977-1979 (in thousands of dollars)

Agency	Studies Concerned Primarily With Lead					Multielement Studies That Include Lead				
	1977	1978	1979	Total	%	1977	1978	1979	Total	%
FWS	—	—	—	0	—	300	150	250	700	57.4
NIEHS	—	—	—	0	—	79	82	82	243	19.9
EPA	—	n.a.	n.a.	0[a]	—	231	n.a.	n.a.	231[a]	19.0
NIH-DRR	—	—	—	0	—	14	15	16	45	3.7
OWRT	3	16	n.a.	19[b]	100	—	—	—	0	—
TOTALS	3	16	—	19	100	624	247	348	1,219	100

[a] EPA totals are for 1977 only; 1978 and 1979 data not available.
[b] OWRT reported amount spent on lead within multielement studies; totals do not include FY 1979.

TABLE B.17 Research Efforts of Federal Agencies on the Interactions Between Lead and Essential Nutrients or Other Toxic Contaminants for FY 1977-1979 (in thousands of dollars)

Agency	Studies Concerned Primarily With Lead					Multielement Studies That Include Lead				
	1977	1978	1979	Total	%	1977	1978	1979	Total	%
NIEHS	314	310	238	862	68.1	—	50	33	83	37.6
FDA	96	100	105	301	23.8	—	—	—	0	—
EPA	10	n.a.	n.a.	10[a]	0.8	116	n.a.	n.a.	116[a]	52.5
NIH-DRR	19	20	21	60	4.7	7	7	8	22	9.9
OWRT	13	19	n.a.	32[b]	2.5	—	—	n.a.	0[b]	—
TOTALS	452	449	364	1,265	100	123	57	41	221	100

[a] EPA totals are for 1977 only; 1978 and 1979 data not available.
[b] OWRT reported amount spent on lead within multielement studies; totals do not include FY 1979.

TABLE B.18   Research Efforts of Federal Agencies on Development of Technological Methods to Control Lead Pollution or Abate Lead Hazards for FY 1977-1979 (in thousands of dollars)

Agency	Studies Concerned Primarily With Lead					Multielement Studies That Include Lead				
	1977	1978	1979	Total	%	1977	1978	1979	Total	%
BM	—	—	—	0	—	1,572	1,379	2,268	5,219	86.4
EPA	—	n.a.	n.a.	0[a]	—	814	n.a.	n.a.	814[a]	13.5
HUD	128	161	100	389	97.5	—	—	—	0	—
NIOSH	—	—	—	0	—	—	10	—	10	0.1
OWRT	5	5	n.a.	10[b]	2.5	—	—	n.a.	0[b]	—
TOTALS	133	166	100	399	100	2,386	1,389	2,268	6,043	100

[a] EPA totals are for 1977 only; 1978 and 1979 data not available.
[b] OWRT reported amount spent on lead within multielement studies; totals do not include FY 1979.

TABLE B.19 Research Efforts of Federal Agencies on Non-Technological Aspects of Prevention of Lead Poisoning for FY 1977-1979 (in thousands of dollars)

Agency	Studies Concerned Primarily With Lead					Multielement Studies That Include Lead				
	1977	1978	1979	Total	%	1977	1978	1979	Total	%
HUD	282	208	100	590	86.9	—	—	—	0	—
NIEHS	—	—	—	0	—	74	18	18	110	100
CDC	27	27	35	89	13.1	—	—	—	0	—
TOTALS	309	235	135	679	100	74	18	18	110	100

TABLE B.20 Research Efforts of Federal Agencies to Evaluate the Effectiveness of Current Programs for FY 1977-1979 (in thousands of dollars)

Agency	Studies Concerned Primarily With Lead					Multielement Studies That Include Lead				
	1977	1978	1979	Total	%	1977	1978	1979	Total	%
HUD	—	633	100	733	100	—	—	—	0	—

TABLE B.21 Research Efforts of Federal Agencies to Develop Improved Analytical Methods for the Determination of Lead in Environmental Samples for FY 1977-1979 (in thousands of dollars)

Agency	Studies Concerned Primarily With Lead					Multielement Studies That Include Lead				
	1977	1978	1979	Total	%	1977	1978	1979	Total	%
USGS	—	—	—	0	—	2,000	2,500	2,800	7,300	72.3
FDA	—	—	—	0	—	752	739	834	2,325	23.0
FWS	—	—	—	0	—	2	170	70	242	2.4
EPA	—	n.a.	n.a.	0[a]	—	120	n.a.	n.a.	120[a]	1.2
NBS	50	40	40	130	68.8	—	—	—	0	—
CDC	28	—	—	28	14.8	—	—	—	0	—
All Others[b]	30	1	—	31	16.4	55	26	27	108	1.1
TOTALS	108	41	40	189	100	2,929	3,435	3,731	10,095	100

[a] EPA totals are for 1977 only; 1978 and 1979 data not available.
[b] Includes NIEHS, DOE, OWRT, and USDA.

TABLE B.22 Research Efforts of Federal Agencies to Develop Sampling Methods and Monitoring Systems to Measure Lead in the Environment for FY 1977-1979 (in thousands of dollars)

Agency	Studies Concerned Primarily With Lead					Multielement Studies That Include Lead				
	1977	1978	1979	Total	%	1977	1978	1979	Total	%
USGS	—	—	—	0	—	300	300	300	900	56.1
EPA	93	n.a.	n.a.	93[a]	47.9	704	n.a.	n.a.	704[a]	43.9
NIEHS	25	26	27	78	40.2	—	—	—	0	—
USDA	23	n.a.	n.a.	23[a]	11.9	—	n.a.	n.a.	0[a]	—
TOTALS	141	26	27	194	100	1,004	300	300	1,604	100

[a] EPA and USDA totals are for 1977 only; 1978 and 1979 data not available.

TABLE B.23 Research Efforts of Federal Agencies on Miscellaneous Topics Related to Lead for FY 1977-1979 (in thousands of dollars)

Agency	Studies Concerned Primarily With Lead					Multielement Studies That Include Lead				
	1977	1978	1979	Total	%	1977	1978	1979	Total	%
BM	—	—	—	0	—	476	1,016	1,071	2,563	100
USDA	21	n.a.	n.a.	21[a]	100	—	—	—	0	—
TOTALS	21	0	0	21	100	476	1,016	1,071	2,563	100

[a] USDA totals are for 1977 only; 1978 and 1979 data not available.

SUPPLEMENT 2

SUMMARIES OF RESEARCH SUPPORTED BY INDIVIDUAL AGENCIES

(Tables B.24 through B.40)

CONTENTS

TABLE B.24 U.S. EPA: Level of Effort in Research on Topics Related to Lead in the Environment Supported by the Environmental Protection Agency in FY 1977 (in thousands of dollars)

Topic	Studies Concerned Primarily With Lead	%	Multielement Studies That Include Lead	%
Sources and Environmental Pathways				
Character of sources and emissions	—		229	6
Transport, fate, geochemical cycling	—		346	9
Levels in environmental media	—		209	6
Levels in biota, foods, housewares	—		—	
Populations with Exposures				
Contributions of specific sources	42	5	—	

Absorption and Pharmacodynamics	67	8	53	1
Biological effects				
Epidemiology	334	41	150	4
Toxicology	276	34	790	21
Ecological effects	—		231	6
Interactions with other substances	10	1	116	3
Pollution Control/Hazard Abatement				
Development of technological methods	—		814	22
Analytical and Measurement Methodology				
Chemical analysis of samples	—		120	3
Sampling and monitoring methods	93	11	704	19
TOTALS	822	100	3,762	100

TABLE B.25 U.S. FDA: Level of Effort in Research on Topics Related to Lead in the Environment Supported by the Food and Drug Administration in FY 1977-1979 (in thousands of dollars)

Topic	Studies Concerned Primarily With Lead					Multielement Studies That Include Lead				
	1977	1978	1979	Total	%	1977	1978	1979	Total	%
Sources and Environmental Pathways										
Levels in biota, foods, housewares	581	597	413	1,591	63	—	—	—	0	—
Populations with Exposures										
Contributions of specific sources	—	20	—	20	<1	—	—	—	0	—
Absorption and Pharmacodynamics	50	50	60	160	6	—	—	—	0	—
Biological Effects										
Epidemiology	20	20	20	60	2	67	66	144	277	11
Toxicology	157	108	130	395	16	—	—	—	0	—
Interactions with other substances	96	100	105	301	12	—	—	—	0	—
Analytical and Measurement Methodology										
Chemical analysis of samples	—	—	—	0	—	752	739	834	2,325	89
TOTALS	904	895	728	2,527	100	819	805	978	2,602	100

TABLE B.26 NIEHS: Level of Effort in Research on Topics Related to Lead in the Environment Supported by the National Institute of Environmental Health Sciences in FY 1977-1979 (in thousands of dollars)

Topic	Studies Concerned Primarily With Lead					Multielement Studies That Include Lead				
	1977	1978	1979	Total	%	1977	1978	1979	Total	%
Sources and Environmental Pathways										
Transport, fate, geochemical cycling	—	—	—	0	—	98	100	100	298	6
Levels in environmental media	—	—	—	0	—	25	26	27	78	1
Populations with Exposures										
Assessment of exposures	—	—	—	0	—					
Contributions of specific sources	28	21	21	70	1	65	60	60	185	4
Absorption and Pharmacodynamics	388	259	207	854	16	145	132	103	380	8
Biological effects										
Clinical studies	228	303	207	738	13	—	—	—	0	—
Epidemiology	93	37	37	167	3	—	—	—	0	—
Toxicology[a]	1,107	885	731	2,723	50	1,094	1,206	1,235	3,535	71
Ecological effects	—	—	—	0	—	79	82	82	243	5
Interactions with other substances	314	310	238	862	16	—	50	33	83	2
Pollution Control/Hazard Abatement										
Non-technological approaches	—	—	—	0	—	74	18	18	110	2
Analytical and Measurement Methodology										
Chemical analysis of samples	—	—	—	0	—	25	26	27	78	1
Sampling and monitoring methods	25	26	27	78	1	—	—	—	0	—
TOTALS	2,183	1,841	1,468	5,492	100	1,605	1,700	1,685	4,990	100

[a] See Table B.27 for detailed breakdown of NIEHS-supported research on toxicology.

TABLE B.27 NIEHS—Toxicology: Subject Matter of Toxicological Research Supported by the National Institute of Environmental Health Sciences in FY 1977-1979 (in thousands of dollars)

Topic	Studies Concerned Primarily With Lead					Multielement Studies That Include Lead				
	1977	1978	1979	Total	%	1977	1978	1979	Total	%
General and comparative toxicology	28	12	12	52	1.9	182	200	200	582	16.5
Cellular effects	47	51	17	115	4.2	68	67	69	204	5.8
Effects on nervous system	615	398	390	1,403	51.5	207	217	220	644	18.2
Teratogenic effects	129	139	140	408	15.0	255	356	376	987	27.9
Behavioral effects	93	59	59	211	7.8	174	195	196	565	16.0
Effects on kidney	71	12	12	95	3.5	48	12	12	72	2.0
Effects on hematopoiesis	65	137	35	237	8.7	—	—	—	0	—
Effects on immune system	—	11	—	11	0.4	127	119	122	368	10.4
Inhalation toxicology	59	66	66	191	7.0	—	—	—	0	—
Effects on skeletal muscle	—	—	—	0	—	33	40	40	113	3.2
TOTALS	1,107	885	731	2,723	100	1,094	1,206	1,235	3,535	100

TABLE B.28 NIH (Except NIEHS): Level of Effort in Research on Topics Related to Lead in the Environment Supported by the National Institutes of Health[a] in FY 1977-1979 (in thousands of dollars)

Topic	Studies Concerned Primarily With Lead					Multielement Studies That Include Lead				
	1977	1978	1979	Total	%	1977	1978	1979	Total	%
Sources and Environmental Pathways										
Transport, fate, geochemical cycling	—	—	—	0	—	31	33	33	97	6
Levels in environmental media	—	—	—	0	—	31	33	33	97	6
Populations with Exposures										
Contributions of specific sources	—	—	—	0	—	13	13	—	26	1
Absorption and Pharmacodynamics	14	15	15	44	3	—	—	—	0	—
Biological effects										
Clinical studies	455	150	37	642	53	61	68	20	149	9
Epidemiology	9	17	9	35	3	63	180	46	289	18
Toxicology	91	166	179	436	36	206	377	331	914	56
Ecological effects	—	—	—	0	—	14	15	16	45	3
Interactions with other substances	19	20	21	60	5	7	7	8	22	1
TOTALS	588	368	261	1,217	100	426	726	487	1,639	100

[a] NIEHS is treated separately. See Tables B.26 and B.27. For a breakdown of efforts by institutes, see Table B.29.

TABLE B.29 NIH (by Institutes): Level of Effort in Research on Topics Related to Lead in the Environment Supported by Five Divisions of the National Institutes of Health in FY 1977-1979 (in thousands of dollars)

Topic	Studies Concerned Primarily With Lead					Multielement Studies That Include Lead				
	1977	1978	1979	Total	%	1977	1978	1979	Total	%
Sources and Environmental Pathways										
Transport, fate, geochemical cycling										
DRR	—	—	—	—	—	31	33	33	97	6
Levels in environmental media										
DRR	—	—	—	—	—	31	33	33	97	6
Populations with Exposures										
Contributions of specific sources										
NHLBI	—	—	—	—	—	13	13	—	26	1
Absorption and Pharmacodynamics										
DRR	14	15	15	44	3	—	—	—	—	—
Biological Effects										
Clinical studies										
NICHD	388	114	—	502	41	61	68	20	149	9

DRR	67	36	37	140	12	—	—	—	—	—
Epidemiology										
NHLBI	9	17	9	35	3	41	41	22	104	7
NCI	—	—	—	—	—	—	116	—	116	7
DRR	—	—	—	—	—	22	23	24	69	4
Toxicology										
NINCDS	62	135	147	344	28	91	215	230	536	33
NICHD	—	—	—	—	—	51	103	91	245	15
NCI	—	—	—	—	—	59	54	5	118	7
DRR	29	31	32	92	8	5	5	5	15	1
Ecological effects										
DRR	—	—	—	—	—	14	15	16	45	3
Interactions with other substances										
DRR	19	20	21	60	5	7	7	8	22	1
Totals by Institute										
NICHD	388	114	—	502	41	112	171	111	394	24
NINCDS	62	135	147	344	28	91	215	230	536	33
NCI	—	—	—	—	—	59	170	5	234	14
NHLBI	9	17	9	35	3	54	54	22	130	8
DRR	129	102	105	336	28	110	116	119	345	21
TOTALS, ALL INSTITUTES	588	368	261	1,217	100	426	726	487	1,639	100

TABLE B.30 NIOSH: Level of Effort in Research on Topics Related to Lead in the Environment Supported by the National Institute for Occupational Safety and Health in FY 1977-1979 (in thousands of dollars)

Topic	Studies Concerned Primarily With Lead					Multielement Studies That Include Lead				
	1977	1978	1979	Total	%	1977	1978	1979	Total	%
Absorption and Pharmacodynamics	—	—	—	0	—	—	—	51	51	20
Biological effects										
Epidemiology	719	193	176	1,088	94	60	28	—	88	35
Toxicology	—	—	75	75	6	—	—	104	104	41
Pollution Control/Hazard Abatement										
Development of technological methods	—	—	—	0	—	—	10	—	10	4
TOTALS	719	193	251	1,163	100	60	38	155	253	100

TABLE B.31 CDC: Level of Effort in Research on Topics Related to Lead in the Environment Supported by the Center for Disease Control[a] in FY 1977-1979 (in thousands of dollars)

Topic	Studies Concerned Primarily With Lead				
	1977	1978	1979	Total	%
Biological Effects Epidemiology	62	75	70	207	64
Pollution Control/Hazard Abatement Non-technological approaches	27	27	35	89	27
Analytical and Measurement Methodology Chemical analysis of samples	28	—	—	28	9
TOTALS	117	102	105	324	100

[a] NIOSH is administered as part of CDC, but is listed separately here (see Table B.30).

TABLE B.32 DOE: Level of Effort in Research on Topics Related to Lead in the Environment Supported by the Department of Energy in FY 1977-1979 (in thousands of dollars)

Topic	Studies Concerned Primarily With Lead					Multielement Studies That Include Lead				
	1977	1978	1979	Total	%	1977	1978	1979	Total	%
Sources and Environmental Pathways										
Character of sources and emissions	—	—	—	0	—	1,227	1,570	1,363	4,160	45
Transport, fate, geochemical cycling	—	—	—	0	—	923	773	759	2,455	27
Levels in biota, foods, housewares	—	—	—	0	—	465	783	840	2,088	23
Absorption and Pharmacodynamics	—	—	—	0	—	136	136	150	422	4
Biological Effects										
Toxicology	1,191	1,026	1,059	3,276	100	100	—	—	—	1
Analytical and Measurement Methodology										
Chemical analysis of samples	—	—	—	0	—	30	—	—	30	<1
TOTALS	1,191	1,026	1,059	3,276	100	2,881	3,262	3,112	9,255	100

TABLE B.33 USBM: Level of Effort in Research on Topics Related to Lead in the Environment Supported by the Bureau of Mines in FY 1977-1979 (in thousands of dollars)

Topic	Multielement Studies That Include Lead				
	1977	1978	1979	Total	%
Sources and Environmental Pathways					
Character of Sources and Emissions	185	207	176	568	7
Pollution Control/Hazard Abatement					
Development of technological methods	1,572	1,379	2,268	5,219	63
Miscellaneous					
Metallurgical research	86	880	961	1,927	23
Mineral commodities studies	95	100	110	305	4
National Research Council studies	295	36	—	331	4
TOTALS	2,233	2,602	3,515	8,350	100

TABLE B.34 USGS: Level of Effort in Research on Topics Related to Lead in the Environment Supported by the Geological Survey in FY 1977-1979 (in thousands of dollars)

Topic	Multielement Studies That Include Lead				
	1977	1978	1979	Total	%
Sources and Environmental Pathways					
Transport, fate, geochemical cycling	1,600	2,100	2,300	6,000	20
Levels in environmental media	4,300	5,200	6,000	15,500	52
Biological Effects					
Epidemiology	—	—	20	20	<1
Analytical and Measurement Methodology					
Chemical analysis of samples	2,000	2,500	2,800	7,300	25
Sampling and monitoring methods	300	300	300	900	3
TOTALS	8,200	10,100	11,420	29,720	100

TABLE B.35   U.S. FWS: Level of Effort in Research on Topics Related to Lead in the Environment Supported by the Fish and Wildlife Service in FY 1977-1979 (in thousands of dollars)

Topic	Multielement Studies That Include Lead				
	1977	1978	1979	Total	%
Sources and Environmental Pathways					
Transport, fate, geochemical cycling	—	—	16	16	2
Levels in biota, foods, housewares	2	25	25	52	5
Biological Effects					
Ecological effects	300	150	250	700	69
Analytical and Measurement					
Methodology					
Chemical analysis of samples	2	170	70	242	24
TOTALS	304	345	361	1,010	100

TABLE B.36   OWRT: Level of Effort in Research on Topics Related to Lead in the Environment Supported by the Office of Water Research and Technology in FY 1977-1979 (in thousands of dollars)

Topic	Amount Spent on Lead[a]			
	1977	1978	Total	%
Sources and Environmental Pathways				
Transport, fate, geochemical cycling	26	114	140	68
Biological Effects				
Toxicology	—	3	3	1
Ecological effects	3	16	19	9
Interactions with other substances	13	19	32	16
Pollution Control/Hazard Abatement				
Development of technological methods	5	5	10	5
Analytical and Measurement Methodology				
Chemical analysis of samples	0	1	1	1
TOTALS	47	158	205	100

[a] OWRT provided an element-by-element breakdown of funds. Data here represent portions of multielement studies that were allocated to lead.

TABLE B.37　NBS: Level of Effort in Research on Topics Related to Lead in the Environment Supported by the National Bureau of Standards in FY 1977-1979 (in thousands of dollars)

Topic	Amount Spent on Lead[a]				
	1977	1978	1979	Total	%
Sources and Environmental Pathways					
Transport, fate, geochemical cycling	—	50	25	75	37
Analytical and Measurement Methodology					
Chemical analysis of samples	50	40	40	130	63
TOTALS	50	90	65	205	100

[a] NBS provided an element-by-element breakdown of expenditures; some studies involved multielement analysis, but amounts here are amounts spent on lead.

TABLE B.38　NOAA: Level of Effort in Research on Topics Related to Lead in the Environment Supported by the National Oceanic and Atmospheric Administration in FY 1977-1979 (in thousands of dollars)

Topic	Multielement Studies That Include Lead				
	1977	1978	1979	Total	%
Sources and Environmental Pathways					
Levels in biota, foods	457	551	460	1,468	100
Biological Effects					
Ecological effects	<1	<1	<1	<1	<1
TOTALS	457	551	460	1,468	100

TABLE B.39   USDA: Level of Effort in Research on Topics Related to Lead in the Environment Supported by the Department of Agriculture in FY 1977 (in thousands of dollars)

Topic	Amount Spent on Lead[a]	%
Sources and Environmental Pathways		
Transport, fate, geochemical cycling	7	3
Levels in biota, foods, housewares	24	11
Biological Effects		
Epidemiology	1	<1
Toxicology	115	52
Analytical and Measurement Methodology		
Chemical analysis of samples	30	14
Sampling and monitoring methods	23	10
Miscellaneous	21	9
TOTALS	221	100

[a] USDA provided an element-by-element breakdown of expenditures. Data here represent portions of multielement studies that were allocated to lead.

TABLE B.40   NSF: Level of Effort in Research on Topics Related to Lead in the Environment Supported by the National Science Foundation in FY 1977-1979 (in thousands of dollars)

Topic	Studies Concerned Primarily with Lead				
	1977	1978	1979	Total	%
Sources and Environmental Pathways					
Transport, fate, geochemical cycling	8	—	—	8	3
Populations with Exposures					
Contributions of specific sources	6	—	—	6	2
Biological Effects					
Toxicology	90	100	110	300	95
TOTALS	104	100	110	314	100

Case Studies of Federal Standard-Setting Activities Pertinent to Lead in the Human Environment

INTRODUCTION

At least eight departments and agencies of the federal government currently administer programs designed to limit human exposure to lead. These programs are authorized under several pieces of federal legislation,[1] and are directed toward reducing or eliminating human lead exposure as it occurs through the air, water, food, and nonfood media. In order to implement their programs, the agencies have promulgated numerous regulations and standards for controlling specific lead exposure pathways. Those control measures are listed in Table C.1.

This appendix presents brief case histories of the processes followed by federal agencies in developing certain lead-related programs and standards. The material here is background for the assessment in Chapter 3 of the interplay between the development of scientific knowledge about lead in the environment and the development of governmental regulations based in part on such knowledge. These case studies summarize the public record of the decision process in each instance, pointing out the requirements of the applicable laws, the rationales used by the agencies, and the major conclusions on scientific and technical issues that were cited in support of the decisions.

We recognize fully the limitations of this approach. For instance, by choosing to rely on public records such as the *Federal Register*, criteria documents, and transcripts of hearings, we have not included the substantially nonpublic parts of the regulatory process that include, for example,

TABLE C.1   Federal Regulatory Actions Governing Human Exposure to Lead

Medium through Which Exposure Occurs	Federal Agency	Specific Exposure Pathway Being Controlled	Federal Regulations	Citation
Nonfood Substances				
Lead paint in housing	Housing and Urban Development	Exposure of children to lead-based paint on surfaces of residential structures.	Notification to purchasers and tenants of HUD-associated housing constructed prior to 1950 of the hazards of lead-based paint poisoning.	24 CFR 35.5
			Prohibition against the use of lead-based paint in HUD-associated housing.	24 CFR 35.14
			Elimination of lead-based paint hazards in HUD-associated housing.	24 CFR 35.24
			Elimination of lead-based paint hazards in federally owned properties prior to sale for residential habitation.	24 CFR 35.56
			Prohibition against the use of lead-based paint in federal and federally assisted construction or rehabilitation of residential structures.	24 CFR 35.62
Lead paint in housing	Health, Education, and Welfare	Exposure of children to lead-based paint on surfaces of residential structures.	Grants to develop local programs for detection and treatment of lead-based paint poisoning and for the identification and elimination	42 CFR 91

Lead in paint, and toys and furniture with painted surfaces	Consumer Product Safety Commission	Exposure of children to lead-based paint on surfaces of residential structures, toys and furniture.	of the hazards of lead paint in residential structures. The following consumer products have been declared as banned hazardous products: (1) paint and other similar surface coatings containing more than 0.06 percent lead. (2) toys and other articles intended for use by children that bear paint containing more than 0.06 percent lead. (3) furniture that bears paint containing more than 0.06 percent lead.	16 CFR 1303.4

Air

Ambient air	Environmental Protection Agency	Exposure of the general population and especially young children (1-5 yrs.) to airborne lead from motor vehicles combusting leaded gasoline.	No gasoline refiner shall exceed an average lead content of 0.5 g Pb/gal after October 1, 1979, averaged over a three-month period.	40 CFR 80.20
Ambient air (including dust and dirt)	Environmental Protection Agency	Exposure of the general population and especially young children (1-5 yrs.) to airborne lead from stationary and mobile emissions sources.	The national primary and secondary ambient air quality standards for lead are 1.5 $\mu g/m^3$, maximum arithmetic mean averaged over a calendar quarter.	40 CFR 50.12

TABLE C.1 *(continued)*

Medium through Which Exposure Occurs	Federal Agency	Specific Exposure Pathway Being Controlled	Federal Regulations	Citation
Water Drinking water	Environmental Protection Agency	Exposure of the general population to lead in drinking water supplied by public water systems.	The interim national primary drinking water maximum contaminant level for lead is 50 $\mu g/l$.	40 CFR 141.11
Food and Eating Utensils Apples, apricots, celery, peaches, pears, strawberries, tomatoes, and several other specific fresh fruits and vegetables	Environmental Protection Agency	Exposure of the general population to lead arsenate pesticide residues in or on raw agricultural commodities.	The tolerance for lead arsenate pesticide residues in or on ten designated raw fruits or vegetables is limited to 7 ppm of combined lead.	40 CFR 180.194
Citrus fruits			The tolerance for lead arsenate pesticide on citrus fruits is limited to 1 ppm of combined lead.	
Ceramic dinnerware, enamelware and pewter	Food and Drug Administration	Exposure of general population to lead that is leachable from pottery glazes.	The action level for leachable lead from ceramic work is 7.0 $\mu g/ml$, 5.0 $\mu g/ml$ and 2.5 $\mu g/ml$ for flatware, small hollow ware, and large hollow ware, respectively.	FDA Administrative Guideline 7417.00

Silver-plated hollow ware	Food and Drug Administration	Exposure of the general population to lead that is leachable from silver-plated hollow ware.	The action level for leachable lead from silver-plated hollow ware for use by adults is 7.0 μg/g. The action level for leachable lead from silver-plated cups intended for use by infants is 0.5 g/ml.	FDA Administrative Guideline 7417.01
Occupational Exposures Occupational exposures to lead in all industries covered by OSHA except construction and agriculture	Occupational Safety and Health Administration	Exposure to airborne lead in the workplace.	50 μg/m averaged over an 8-hour period.	29 CFR 1910.1025

the development and revision of drafts, arguments, pressures, negotiations, and compromises that are a vital part of any decision-making sequence. Unfortunately, effective documentation of every part of the decision process was too ambitious a task for our purposes; we therefore restricted ourselves to reviewing the agencies' own descriptions of their intent, the procedures they followed, and the basis for their decisions. The resulting case histories consequently are less than complete explanations of the reasons for specific decisions. However, they do meet our need, which is to provide a context in which to examine the policy-related importance of what is known and unknown about lead in the human environment.

U.S. DEPARTMENT OF HEALTH, EDUCATION, AND WELFARE: LEAD-BASED PAINT POISONING DETECTION AND HAZARD ELIMINATION

LEGISLATIVE AUTHORITY

The Lead-Based Paint Poisoning Prevention Act as amended authorizes the Department of Health, Education, and Welfare (HEW) to provide grants to local governments and nonprofit organizations for purposes of establishing lead paint poisoning detection and treatment programs and lead paint hazard elimination programs. Congress first passed lead paint poisoning control legislation in 1971 in order to reduce the alarmingly high incidence of lead poisoning and elevated blood lead levels among inner-city children.[2] In the hearings on the 1971 act and its subsequent amendments,[3-5] Congress acknowledged that the removal of all lead paint from housing would be necessary in order to eliminate completely any probability of childhood lead-based paint poisoning.

In spite of this pronouncement, the current lead paint poisoning prevention legislation does not articulate a clear priority for efforts in implementing detection/treatment programs over paint removal programs, or vice-versa.

Section 101 of the current law authorizes HEW, through the Center for Disease Control (CDC), to underwrite the costs of developing and carrying out local lead-based paint poisoning detection and treatment programs. In order to qualify for federal assistance, detection programs must include:

1. Educational programs that communicate to parents, educators and health officials information concerning the health danger and prevalence of lead-based paint poisoning among children in inner-city areas.[6]

2. Intensive community testing programs designed to detect incidents of lead-based paint poisoning and to ensure prompt medical treatment for afflicted individuals.[7]

3. Intensive follow-up programs to ensure that identified cases of lead-based paint poisoning are protected against further exposure to lead-based paints in their living environments.[8]

Follow-up programs must include the elimination of lead paint hazards from surfaces in and around the residences of children diagnosed as having lead poisoning and must include financial assistance to the owners of such residences who are unable to afford the costs of paint removal.

Section 201 of the act authorizes CDC to make grants to local public agencies for the purposes of (a) identifying high-risk areas that pose potential health hazards to residents because of the presence of lead-based paint, and (b) carrying out programs to eliminate the hazards of lead-based paint poisoning. To obtain these grants, local programs should include:

1. Comprehensive testing programs to detect the presence of lead-based paint on the surfaces of residential housing.[9]

2. Paint removal programs to remove from exposure to young children all interior and exterior housing surfaces which are hazardous to health because of the presence of lead paint.[10]

These grants are not limited with respect to the fraction of local program costs that can be covered, and they can be used for lead paint hazard elimination in any kind of housing, federally assisted or otherwise. Some potential overlap, therefore, exists with HUD's authority to eliminate lead paint hazards in HUD-associated housing (see HUD case study, below).

The legislative hearings for the 1971 act and the amendments of 1973 and 1976 clearly indicate that Congress' overriding intent was to establish categorical programs for inner-city lead paint poisoning detection and treatment and lead paint removal.[11-13] Administration representatives from HEW and HUD testified that other existing legislation provided authority to carry out broad-based lead paint poisoning control programs. (Indeed, prior to 1971, HEW had funded detection programs under the Public Health Service Act.) However, Congress, and Senator Edward M. Kennedy in particular, sought to designate specific resources for fighting these problems and giving them greater public visibility.

The 1971 act developed as a compromise measure between two very similar bills.[14] Legislation passed by the House (H.R. 19172) contained provisions authorizing HUD to assist in initiating lead paint removal programs and HEW to assist in establishing lead poisoning detection programs; legislation introduced into the Senate (S. 3216) contained provisions authorizing HEW to implement both the paint removal and poisoning detection programs. The House bill also contained provisions directing HUD to undertake a research program to determine the extent of lead-based paint poisoning in the United States and to prohibit the use of lead-based paint in future federally assisted construction (see HUD case study). The compromise bill that eventually passed both houses gave all program and regulatory authority to HEW and research authority to HUD.

In 1971, Congress did not establish any priority for implementing lead paint removal programs over lead poisoning detection and treatment programs or vice-versa. The hearing record indicates that Congress regarded both kinds of programs as critical needs.[15] Congress gave HEW sole jurisdiction over implementation of paint removal and poisoning detection programs in order to facilitate the awarding of grants to local governments.[16] Congress gave HUD research responsibility because certain basic information needs, such as the extent of the lead paint poisoning problem and the cost-effectiveness of paint removal, were related primarily to housing.

Although the 1973 amendments authorized larger appropriations for both detection/treatment and hazard elimination programs, Congress has appeared to place a greater priority on detection programs, increasing the maximum federal share of grants for community-based detection programs from 75 to 90 percent, and recently eliminating even the 10 percent matching requirement. Congress also extended HEW's authority to award detection program grants to community agencies and other private, nonprofit organizations. Congress was impressed by the large amounts of funding that local communities were requesting for detection programs and emphasized that a critical phase of the attack on the childhood lead poisoning problem was the search for children with elevated blood lead levels.[17]

The 1976 amendments emphasized hazard elimination, particularly in the residences of children with lead poisoning or elevated blood lead levels. With the 1976 amendments, Congress made it mandatory for local agencies to include educational and follow-up activities in programs under Section 101. With respect to follow-up, Congress recognized that it was ineffective to treat sick children and then return them to the hazardous conditions that caused lead poisoning in the first place. Unless abatement measures were initiated to remove lead paint from surfaces in and around the residences of children diagnosed as having lead poisoning, the children were likely to remain at risk.

HEW'S PROGRAMS

In January 1972, HEW proposed rules to govern the application and awarding of grants under Sections 101 and 201 of the Lead-Based Paint Poisoning Prevention Act.[18] The proposed rules combined grant application procedures for detection and treatment activities with procedures for hazard elimination activities into a single program for CDC to administer. HEW did not give its rationale for the decision to implement the law in this manner, nor describe grant application procedures. No public comments on the rules were received, and the regulations were promulgated in final form in May of 1972.[19]

The main element of information that local units of government must develop in an application is a description of the proposed lead-based poisoning prevention program. This description must include:[20]

1. A description of the nature and extent of the actual and potential lead-based paint poisoning problem in the community.

2. A description of the overall objectives of the program appropriate to the solution of the lead-based paint poisoning problem.

3. A description of a comprehensive program for detection and treatment of incidents of lead-based paint poisoning and for the identification and elimination of hazards of lead-based paint poisoning.

Specifically, a comprehensive program description must include:

1. Effective informational programs to develop an awareness of the problem in the community.

2. Community self-help programs to enable residents to remove lead-based paint poisoning hazards from residences.

3. Training, education, and employment opportunities in the program for residents of the community affected by lead-based paint hazards.

4. The establishment of lead-based paint screening services.

5. An intensified community follow-up program to ensure that children with blood lead levels of more than 40 μg/100 ml are followed under a program of medical surveillance or treatment.

6. A comprehensive program to detect the presence of lead-based paints in residential housing.

7. A comprehensive program requiring landlords to remove unacceptable levels of lead paint from surfaces accessible to children.

Although local governmental units must propose to carry out both lead paint poisoning detection and treatment and lead paint hazard identification and elimination activities, HEW regulations state that a (comprehensive) program shall emphasize screening and detection activities. In addition, the regulations greatly restrict the use of grant funds for the medical treatment of children and the deleading of residences. According to the regulations, the department will grant funds for treatment activities only on an emergency basis, and for hazard elimination activities only when the presence of lead paint on interior surfaces presents an imminent danger to health. However, in both instances federal funds can be used only when the grant applicant demonstrates that no other funds are reasonably available.[21]

BASIS FOR HEW'S DECISIONS

Although the promulgation notice in the *Federal Register* did not present a rationale for HEW's decision to emphasize detection/treatment activities over hazard elimination activities, reasons for the department's policy can be found in the lead-based paint poisoning prevention legislative hearing record and in statements by the Surgeon General.[22,23] These reasons fall primarily into four categories: (1) HEW's view of its mission in lead-based paint poisoning prevention; (2) the budgetary realities of meeting departmental objectives in this area; (3) political attitudes toward federal health and welfare programs in the early 1970s; and (4) changing practices in lead paint poisoning detection and treatment. It is beyond the scope of this discussion to examine in detail the influence of each of these factors on the manner in which HEW has implemented Sections 101 and 201 of the Lead-Based Paint Poisoning Prevention Act.

HEW regards its mission as one of preventing undue lead absorption and lead paint poisoning through screening, diagnosis, treatment, and follow-up of children in high-risk areas. In this regard, HEW has consistently viewed lead paint hazard elimination as an essential element of prevention, especially among children confirmed as having lead poisoning or undue lead absorption.[24,25] HEW has emphasized that the identification of lead hazards and the reduction of lead intake of these children is as much a medical necessity as is clinical management. HEW also has stated that the ultimate way in which to prevent undue lead absorption and lead poisoning is to identify and remove lead paint hazards before they harm children, but that until this can be accomplished it will be necessary to continue screening, diagnosis, treatment, and environmental management activities.[26]

One obvious reason HEW has maintained a screening orientation in its prevention program is budgetary. The department simply has not had sufficient resources to complete the Section 101 responsibilities of finding and treating children who may be, in terms of health status, dangerously exposed to deteriorating lead paint conditions. Initially, Congress authorized large levels of funding for Section 101 ($25 million for fiscal years 1974 and 1975), but appropriations were significantly less than authorizations ($9 million for fiscal years 1974 and 1975) and have declined somewhat since the 1975 peak.[27]

Although Congress was willing to appropriate more for lead paint poisoning detection and hazard elimination, the administration wanted smaller programs in this area. In general, the "New Federalism" of the Nixon–Ford Presidential years was aimed at de-emphasizing the role of the federal government and increasing the roles of state and local governments in implementing health and welfare programs. When translated into political action, this policy often meant resisting any increase in the number of new programs while seeking reductions in the scope and level of funding of existing programs. This policy is very apparent in testimony by Dr. David J. Sencer of HEW, opposing proposed 1975 amendments that would have greatly expanded CDC's lead-based paint hazard elimination responsibilities under Section 101.[28] Dr. Sencer testified:

First, we object to increased Federal responsibilities for elimination of lead paint hazards in homes, since this task is primarily a local responsibility that can be adequately addressed through local housing ordinances. The Federal role of limited research and demonstration of new and effective techniques for removal should continue.

Moreover, increased investments in lead hazard elimination under Title I (Section 101) child screening grants could also have the effect of severely reducing the number of children identified as suffering from undue lead absorption and subsequently being placed under pediatric management. Total elimination of lead-based paint hazards in the homes of children who have elevated blood lead levels will be a costly venture, and this will inevitably reduce the amount of funds available for screening and pediatric management. In addition, there are other effective methods of preventing re-exposure.

The success of the Childhood Lead Poisoning Prevention Programs has been due in large measure to the adaptability and ingenuity of local communities in meeting their needs. Often this has meant finding alternate housing for the affected family rather than remodeling the house. The provisions of this bill would remove that option. In addition, in many instances the hazard of undue lead absorption can be markedly reduced without the total elimination of all lead painted surfaces. The awareness of other family members of the dangers of pica in a young child and the control of flaking paint and dust can reduce the risk of exposure. We have recommended that hazard removal be undertaken based upon consideration of the risk to the child as determined by the screening procedures. The bill ties the removal of paints so closely to case finding and medical evaluation that no flexibility is available for local managers to deal with the problem without embarking on a multi-million dollar renovation program. There is little question that grant resources will become a major source of supporting this renovation since the disease occurs most often in areas where using is in poor and dilapidated condition and rental units are marginally profitable. Therefore, the majority of housing rentals would fall into the category "when the owner of said units or houses is unable to eliminate such lead-based paint surfaces."

Dr. Sencer's remarks concerning the proposed amendment's impact on the extent and flexibility of screening activities undoubtedly also reflected the fact that the administration had requested a 60 percent reduction in funding for Section 101.[29]

Finally, the detection and management of children with elevated blood lead levels is a rapidly changing field, and HEW has used new data from clinical, epidemiological, and experimental studies in efforts to improve the effectiveness of its programs.[30] Specifically, HEW has used this new information to develop priorities for screening to locate children who are at greatest risk in the target population; to give precise operational meaning to the terms elevated blood lead level, lead toxicity, undue lead absorption, and lead poisoning; and to establish criteria for classifying screening results into risk categories that reflect priorities for medical evaluation and lead hazard elimination. In terms of program effectiveness, the importance of establishing priorities for screening, treatment, and environmental management activities is accentuated by the fact that the large-scale screening studies of children without clinical symptoms of lead poisoning have demonstrated that the number of children with undue lead absorption is greater than previously anticipated.[31] In conclusion, the reasons discussed above provided some of the basis for HEW's decision to emphasize detection and treatment activities, and the last item is the chief reason for the department's continued emphasis in the detection area.

U.S. DEPARTMENT OF HOUSING AND URBAN DEVELOPMENT: LEAD-BASED PAINT HAZARD ELIMINATION PROCEDURES

LEGISLATIVE AUTHORITY

The Lead-Based Paint Poisoning Prevention Act, as amended, provides the Department of Housing and Urban Development (HUD) with regulatory and research responsibilities for eliminating the hazards of lead-based paint poisoning in HUD-associated and certain other housing.[32] The overall objective of the act is to eliminate childhood lead poisoning caused by the ingestion of lead paint in residential structures. The law provides HUD with three specific regulatory avenues for protecting children from exposure to such ingestion of paint:

1. Establishing procedures to eliminate, as far as practicable, the hazards of lead-based paint poisoning in HUD-associated housing and in federally owned properties that are sold for residential habitation.[33]

2. Establishing procedures to notify purchasers and tenants of HUD-associated housing of the hazards of lead-based paint.[34]

3. Prohibiting the use of lead-based paint in HUD-associated housing or in any federal or federally assisted construction or rehabilitation of residential structures.[35]

Section 302 of the 1973 Amendments to the Lead-Based Paint Poisoning Prevention Act mandated HUD to implement lead paint hazard elimination procedures. HUD had administratively implemented lead paint removal procedures in 1972.[36] The 1973 amendments sought to improve such procedures generally and to increase resources available for eliminating lead paint hazards. With respect to HUD, Congress intended that the department should establish procedures that would apply as a condition for Federal Housing Authority acceptance of applications for mortgage insurance or housing assistance payments.[37]

As a minimum, the 1973 amendments require HUD to establish practicable procedures for eliminating immediate hazards of lead paint to children living in housing that is owned or financially assisted by HUD. In addition, HUD must notify purchasers and tenants in such housing of the hazards of lead paint, of the symptoms and treatment of lead poisoning, and of the importance and availability of techniques for eliminating such hazards. HUD must carry out these programs for all HUD-associated housing constructed prior to 1950 and for any housing constructed after 1950 that, in the Secretary's judgment, contains lead-based paint hazards.

Section 401 of the amended act requires HUD to establish procedures for prohibiting the use of lead-based paint in HUD-associated housing or in any federally assisted housing. The 1976 amendments to the act transferred to HUD from HEW the responsibility for implementing this section, which had been included in the original 1971 law.

The intent of Section 401 is to prevent the occurrence of childhood lead paint poisoning in the future by prohibiting the construction or maintenance of the kind of housing environment that is presently causing this problem. To achieve that objective, Section 501 of the act as amended defines lead-based paint as paint containing more than 0.06 percent lead by weight. In 1976, Congress provisionally established the 0.06 percent level as being "safe," subject to the Consumer Product Safety Commission's determination (within 6 months after enactment) that a higher concentration of lead in paint was also safe.[38] In 1977, the CPSC reported that it could not recommend that a lead concentration in excess of 0.06 percent would be safe (see CPSC case study, below).

HUD'S PROGRAMS

HUD interpreted the mandate in the 1973 amendments as requiring the practicable elimination of lead-based paint hazards in housing subject to the act without regard to any quantifiable risk factor.[39] In other words, the department believed that it could carry out the hazard elimination program without establishing a lead paint poisoning detection program. Hazardous paint conditions would be determined only by inspection of residences.

In proposing procedures to carry out the 1973 mandate, HUD distinguished between two alternative solutions to the lead paint hazard problem: the "health approach" and the "housing approach."[40] The health approach would involve an initial screening of children to determine their blood lead levels; removal of lead from the homes would follow for those children found to have elevated blood lead levels. In contrast, the housing approach would involve the inspection of all HUD-associated housing for lead-based paint and the removal of such paint, regardless of the ages or blood lead levels of the inhabitants.

In evaluating the two approaches, HUD considered a number of health and cost-related issues concerning lead-based paint poisoning control. These included the relative importance of lead paint as a cause of lead poisoning; local procedures for controlling lead-paint poisoning; the cost-effectiveness of available methods for detecting and eliminating lead-based paint hazards; the outlook for technological improvements in these methods; and the impact of hazard elimination procedures on the supply of housing available to low- and moderate-income families. This evaluation focused on determining the most cost-effective and practicable methods for achieving the Congressional intent of Section 302.

With respect to the housing approach, HUD determined that cost considerations made impractical the removal of all lead paint in existing HUD-associated housing.[41] When revised removal procedures were promulgated in 1976, the department reasoned:[42]

While completely removing all lead-based paint for all housing could substantially eliminate one source of lead poisoning, the potential costs involved would be prohibitive. In addition, such costs could adversely affect the value of the housing involved and could also substantially reduce the supply of otherwise standard housing available to low and moderate income families.

The department further stated that cost-effective solutions to lead-paint hazard prevention were highly sensitive to technological developments. In this regard, HUD indicated that its research efforts would be directed toward developing improved and less costly methods for lead paint detection and removal (see Appendix B). HUD noted that current (1976) methods of detection were time-consuming, inefficient, and unreliable for detecting low levels of lead paint on walls, and it pointed to a need for further testing of new paint removal techniques.

Because of these considerations, HUD concluded that in line with its mandate, the most practicable lead paint hazard elimination program that it could then implement was to concentrate on the correction of defective paint conditions in HUD-associated housing. A "defective paint condition" was defined as any paint—with or without lead—that is cracking, scaling, chipping, peeling, or loose on interior surfaces and on those exterior surfaces that are readily accessible to children under 7 years of age.

HUD concluded that defective paint conditions presented an "immediate hazard." In this manner the department distinguished between paint (which may or may not contain lead) that is in sound, tight condition on applicable surfaces, and paint that is not. HUD defined intact paint as being a "potential hazard" and, hence, without immediate need for removal.

Based on the rationale just stated, HUD adopted procedures for eliminating immediate lead paint hazards, as follows:

First, HUD-associated housing is inspected to determine whether defective paint conditions are present. If such conditions are present, treatment to eliminate them must as a minimum include sufficient washing, scraping, and brushing to remove all defective paint on applicable surfaces. These surfaces must then be repainted with two coats of suitable nonleaded paint. If the integrity of surfaces bearing defective paint cannot be maintained, the paint must be removed completely or covered with a suitable material such as wallboard, plywood, or plaster before repainting.

Inspection for defective paint conditions is required only prior to occupancy. Consequently, only those HUD-associated housing units that change hands are examined for lead paint hazards. HUD did not believe that it was necessary to provide uniformly for periodic inspection for and removal of defective paint conditions. Each assistant secretary was directed to implement lead paint elimination procedures that were most appropriate for the particular HUD programs within his administrative jurisdiction.

HUD's lead paint hazard notification procedures for current occupants of HUD-associated housing consist of providing residents with brochures that: (a) indicate that the property may contain lead paint; (b) describe the immediate and potential hazards of lead-based paint; (c) describe the symptoms and treatment of lead-based paint poisoning; and (d) discuss the precautions that can be taken to avoid lead paint poisoning. The brochures are printed in English and Spanish; steps that must be taken to ensure their distribution have been left to the assistant secretaries to establish, in accordance with local programs. These procedures were adopted on an interim basis in 1975[43] and promulgated in 1976[44] without discussion.

Although HUD adopted the "housing approach" as a cost-effective solution, the department indicated that the "health approach" also would be effective. HUD noted that, given the vast number of housing units containing lead paint, the high costs of present methods of lead paint removal, and the fact that excessive lead absorption occurs in only a small percentage of children, population screening offers a way to direct resources to individuals who are adversely affected, rather than to generalized abatement. In addition, the department indicated that the health approach is used almost universally in local programs, and provides a basis for initiating lead paint removal in communities with abatement requirements. In spite of these considerations, HUD did not incorporate child screening into its procedures, because the department believed it lacked the capability and authority to do so,[45] and because the Department of Health, Education, and Welfare supports many local screening programs (see previous section).

In 1977, HUD promulgated regulations[46] that implemented Section 401 prohibitions against the use of lead paint in federally assisted housing. These regulations direct federal agency heads to prohibit in federally assisted residential construction or rehabilitation the use of lead-based paint on interior and exterior surfaces that are readily accessible to children. In addition, contracts and subcontracts for this type of construction or rehabilitation are to include these prohibitions and provisions for their enforcement. In accordance with the 1976 amendments, the *Federal Register* notice simply substituted HUD in the place of HEW as having the authority to enforce a set of previously promulgated HEW prohibitions on the use of lead paint.[47]

BASIS FOR HUD'S DECISIONS

To assist in its evaluation of the proposed hazard elimination procedures, HUD held 4 days of public hearings and gathered testimony from many expert witnesses. The transcript of these hearings and various reports completed under HUD's lead paint hazard elimination research program[48] were apparently used as background documents in this evaluation. It is difficult to determine what information HUD used in developing the different elements of its rationale, however, because the published (*Federal Register*) accounts of the department's evaluation were poorly organized and referenced background materials inadequately.

The public hearings provided HUD with information on the multimedia nature of human lead exposure. The testimony pointed out that lead-based paint is only one source of lead in the environment. Experts indicated that other sources such as dust, dirt, and airborne particles from combustion of gasoline also contribute to the total amount of lead in the environment, but that the extent to which these other sources contribute to childhood lead poisoning is unclear.

In its statements of proposed and promulgated hazard elimination procedures,[49] HUD did not provide quantitative information on the extent of lead-based paint hazards or on the costs of alternative solutions. No estimates were made of the number of HUD-associated housing units containing defective paint conditions. The department simply adopted the definition of immediate hazard, which is central to the elimination program, directly from its own 1972 administrative procedures, without discussion of whether that definition conformed to Congress' intent in Section 302 of the legislation. Finally, no cost estimates were presented to justify IIUD's selection from among the different alternatives considered: inspection and elimination of lead paint hazards in vacant housing units; periodic inspection and elimination in housing regardless of occupancy; and population screening, followed by inspection and elimination.

In summary, although HUD must notify all occupants of HUD-associated housing of the hazards of lead-based paint, the department's hazard elimination program applies only to units that are changing occupancy or are about to be occupied for the first time. Prior to occupancy by new residents, these units must be inspected, and any defective paint conditions must be removed. As a result, HUD's hazard elimination program affects only that pre-1950 housing that has defective paint conditions and is changing occupants.

CONSUMER PRODUCT SAFETY COMMISSION: CONTROLS ON LEAD-BASED PAINT AND TOYS AND FURNITURE BEARING LEAD-BASED PAINT

LEGISLATIVE AUTHORITY

The Consumer Product Safety Act (CPSA) provides general authority to the Consumer Product Safety Commission (CPSC) to ban as hazardous any consumer product that presents an unreasonable risk of injury.[50] Under this authority, the commission has banned from sale in interstate commerce paint and surface coatings containing more than 0.06 percent lead, toys with painted surfaces containing more than 0.06 percent lead, and furniture with painted surfaces containing more than 0.06 percent lead. These controls, which became effective in February 1978, were adopted in order to eliminate or reduce the unreasonable risk of personal injury or serious or frequent illness associated with lead poisoning in children.[51]

CPSC chose to regulate these consumer-related uses of lead paint under the broader authority of the CPSA, even though the 1976 Amendments to the Lead-Based Paint Poisoning Prevention Act had mandated the commission to take action prohibiting the application of lead paint to any toy or article of furniture.[52] The 1976 amendments also had selectively prohibited the use of lead-based paint in federal and federally assisted housing and on cooking utensils, but CPSC believed that because Congress had deemed unsafe certain uses of lead paint it had intended to establish general control over all consumer-related uses of paint containing unsafe amounts of lead. Accordingly, the commission decided to expand the mandated prohibitions and include other consumer and nonhousing uses of lead paint.[53]

In addition to requirements to prohibit certain uses of lead paint, the 1976 Amendments to the Lead-Based Paint Poisoning Prevention Act also required CPSC to determine a safe level of lead in paint.[54] The amendments defined lead-based paint as any paint containing more than 0.5 percent lead by weight in the total nonvolatile content of the paint or in the dried film of paint already applied. The act ordered CPSC to determine—within 6 months of enactment and on the basis of available scientific information and data and consultation with the Center for Disease Control of the Department of Health, Education, and Welfare and with the National Academy of Sciences—whether a level of lead greater than 0.06 percent but less than 0.5 percent was safe. If CPSC made such a determination, then a new definition of lead-based paint would be established in accordance with the designated safe level. If CPSC did not make such a determination, then a new definition of lead-based paint as any paint containing more than 0.06 percent lead would be automatically established 12 months after enactment.

BASIS FOR CPSC'S DECISION ON SAFE LEVEL OF LEAD IN PAINT

The amendments gave CPSC the burden of proving that a level of lead in paint greater than 0.06 was safe, a considerably more demanding requirement than determining a safe level of lead in paint in the 0.06 to 0.5 percent range. CPSC had been required to do the latter by the 1973 Amendments to the Lead-Based Paint Poisoning Prevention Act, and had concluded in a report to Congress in 1974[55] that on the basis of certain animal studies[56,57] the 0.5 percent level was safe. According to CPSC, this level provided a reasonable assurance that with expected exposures there would be no serious toxic effects.[58]

In making a determination of a safe level of lead in paint under the 1976 act, the commission followed the recommendations of the National Research Council[59] and rejected the animal study findings as insufficient for this purpose.[60] The NRC study had concluded:[61]

. . . since the CPSC studies did not adequately simulate the conditions found in young children, particularly in relation to age and diet, we were unable, on the basis of these studies, to determine that 0.5 percent lead in paint was safe.

The NRC committee also found that a 0.5 percent level of lead in paint represents a hazard to a child with pica for paint, and specifically recommended:[62]

. . . that the deliberate addition of lead to paint for residential buildings or other surfaces accessible to young children be immediately discontinued and that a level not to exceed 0.06 percent lead in the final dried product be set for regulatory purposes.

The recommendations of the Center for Disease Control and the American Academy of Pediatrics generally supported those of the NRC. The National Paint and Coatings Association and toy industry representatives proposed levels of 0.2 and 0.25 percent, respectively, but did not provide toxicity data to support their assertions that the suggested levels were safe. As a result, the commission concluded that available information was insufficient to support a finding that a level of lead in paint above 0.06 percent was safe.[63]

CPSC did not indicate in the *Federal Register*[64] that it had followed a specific rationale in determining a safe level of lead in paint, other than its evaluation of the aforementioned animal studies. The rationale followed by the NRC committee that advised the CPSC is described in Appendix A of this report, where the NRC's report to the CPSC is summarized. The commission did hold public hearings on the matter and in addition to comments related to lead paint toxicity received testimony related to the economic and technical effects of lowering the level of lead in paint. These issues appear to have been of secondary interest to the CPSC, however, and the determination of a "safe" level of lead in paint was based principally on toxicity and safety considerations.

The determination of a "safe" level of lead in paint obviously influenced CPSC's decisions regarding which lead levels to ban as hazardous in paint and on painted toys and furniture. In proposing the ban, the CPSC had stated that it would adopt the level determined under the Lead-Based Paint Poisoning Prevention Act as the "safe level" of lead for products.[65]

RATIONALE AND BASIS FOR CPSC'S REGULATIONS

Prior to 1978, CPSC had limited the level of lead in paint for use in houses and on toys to 0.5 percent, under the Federal Hazardous Substances Act (FHSA). Through a series of extensions, the commission had kept in force controls that had been promulgated in 1972 by the Food and Drug Administration[66] and redesignated to CPSC in 1973 with the enactment of the CPSA.[67]

In proposing the more stringent controls on lead in paint and on painted products in 1976, the commission chose to act under CPSA instead of FHSA primarily because of the former law's simpler requirements for public hearings and broader provisions for product coverage.[68] Under the CPSA, the commission must find it in the public interest to ban for risk of injury any products which could also be controlled under FHSA.[69] The commission made such a finding, based on its desire to avoid the lengthy FHSA evidentiary hearing requirements, which would have constrained opportunities for public participation and delayed resolution of the issue.[70]

The general procedure which CPSC must follow in promulgating any rule declaring a consumer product a banned, hazardous product is clearly defined by the CPSA.[71] For any consumer product that the commission finds as presenting an unreasonable risk of injury, it must determine:

1. The degree and nature of the risk of injury which the consumer products ban is designed to eliminate or reduce.

2. The approximate number of types of consumer products subject to such a ban.

3. The public's need for the banned consumer products and the probable effect of the ban on the utility, cost or availability of such products to meet this need.

4. Any means of achieving the objective of the ban while minimizing adverse effects to competition, manufacturing, or other commercial practices. In making these determinations, CPSC must consider relevant available product data, including the results of research, development, and testing.

This procedure outlines the basic rationale that CPSC followed in banning paint and painted surfaces containing more than 0.06 percent lead on toys and furniture. The commission's findings for each step in the procedure are the major conclusions drawn by the agency in reaching its decision.

With respect to the nature and extent of the risk of injury, CPSC concluded that lead paint is the main source of lead poisoning in children; that paint that flakes and peels from walls is sometimes eaten by children, especially those with pica; and that certain surfaces containing lead paint, such as toys or furniture, are also easily accessible to children.[72] These findings did not originate with CPSC, but rather were basic tenets of the 1971 Lead-Based Paint Poisoning Prevention Act, which was amended in 1976 to require the CPSC action on paints and painted products.

The commission summarized information on the adverse health effects of lead poisoning[73] and relied on the NRC's report[74] for evidence of the seriousness of the problem. CPSC emphasized that children with pica were of special concern, and concluded that this habit occurs in 50 percent of children in the high-risk ages between 1 and 3. The commission also cited estimates by the the U.S. Surgeon General[75] and the National Bureau of Standards,[76] respectively, that 400,000 and 600,000 preschool children had elevated blood lead concentrations. Finally, the commission noted that because lead paint poisoning injuries result from chronic rather than acute hazards, they are not reported through the National Electronic Injury Surveillance System, which monitors only emergency room treatment; there is therefore no systematic national record of the incidence of such injuries.

The commission banned as hazardous all interior and exterior household paints and coating materials—including varnishes, lacquers, stains, enamels, and primers—containing more than 0.06 percent lead. All toys and other articles intended for use by children and furniture articles with surface coatings containing more than 0.06 percent lead also were banned. Some major product categories were exempted from control, including agricultural and industrial equipment coatings, motor vehicle coatings, artist's paints, other specialized coatings, household appliances, and certain household items such as window shades and wall hangings.

In determining whether a specific risk of injury is unreasonable, CPSC attempts to balance the risk and gravity of potential injury against the impact of a product ban on the utility, cost, and availability of such products. With respect to utility, the commission acknowledged that the primary economic impact of the regulations would be to eliminate the use of lead driers in paints, since lead pigments were already precluded under FHSA control levels.[77] The commission concluded that this impact would not be severe because nearly 70 percent of oil-based paints intended for consumer use already had levels of lead at or below 0.06 percent.[78] (Lead driers are not used in latex paints.)

The commission estimated that the added costs to the consumer for paints affected by this rule would not exceed 5 to 10 cents per gallon.[79] These increases would be caused by the need for manufacturers to use more expensive driers and to adopt more stringent housekeeping and process control measures. Costs to consumers for furniture and toys were not expected to increase as a result of compliance with the regulations.

With regard to availability, the commission noted that there was limited need by consumers for paint containing more than 0.06 percent lead. With the exception of certain special paint products, substitutes were available at prices comparable to those for the banned products.[80]

In summary, CPSC's decision to ban as hazardous lead paint and certain products bearing lead paint was based on conclusions that: (a) the main source of lead in childhood lead poisoning is lead-containing paint; (b) paint containing more than 0.06 percent lead on walls poses a hazard if ingested by children with pica; and (c) paint containing more than 0.06 percent lead on toys and other objects also poses a hazard if chewed by children. Because CPSC's jurisdiction is product safety, which in this instance has a narrower focus than the issue of health risk due to lead exposure, the commission did not consider potential health risks due to lead exposure from sources other than paint, nor did it attempt to estimate the relative importance of lead in paint as a source of exposure. Finally, the commission concluded that the injury-reducing benefits of lead paint restrictions more than offset any associated cost impacts to consumers.

U.S. ENVIRONMENTAL PROTECTION AGENCY: LEAD IN FUELS

LEGISLATIVE AUTHORITY

Section 211 of the Clean Air Act of 1970 authorized the Administrator of the Environmental Protection Agency to control or prohibit the manufacture and sale of motor vehicle fuels or fuel additives if their emission products (a) "will endanger the public health or welfare," or (b) "will impair to a significant degree the performance of any emission control device or system which is in general use, or which the Administrator finds has been developed to a point where in a reasonable time it would be in general use were such regulations to be promulgated."[81] Under the first condition, all relevant medical and scientific evidence, as well as feasible alternatives, must be considered. Under the latter condition, consideration of scientific data and cost–benefit analysis of alternative emission control devices is required.

The EPA has promulgated two sets of regulations that restrict the use of lead additives in gasoline. In the first case, EPA ordered major gasoline retailers to sell at least one grade of "unleaded" gasoline, defined as containing no more than .05 grams per gallon (gpg), beginning July 1, 1974.[82] The purpose of this regulation was to provide for the general availability of lead-free gasoline to protect lead-intolerant catalytic emission control systems that were installed on 1975 and later model cars to meet federal automobile emission standards. In the second set of regulations, EPA established a 5-year, phased-reduction schedule beginning January 1, 1975, that incrementally reduced the maximum allowable lead content of leaded grades of gasoline to an average of 0.5 gpg by January 1, 1979.[83] EPA's purpose in phasing down the lead content of leaded grades of gasoline was to reduce automotive lead emissions, which EPA considers a hazard to public health.

UNLEADED GASOLINE

In order to meet the 1975 federal emission standards, automobile manufacturers adopted an add-on control strategy that required the use of catalysts that are rendered inoperative by lead. Given the time and economic constraints imposed by the 1970 amendments to the Clean Air Act, an add-on strategy provided the only feasible means of meeting 1975 standards on schedule; and the catalytic converter had demonstrated technical advantages over other alternatives. Therefore, EPA ordered the general availability of unleaded gasoline, proposing regulations on February 23, 1972,[84] with final promulgation on January 10, 1973.[85] The rationale for this regulation was based primarily on engineering and economic considerations. EPA stated that without regulatory action requiring retail outlets to market at least one grade of lead-free gasoline, supplies would be uncertain and insufficient.[86]

LEAD PHASE-DOWN

The Clean Air Act of 1970 provided EPA alternative avenues for regulating human exposure to airborne lead. Under Sections 108 and 109, EPA could identify lead as a hazardous pollutant, issue air quality criteria, and establish national ambient air quality standards for lead. However, the Administrator recognized this alternative as discretionary[87] and determined that since "research has not documented beyond reasonable doubt the levels of airborne lead in ambient air at which health effects in persons would be caused . . . we do not have a basis on which . . . (such standards) . . . could properly be established at this time."[88] Although EPA could have imposed a lead emission standard for motor vehicles under Section 202 of the Clean Air Act, this alternative was rejected as infeasible.[89] Consequently, EPA chose to address the health hazards of automobile-emitted airborne lead under Section 211 (c)(1) of the act, by controlling lead additives directly. "In EPA's opinion, lead in gasoline is the most important remaining source of *controllable* lead entering the environment."[90]

The phase-down regulation, designed to achieve a 60 to 65 percent reduction from 1971 levels of lead in the air, was proposed January 10, 1973, and promulgated November 28, 1973. The final regulation[91] contained a schedule of lead reduction requiring quarterly average lead concentrations over all grades of gasoline of 1.7 gpg after January 1, 1975; 1.4 gpg after January 1, 1976; 1.0 gpg after January 1, 1977; 0.8 gpg after January 1, 1978; and 0.5 gpg after January 1, 1979. Because of subsequent litigation and to avoid possible shortages of gasoline, EPA suspended the timetable through 1977. In addition, because meeting the 0.8 gpg level for 1978 required about the same amount of refinery construction time as meeting the 0.5 gpg standard for 1979, EPA suspended the 1978 phase-reduction level for those refiners who have made sufficient progress in procuring and installing new capacity so as to meet the 0.8 gpg level at the earliest practicable date. The 0.5 gpg standard was scheduled to go into effect on October 1, 1979.[92] However, once again considerations related to a fuel shortage and political pressures resulted in another postponement and relaxation of the regulations. In June 1979, EPA suspended enforcement of the lead phase-down until October 1, 1979, and postponed the effective date of the 0.5 gpg standard until October 1, 1980.[93]

In contrast to the technical basis for ordering unleaded gasoline, the rationale for the implementation of the phased-reduction schedule was based entirely on public health considerations. On the basis of an evaluation of available scientific and medical information, EPA concluded that environmental lead exposure is a major public health problem, with present levels of lead exposure constituting a sufficient risk of adverse physiological effects for a small but significant portion of the urban adult population and up to 25 percent of the children in urban areas.[94]

EPA also concluded that the combustion of leaded gasoline contributes the largest fraction of lead currently reaching the environment, and that automotive lead emissions account for at least 90 percent of airborne lead. Lead from gasoline is ubiquitous, and people may be exposed directly through inhalation and indirectly through ingestion of lead contaminated dust and dirt, especially in urban areas. The agency recognized that lead exposure results from a combination of sources, including lead in the air, food, water, leaded paint, and street dust, and that it is difficult to determine which source is the most significant from a health standpoint. Although ingestion of lead-based paint chips is regarded as the major cause of overt lead poisoning in children in EPA's judgment sources of lead other than paint may play an important role in childhood lead exposure, especially at subclinical levels of lead toxicity.

With respect to lead in dust and dirt, EPA concluded that these sources contribute to increased lead levels in human beings, both through inhalation of resuspended dust and, in children, through ingestion of dust and dirt. The agency concluded that the availability of lead from this source significantly reduces the quantity of lead required to produce clinical lead poisoning in a child who is exposed to other sources of lead. Finally, because automotive lead is a major contributor to lead in dust and dirt, and because lead in dust and dirt has been related to undue absorption of lead in children, EPA concluded that lead in gasoline should be reduced to the greatest degree possible.

In the preamble to its final phased-reduction regulations, issued in 1973, EPA stated that the rationale for the original proposal, which had concluded that airborne lead levels of about 2 $\mu g/m^3$ were associated with risk of adverse health effects, was not valid, since available information was insufficient to establish a precise level of airborne lead as a basis for a control strategy.[95] A revised evaluation of health effects, contained in the document "EPA's Position on the Health Implications of Airborne Lead," served as the health basis for the regulation. However, EPA concluded that information was still insufficient in several areas, including: (a) relative quantitative significance of various routes of exposure, (b) precise correlation of air lead and blood lead levels, and (c) significance of subclinical effects of lead exposure.

U.S. ENVIRONMENTAL PROTECTION AGENCY: NATIONAL AMBIENT AIR QUALITY STANDARD FOR LEAD

LEGISLATIVE AUTHORITY AND INTENT

The Clean Air Act as amended requires the Administrator of the U.S. Environmental Protection Agency (EPA) to promulgate national primary (health) and secondary (welfare) ambient air quality standards for air pollutants that endanger public health and welfare. On October 5, 1978, in accordance with these provisions, EPA promulgated a primary ambient air quality standard of 1.5 μg Pb$/m^3$. This standard addresses the problem of human exposure to lead emitted into the atmosphere from various stationary and mobile sources. Under provisions of the Clean Air Act, the states must develop implementation plans for attaining the standard by 1982.

Sections 108 and 109 of the Clean Air Act govern the development of and timetable for the establishment of national ambient air quality standards. Section 108 requires EPA to list any air pollutant that may reasonably be anticipated to endanger public health or welfare.[96] Within 12 months after listing, the Administrator must issue air quality criteria that reflect the latest scientific knowledge useful in indicating the nature and extent of all identifiable effects from varying airborne concentrations of the pollutant on public health and welfare.[97] Simultaneously with the issuance of these criteria, the Administrator must also issue emission control information for the pollutant, including estimates of the costs of installation and operation of controls, and the emission reduction potential and energy and environmental impacts of controls.[98]

Section 109 addresses the actual setting of the standard. At the same time that the Administrator issues the air quality criteria, he must also propose a national ambient air quality standard for the pollutant in question. Primary standards must be set at a level which in the judgment of the Administrator is sufficient to protect the public health, allowing for an adequate margin of safety.[99] Final standards must be promulgated within 90 days after the proposed standards have been issued.[100]

It is apparent from these provisions that Congress intended for the EPA to enact measures to protect public health as expediently as possible, once the agency has identified air pollutants that are potential hazards to public health. EPA's decision to list lead as a hazardous pollutant was made in response to a court order stemming from a suit brought against the agency by the Natural Resources Defense Council.[101] This suit followed EPA's efforts to control airborne lead by a phased reduction of the allowable lead concentration of gasoline (see previous case study) without establishing an ambient standard for lead.

Congress intended the language of Section 108 to emphasize the preventive or precautionary nature of the act. The provision allowing the Administrator to control air pollutants that in his judgment "may reasonably be anticipated to endanger public health" was added in 1977, in order to allow regulatory action to prevent harm and to emphasize the predominant value of protecting public health.[102] This aspect of the legislative intent was extremely important in EPA's determination of a health basis for the ambient air quality standard for lead.

In following the legislative requirements of Section 109, EPA based its determination of the maximum allowable level of lead in air on scientific information presented in a criteria document[103] summarizing the health and welfare implications of airborne lead. (A synopsis of that document appears in Appendix A of this report.) The agency interpreted the requirement to provide a margin of safety to mean that the air quality standard should be set at a point below the airborne concentration associated with demonstrable adverse health effects:[104]

It is clear from section 109 the agency should not attempt to place the standard at a level estimated to be at the threshold for adverse health effects, but should set the standard at a lower level in order to provide a margin of safety. EPA believes that the extent of the margin of safety represents a judgment in which the agency considers the severity of reported health effects, the probability that such effects may occur, and uncertainties as to the full biological significance of exposure to lead.

The Clean Air Act requires EPA to use health criteria as the entire basis for setting air quality standards. Unlike other sections of the act, the agency is not required to consider the economic costs and technical availability of air pollution control systems or the potential economic benefits of improvements to public health that can accrue from setting ambient standards. Although recent executive orders[105] compelled EPA to conduct a general analysis of the economic impacts that might result from the implementation of lead regulations, this analysis was not intended for use in deriving a numerical value for the standard and was issued solely for informational purposes.[106]

EPA'S RATIONALE

As outlined in the proposed air quality standard,[107] EPA's basic rationale required judgments in five key areas: (1) determining the critically sensitive population; (2) determining the health significance of subclinical effects and thresholds for these effects; (3) determining a maximum safe level of total lead exposure for the sensitive population as indicated by blood lead concentrations; (4) determining the relationship between airborne lead exposure and resulting blood lead concentration; and (5) determining the allowable blood lead increment from airborne lead, including an estimate of the contribution to blood lead levels caused by other sources.

Critically Sensitive Population

Although a number of other high-risk population subgroups were identified, EPA concluded that young children 1 to 5 years of age are the foremost critically sensitive population to lead exposure. Children have a lower threshold for adverse physiological effects because of: (a) potentially greater intake per unit of body weight; (b) proportionally greater absorption and retention of ingested lead; (c) greater physiological sensitivity to lead due to rapid growth; (d) incomplete development of a metabolic defense system; and (e) greater sensitivity of other developing systems. In addition, children have a greater risk of exposure to lead from sources other than air, food, or water, by normal mouthing activity or by abnormal ingestion of nonfood items (pica).[108-110]

Health Significance of Subclinical Effects

In establishing the health basis for the standard, EPA used the level of lead in blood as an indicator of exposure and internal dose, and identified a range of effects associated with various blood lead levels. Although anemia is clinically detectable in children at 40 μg Pb/100 ml, EPA also was concerned about subclinical effects of lower levels. The criteria document reports that at blood lead levels above 15 to 20 μg/100 ml there is an elevation of erythrocyte protoporphyrin (EP).[111] An increase of protoporphyrin in red blood cells indicates an interference with the iron insertion process in the formation of heme, such that "protoporphyrin, rather than heme, is incorporated in the hemoglobin molecule where it remains throughout the erythrocyte life span (120 days)."[112]

From a review of its criteria document, EPA concluded that the effects of lead on the cellular synthesis of heme as indicated by elevated EP are potentially adverse to the health of young children.[113,114] In response to challenges on the significance of elevated EP as the health basis for the standard, EPA indicated that the initial elevation of EP as a result of exposure to lead may not be a disease state or seen as a clinically detectable decline in performance; however, impairment of heme synthesis increases progressively with lead dose, or as pointed out in the criteria document[115] and cited by EPA:[116]

The hematological effects described above are the earliest physiological impairments encountered as a function of increasing lead exposures as indexed by blood lead elevations; as such, those effects may be considered to represent critical effects of lead exposure. Although it may be argued that certain of the initial hematological effects (such as ALAD inhibition) constitute relatively mild, nondebilitating symptoms at low blood levels, they nevertheless signal the onset of steadily intensifying adverse effects as blood lead elevations increase. Eventually, the hematological effects reach such magnitude that they are of clear-cut medical significance as indicators of undue lead exposure.

Maximum Safe Exposure for Children

EPA made a clear distinction between a safe blood lead level for an individual child and a safe mean blood lead level for the target population.[117] From a review of information provided in the criteria document, EPA concluded that the maximum safe blood lead level for an individual child is 30 μg/100 ml. This conclusion was based on the following factors:[118]

1. The maximum safe blood lead level should be somewhat lower than the threshold for a decline in hemoglobin levels (40 μg Pb/100 ml).
2. The maximum safe blood lead level should be at an even greater distance below the threshold for risks of nervous system deficits (50 μg Pb/100 ml).
3. The maximum safe blood lead level should be no higher than the blood lead range characterized as undue exposure by the Center for Disease Control of the Public Health Service, as endorsed by the American Academy of Pediatrics, because of elevation of erythrocyte protoporphyrin (> 30 μg Pb/100 ml).
4. The maximum safe blood lead level for an individual need not be as low as the detection point for the initial elevation of EP (15–20 μg Pb/100 ml).

Using standard statistical techniques, EPA estimated the mean population blood lead level that would place a given percentage of the population below the selected maximum safe childhood blood level of 30 μg/100 ml.[119] The agency used data from epidemiological studies that showed that the logarithmic values of measured blood lead levels in a uniformly exposed population are normally distributed with a geometric standard deviation of 1.3 to 1.5.[120] EPA then selected a standard deviation of 1.3, and estimated that a population geometric mean of 15 μg Pb/100 ml would be necessary in order to place 99.5 percent of the children in the U.S. below 30 μg Pb/100 ml.[121]

EPA elected to use margin-of-safety considerations in estimating the percentage of the target population to be placed below the maximum safe blood lead level.[122] In this regard, EPA viewed the 99.5 percent range as precautionary and not excessive. The agency pointed out that in 1970 there were approximately 20 million children under 6 years of age, 12 million in urban areas and 5 million in central cities where lead exposure is potentially high. Based on the fact that there are special high-risk groups of children within the general population, the agency believed that it could not consider lower percentages.[123]

Airborne Lead Exposure and Blood Lead Levels

On the basis of its review of epidemiological studies discussed in the criteria document, EPA selected a ratio of 1.0 to 2.0 for estimating the impact of air lead levels on blood lead levels in children; that is, EPA assumed that each μg Pb/m^3 in the air contributes 2 μg Pb/100 ml to blood lead level. In this regard, EPA was particularly influenced by a study of adults by Azar et al. (1975).[124] According to the agency, the data from this study indicate that at an airborne lead concentration of 1.5 μg/m^3, the (air lead)/(blood lead) ratio is 1.0/1.8.[125]

Because children are known to have greater net absorption and retention of lead than adults, EPA chose a ratio of 1 to 2 as the basis for its standard. The agency also noted that the (air lead)/(blood lead) ratio is nonlinear, with higher ratios occurring for lower air lead levels.[126]

Allowable Blood Lead Increment from Airborne Sources

In promulgating an air quality standard for lead, EPA took into account the multimedia nature of human lead exposure and attempted to quantify the fractions of total body burden of lead that could be attributed to airborne and nonairborne pathways, respectively. The agency based its calculation of the ambient standard on the assumption that the lead contribution from nonair sources to blood lead should be subtracted from the estimate of the safe mean population blood lead.[127]

The agency noted that the level of the standard is strongly influenced by judgments regarding the nonair contribution to total exposure. The studies reviewed in the criteria document[128] do not provide detailed or extensive information about the the relative contributions of various sources of lead to children's blood lead levels. In spite of these difficulties, EPA attempted to estimate the relative contributions to population blood lead levels from air and nonair sources on the basis of available information. The evidence used included general epidemiological studies, studies showing declines of blood lead levels with decreases in air lead, and isotopic tracing studies. Ultimately, the agency based its determination of the contribution of nonair sources to children's blood lead on inference from empirical studies that usually involved adults.[129]

Allowable Level of Airborne Lead

In the absence of more precise information, EPA calculated the air quality standard by assuming that on the average 12.0 μg Pb/100 ml of the blood lead levels in children could be attributed to nonair sources. The agency concluded that to use a larger estimate of the nonair contribution to blood lead would result in an exceptionally stringent air standard.[130]

In summary, EPA's determination of the national ambient air quality standard of 1.5 μg Pb/m^3 was based on the following conclusions:[131]

1. The most sensitive population is children aged 1–5.

2. The maximum safe blood lead level for individual children is 30 μg/100 ml, based on concern for impaired heme synthesis above 30 μg Pb/100 ml, margin of safety for anemia above 40 μg Pb/100 ml, and nervous system deficits above 50 μg Pb/100 ml.

3. The maximum safe geometric mean blood lead for children, which would place 99.5 percent of the sensitive population below the 30 μg/100 ml level of concern, is 15 μg/100 ml.

4. The estimated blood lead level attributed to nonair sources is 12 μg/100 ml.

5. The allowable contribution to blood lead from air that meets the standard is therefore 15 μg Pb/100 ml $-$ 12 μg Pb/100 ml $=$ 3 μg Pb/100 ml.

6. Finally, the air lead concentration consistent with blood lead contribution of 3 μg/100 ml from air sources is 1.5 μg/m^3, based on the (blood lead)/(air lead) ratio of 2.0.

U.S. ENVIRONMENTAL PROTECTION AGENCY: NATIONAL PRIMARY DRINKING WATER REGULATIONS FOR LEAD

LEGISLATIVE AUTHORITY

The Safe Drinking Water Act of 1974 requires the EPA to promulgate national primary and secondary drinking water regulations for the purposes of protecting public health and welfare. The objective of the act is to control the quality of drinking water in public water systems, and the law establishes a three-stage mechanism for achieving this goal:

1. Promulgation of national interim primary drinking water regulations.[132]

2. Completion of a study by the National Academy of Sciences (NAS), within 2 years of enactment, on the human health effects of exposure to contaminants in drinking water.[133]

3. Promulgation of revised national primary drinking water regulations based upon the NAS study.[134] With respect to lead, the regulations would limit and in some cases reduce the daily intake and consequent contribution to total body burden of lead from drinking water.

For any drinking water contaminant that may have an adverse effect on public health, the act defines a primary drinking water regulation as specifying a maximum contaminant level (MCL) that is permissible in water delivered to any user of a public system.[135] Primary drinking water regulations shall require treatment necessary to prevent known or anticipated adverse effects on the health of persons to the extent feasible. To this end, primary regulation must be achieved with the use of the best technology, treatment techniques, or other means which the Administrator finds to be generally available, taking cost into consideration.[136] Primary regulations are applicable to all public water systems and are enforceable by EPA or the states that have accepted primacy responsibilities.

A secondary drinking water regulation is defined as specifying the maximum contaminant level that may have an adverse effect on public welfare (fish, wildlife, recreation). In addition to contaminants, secondary regulations may apply to pH, corrosiveness, odor or appearance. Secondary regulations are not federally enforceable and are intended as guidelines for the states.

The Safe Drinking Water Act mandated EPA to propose within 90 days and to promulgate within 180 days of enactment national interim primary drinking water regulations. Congress intended that the interim regulations be promulgated as soon as possible in order to provide the public with minimal protection during the period in which NAS was preparing its report. Interim regulations protect the public health to the extent that it is feasible, using generally available water treatment techniques. For inorganic contaminants such as lead, this criterion is generally less stringent than the detection criterion of the MCL.

EPA promulgated interim primary drinking water regulations in December 1975.[137] Because of the short period available for development of a basis for setting standards, the regulations were based heavily on the Drinking Water Standards adopted in 1962 by the U.S. Public Health Service. The interim MCL for lead was the same as the PHS standard, 50 μg/l.

BASIS FOR EPA'S ACTIONS

EPA's rationale for setting the interim standard for lead at 50 μg/l was based on three major considerations: (1) adverse health effects, (2) relationship of the contribution from drinking water to the total dietary in take of lead, and (3) the current attainability of the standard. The discussion of these is included in EPA's "Statement of Basis and Purpose," issued in support of the standards. This "Statement" was not reported in the *Federal Register* promulgation notice but was published subsequently as an appendix in *National Interim Primary Drinking Water Regulations.*[138]

In discussion of health hazards of lead, EPA's "Statement" identified young children as an especially sensitive group. The agency pointed out that young children are at increased risk because their food and air intakes are proportionally greater than those of adults in relation to body size, and because they absorb larger percentages of lead from the gut, perhaps as much as 50 percent of ingested lead.[139] On the basis of these findings, EPA concluded:[140]

With the widespread prevalence of undue exposure to lead in children, its serious potential sequelae (chronic brain or kidney damage, as well as acute brain damage) and studies suggesting increased lead absorption in children, it would seem wise at this time to continue to limit the lead in water to as low a level as practicable.

EPA stated that interim drinking water regulations for inorganic chemicals are based upon possible health effects that may occur after a lifetime of exposure.[141] Although the "Statement of Basis and Purpose" discusses various health effects associated with blood lead levels, neither a specific health effect nor a specific blood lead level was clearly identified as a target for prevention. However, the discussion did indicate that 40 μg Pb/100 ml is suggestive of undue lead absorption and associated adverse health effects,[142] a conclusion which was based on the 1971 PHS guideline[143] and the 1972 NAS airborne lead study.[144]

With respect to drinking water's contribution to total dietary intake of lead, the "Statement" points out that lead in drinking water could potentially contribute a significant fraction of total daily intake. Assuming an average daily adult dietary intake of 100 to 300 μg Pb/day, an adult who drinks 2 l of water per day containing 50 μg Pb/l would receive 33 percent of dietary lead from water. Assuming a scaled-down dietary intake and water consumption of 1 l per day, a child would receive between 25 and 33 percent of ingested lead from water containing 50 μg/l.[145]

Other routes of exposure were mentioned, including air, dust, paint, and other materials. Taking all sources into consideration, EPA concluded that because of the narrow range between average daily lead exposure levels and exposure levels that are considered excessive (especially in children), it was imperative that lead in water be maintained below rather strict limits.[146] However, no specific maximum safe daily dietary intake of lead for children was identified.

EPA determined that it was economically and technologically feasible by available methods to monitor drinking water for contaminants at the levels stated in the interim primary drinking water regulations.[147] Several references cited in the "Statement of Basis and Purpose" indicated that most existing raw and finished water supplies are already below the standard for lead (see Chapter 2 of this report); EPA concluded, therefore, that a lead concentration of below 50 μg/l can be attained in most drinking water supplies.[148]

SCIENTIFIC FINDINGS BY THE NATIONAL ACADEMY OF SCIENCES

The Safe Drinking Water Act required a study by the National Research Council of the National Academy of Sciences to determine the health effects of contaminants of drinking water, to provide EPA with a basis for setting maximum contaminant levels. The NRC study attempted to provide health goals, i.e., to specify the levels at which there are no known adverse health effects.[149] EPA has viewed the conclusions of the NRC study as advisory: the agency feels that the Administrator may modify the study's recommendations by incorporating safety factors, by taking economics into account, or for other reasons.[150]

The NRC study concluded that the current drinking water standard of 50 μg Pb/l should be reduced to 25 μg Pb/l, to provide a margin of safety against adverse health effects.[151] As evidence of the need to reduce the maximum allowable concentration of lead in drinking water, the NRC report referred to reports of increased blood lead levels in children in Boston using a water supply that contained 50 to 100 μg/l of lead. In addition, the report noted that at 50 μg/l, a typical 12-kg child would receive more lead from water alone than the World Health Organization's recommended maximum safe intake of 5 μg of lead per kilogram of body weight per day.

EPA published the recommendations of the NRC study in the *Federal Register*[152] in accordance with requirements of the Safe Drinking Water Act. The agency has not yet proposed any revised national primary drinking water regulations, although the deadline mandated by the act has passed.

In March 1977, EPA proposed national secondary drinking water regulations[153] for several contaminants, including corrosivity and pH. In the proposal, the agency noted that because of corrosion products such as cadmium and lead, the corrosivity standard had health as well as welfare significance. Final promulgation of these secondary regulations was expected in mid-1979.

In summary, EPA's decision to use 50 μg/l as the interim primary drinking water regulation for lead was based on considerations of health and economic and technical feasibility. Within the time frame allowed for promulgating these regulations, the agency had little choice but to adopt the 1962 PHS drinking water standards. EPA has not yet indicated whether it will follow the NRC's recommendation to lower the primary drinking water standard to 25 μg/l.

WATER QUALITY CRITERIA AND DRINKING WATER STANDARDS

EPA recently published for public comment an ambient water quality criterion for human health of 50 μg/l for lead.[154] The criterion is intended to be the best estimate of an ambient concentration of lead that does not pose an undue risk to humans who drink water without further treatment, or eat fish or shellfish from the water. This action was taken under the provisions of Section 304(a) of the Clean Water Act,[155] which authorizes EPA to publish and update water quality criteria that reflect the latest scientific knowledge on the identifiable effects of pollutants on public health and welfare, aquatic life, and recreation. When published in final form after public comment, water quality criteria may serve as the basis for developing enforceable standards under the Clean Water Act or the Safe Drinking Water Act.

Because of different legal requirements, health-based water quality criteria may not be the same as standards issued by EPA under the Safe Drinking Water Act. The mandate for establishing national primary drinking water standards, for instance, expressly requires consideration of economic and technical feasibility, whereas feasibility is not a factor in developing Section 304 water quality criteria. Future EPA rulemaking proceedings for drinking water may, however, make use of health-based Section 304 criteria. For this reason a brief summary of EPA's rationale for the health-based lead criterion is included here.

In assessing the impact of lead in water on human health, EPA used basically the same approach it took for lead in air.[156] This approach involves, first, identifying a critical target organ or system with respect to the health effects of lead. Then, the highest internal dose of lead that the target organ could tolerate without injury is determined. Finally, the fraction of the maximum tolerated internal dose that is attributable to lead in water is estimated, and the likely consequences of specific reductions in the maximum allowable concentration of lead in water are calculated.

EPA selected blood lead (PbB) as an index of internal dose, and reviewed summaries by EPA[157] and the World Health Organization[158] of the lowest PbB's associated with observed biological effects in children. In order to minimize risk to a single individual, EPA determined that the maximum safe PbB concentration for a given child should not exceed 30 μg/100 ml, a level below that at which the hemoglobin level begins to decline (40 μg/100 ml). In order to minimize risk for the entire population, EPA used epidemiological evidence and statistical considerations to estimate that if the geometric mean PbB were kept at 15 μg/100 ml, 99.5 percent of children would have PbB's below the designated safe level of 30 μg/100 ml. EPA concluded that this goal would provide a substantial margin of safety that would accommodate minor excursions in lead exposure due to adventitious sources.[159]

In order to estimate the relative contribution of lead in water to total absorption of lead, EPA assumed (as did the agency's air quality criteria document) that, at an average PbB of 15 μg/100 ml, 12 μg/100 ml is attributable to lead in food and water. EPA presented evidence from three studies on the relationships between PbB and lead in drinking water, and, using a regression equation based on those data, estimated that the present national average concentration of about 10 μg Pb/l in drinking water contributes about 5 μg/100 ml to blood lead. EPA used the same regression equation to calculate that water containing 50 μg Pb/l would contribute approximately an additional 3.4 μg/100 ml to PbB. EPA estimated that a total PbB of 15.4 μg/100 ml, or approximately the geometric mean PbB compatible with keeping 99.5 percent of the population under a PbB of 30 μg/100 ml, would be associated with a level of 50 μg Pb/l in drinking water. Based on this analysis, the agency concluded:[160]

. . . the present water standard of 50 μg Pb/l may be viewed as representing the upper limit of acceptability.

OCCUPATIONAL SAFETY AND HEALTH ADMINISTRATION: OCCUPATIONAL HEALTH STANDARD FOR LEAD

LEGISLATIVE AUTHORITY

Under the provisions of the Occupational Safety and Health (OSH) Act of 1970,[161] the Occupational Safety and Health Administration (OSHA) of the U.S. Department of Labor in November 1978 promulgated regulations to lower occupational exposures to airborne lead from 200 μg/m^3 to 50 μg/m^3, averaged over 8 hours.[162] In addition to the 50 μg Pb/m^3 permissible exposure limit (PEL), the regulations establish 30 μg Pb/m^3 as an "action level" above which employers must initiate environmental monitoring, record keeping, education and training, medical surveillance, and medical removal protection (MRP) of exposed employees. The new PEL is designed to protect workers in all industries covered by the OSH Act, except construction and agriculture, from undue occupational exposures to airborne concentrations of metallic lead, all inorganic lead compounds, and organic lead salts. The provisions for MRP are designed to increase worker protection by requiring temporary removal from the workplace of employees who experience certain combinations of air lead exposures and blood lead responses. The regulations establish a 10-year period for achieving full compliance. During this time, the major lead production and fabrication industries must meet a phased schedule of increasingly stringent interim exposure levels.

The overall objective of the Occupational Safety and Health Act is to assure "so far as possible" that employees of industries engaged in interstate commerce have safe and healthful working conditions.[163] To achieve this goal, the law authorizes OSHA to implement mandatory work safety and health standards. These standards require employers to establish working conditions, practices, or processes that are "reasonably necessary or appropriate" to provide safe and healthful places of employment.[164]

More specifically, for toxic materials, the act requires that mandatory health standards must establish maximum permissible occupational exposure levels (PELs) that most adequately assure, "to the extent feasible," that no employee will suffer material impairment of health or functional capacity.[165] A PEL must be based on best available evidence concerning health effects associated with various levels of exposure to a toxic material, and it must protect the employee for the duration of the individual's working life. In determining a maximum PEL for a toxic material, OSHA must take into account the feasibility of achieving the desired standard as well as the protection of health.

Although the OSH Act did not establish a specific timetable for promulgating mandatory health standards, the law did require OSHA to adopt so-called national consensus health standards within 2 years after enactment.[166] National consensus standards refer to occupational health standards that had been endorsed by nationally recognized industrial hygiene and safety organizations and in some cases had been vigorously enforced by states, but were not legally enforceable at the federal level under previous legislation. With this provision, Congress intended to establish as rapidly as possible standards that would provide at least minimal protection of worker health.[167] To meet this minimal safety requirement for inorganic lead, in 1971 OSHA adopted the 8-hour time-weighted average exposure limit of 200 μg Pb/m^3, which was recommended by the American National Standards Institute.[168]

Under the OSH Act, a mandatory standard-setting process may be initiated in a number of different ways, including the publication of occupational health criteria by the National Institute for Occupational Safety and Health (NIOSH). Although NIOSH is generally considered the research arm of OSHA, it is an independent agency under the Department of Health, Education and Welfare, and, in this regard, represents the only institutional arrangement for federal decision making concerning human lead exposure in which the scientific basis for regulatory action is developed independently of the standard-setting process.

OSHA'S STANDARDS

In January 1973, NIOSH issued a criteria document that recommended lowering the existing airborne lead exposure limit to 150 $\mu g/m^3$. In August 1975, following a joint review by OSHA and NIOSH of the health effects of occupational lead exposure, the director of NIOSH recommended that the PEL limits be reduced from 150 μg Pb/m^3 to lower ranges. NIOSH continued to review and evaluate scientific information published after the original criteria document was issued, and in May 1978 the agency published a new criteria document[169] that recommended lowering the PEL to 100 μg Pb/m^3 (NIOSH 1978).[170]

In response to the initial NIOSH criteria document and joint review, OSHA proposed an 8-hour average maximum permissible occupational exposure to airborne inorganic lead of 100 $\mu g/m^3$ in October 1975.[171] In so doing, the agency interpreted its legislative mandate as requiring the implementation of necessary protective standards based on the best available knowledge, even though medical and scientific evidence of human health effects associated with various exposures to lead might be inconclusive.[172] OSHA's interpretation of the law matched Congress' intent that the agency should use medical or scientific evidence that was still under debate or on the frontiers of scientific knowledge.[173] This aspect of the law has been upheld by the courts in reviewing OSHA's standards for vinyl chloride[174] and asbestos.[175]

BASIS FOR OSHA'S ACTION

OSHA's rationale for determining a maximum PEL for lead involved balancing the amount of worker protection that would be achieved at various exposure levels against the feasibility of meeting those levels. In arriving at the 50 μg Pb/m^3 limit, the agency evaluated scientific evidence in each of four areas: (1) the nature and extent of adverse health effects associated with blood lead levels in occupationally exposed individuals, (2) the correlation between blood lead levels associated with adverse health effects and various airborne lead exposure levels, (3) the feasibility and benefits of using medical removal protection, and (4) the technological and economic limitations associated with each industry's ability to meet the standard.

Adverse Health Effects of Lead

In evaluating health effects, OSHA adopted the view that the adverse health effects of lead exposure should be viewed as occurring along a continuum rather than separated into categories of clinical and subclinical effects.[176] According to the agency, the lead-induced disease process is composed of five stages: normal, physiological change of uncertain significance, pathophysiological change, overt symptoms of morbidity, and mortality. Incapacitating illness and death represent one extreme of a spectrum of human responses to continued lead exposure, and biological effects such as metabolic or physiological changes that are precursors or sentinels of disease represent the other. Within the disease process, OSHA concluded, there are no sharp distinctions, and the boundaries between the five stages overlap due to the variation of individual susceptibilities and exposures in the working population.

For the purpose of standard setting, OSHA concluded that the adopted standard must prevent pathophysiological changes.[177] The agency adopted the position that although these changes may precede the actual beginnings of illness, they do indicate important health effects. Therefore, the standard must be selected to prevent these earlier points of measurable change because: (a) pathophysiological changes are the initial stages of a disease process that would grow worse with continued lead exposure; and (b) prevention of pathophysiological changes will prevent the onset of more serious and potentially irreversible and debilitating manifestations of disease. OSHA applied this line of reasoning in determining the blood lead levels associated with measurable changes preceding the occurrence of adverse effects in each of four bodily systems: heme synthesis, neurological, renal, and reproductive.

The evidence of biological effects of lead in adults with occupational exposures is reviewed in Chapter 2. OSHA's judgments on effects of each kind are discussed extensively in the *Federal Register*, and are summarized here. With respect to heme synthesis, OSHA concluded that the earliest demonstrated effects of lead on heme synthesis are early stages of a disease process that eventually results in the clinical symptoms of lead poisoning, and that the disruption of heme synthesis over a working lifetime should be considered a material impairment of health.[178] Based on evidence that 20 percent of the population would have 70 percent inhibition of ALAD at blood lead concentrations of 40 μg/100 ml (see Chapter 2), OSHA determined that blood lead levels should ideally be kept below 40 μg/100 ml in order to minimize the effects of heme synthesis inhibition. In addition, OSHA concluded that lowered hemoglobin is clinically apparent at blood lead concentrations as low as 50 μg/100 ml, and that heme synthesis is inhibited by lead not only in blood, but in other tissues as well. For regulatory purposes, the agency stated:[179]

Such a pervasive physiological disruption must be considered as a material impairment of health and must be prevented. PbB (blood lead) levels greater than 40 μg/100 g should, therefore, be prevented to the extent feasible.

Concerning adverse neurological effects of lead, OSHA concluded that lead-induced central nervous system (CNS) disease in the form of behavioral disorders and CNS symptoms have been confirmed in workers whose blood lead levels are below 80 μg/100 ml, and that peripheral nervous system effects occur at blood lead levels of 50 μg/100 ml and above. From testimony given at hearings on the proposed standard, OSHA concluded that the incidence of kidney disease from occupational exposure to lead was probably more prevalent than previously believed,[180] and that maintenance of blood lead levels at or below 40 μg/100 ml was required to prevent renal damage. Finally, OSHA determined that occupational exposures to lead can have profoundly adverse effects on the reproductive systems in both males and females.[181] To protect persons either pregnant or planning pregnancies, OSHA concluded that blood lead levels should be maintained below 30 μg/100 ml.

In summary, OSHA concluded that recent scientific evidence demonstrates that workers exposed to lead experience material impairment of health at blood lead levels below those previously considered hazardous, and that to the extent feasible blood lead levels should be kept at or below 40 μg/100 ml.

Relationship Between Air Lead and Blood Lead

In setting the lead standard OSHA adopted the position that compliance with a PEL, which would accomplish the intended goal of minimizing the probability of employee blood lead concentrations exceeding 40 μg/100 ml, could be based primarily on measurement of air lead levels.[182] The Lead Industries Association (LIA) had recommended that OSHA adopt a biological limit as the basis for enforcement instead of using a specific air lead level. Industry maintained that blood lead levels cannot be correlated with or predicted from air lead concentrations. However, OSHA concluded that scientific evidence of the relationship between air lead levels and population-average blood lead levels was sufficiently strong to use air lead levels as a basis for protecting worker health.

OSHA used a physiological dose–response model to predict the effect of long-term exposure to various air lead levels on blood lead levels. A model was needed because, although there is considerable evidence of a correlation between blood lead and air lead levels, insufficient epidemiological data exist to establish a definite relationship between long-term blood lead levels and varying air lead exposures. The specific model used by OSHA takes into account relationships between airborne lead particle sizes, different job tenure exposures, and blood lead concentrations.[183]

OSHA used this model to estimate the number of workers who would exhibit blood lead levels in excess of 40, 50, and 60 μg/100 ml at various exposure levels, and used the difference in the numbers of workers exceeding these limits at 50 μg Pb/m³ and higher air lead concentrations as a measure of the incremental benefits derived from the PEL. OSHA estimated that nearly 51,000 fewer workers would have blood leads over 40 μg/100 ml at a PEL of 50 μg Pb/m³ compared with a PEL of 200 μg Pb/m³.[184]

Medical Removal Protection

As part of its regulations, OSHA included provisions for temporarily removing from the workplace workers who were discovered through medical surveillance to be at risk of sustaining material impairment to health from continued exposure to lead.[185] The regulations require medical removal protection (MRP) for any worker whose blood lead exceeds 60 μg/100 ml at any one test, or any worker whose blood lead is at or above 50 μg/100 ml for 6 months. During the period of temporary MRP, the employer must maintain the worker's earnings, seniority, and other employment benefits.

OSHA regards MRP as an indispensible part of the lead regulations, for several reasons. First, according to the agency, the PEL of 50 μg Pb/m³ provides little margin for safety. Even with full employer compliance with that standard, OSHA estimated that approximately 6 percent of exposed workers are likely to have blood lead levels in excess of 50 μg/100 ml.[186] OSHA believes that temporary medical removal is the only way to protect these workers from health impairment. Second, OSHA concluded that some segments of the lead industry will require several years to attain the PEL.[187] Although employees use respirators to reduce exposure, this is an inadequate means of worker protection, in OSHA's judgment, and temporary removal provides a fall-back mechanism for protecting workers when other protective means are insufficient. Finally, OSHA believes that MRP provides an economic incentive for employers to comply with the final standard.[188]

Technological and Economic Feasibility

In promulgating the final standard, OSHA evaluated the technological feasibility, cost data, and economic impact assessments for each approach that the major lead production and fabrication industries could use to meet the PEL.[189] OSHA concluded that the use of respirators could reduce the lead content of inhaled air to less than 50 μg/m³ where engineering and administrative controls were not sufficient. The primary feasibility issue, therefore, was whether the PEL and interim levels could be achieved within the required timetables solely through the use of engineering and work practice controls.

From a survey of practices within the industry, OSHA concluded that the standard of 50 μg Pb/m^3 was achievable entirely through engineering and work practice controls that employed technology that is presently available or likely to be available in the immediate future. According to OSHA, industries that will face the greatest difficulties in implementing engineering controls include primary and secondary smelters, pigment manufacturing, brass/bronze foundries, and battery manufacturing. For this reason the agency developed a phased implementation schedule, with extended periods of time alloted for compliance by those industries.

In summary, OSHA proposed a maximum occupational exposure level of 100 μg Pb/m^3, but adopted a much more stringent standard of 50 μg/m^3. Evidence presented at hearings on the proposed standard led the agency to conclude that the more stringent standard was necessary to assure, to the extent feasible, that the largest number of lead-exposed employees would not suffer material impairment of health. OSHA based this conclusion in part on its finding that to protect against adverse effects on health, the blood lead levels of lead industry workers must be kept below 40 μg/100 ml. Using a model of the relationship between various airborne lead levels and long-term blood lead responses, the agency estimated that about 70 percent of lead workers would have blood lead concentrations below 40 μg/100 ml at the 50 μg Pb/m^3 exposure limit. The agency further determined that most of the remaining 30 percent could be adequately protected through the use of medical removal protection.

Immediately after the promulgation of OSHA's standards, petitions were filed in several U.S. Courts of Appeal challenging its validity. The petitions were transferred to the U.S. Court of Appeals for the District of Columbia, and consolidated. On March 1, 1979, in a decision on motions to stay the standard, the Court ordered stayed certain provisions of the standard and denied the stay motions on others.[190] Although the Court left intact many of the regulation's major provisions, including the 50 μg Pb/m^3 standard and medical removal protection, OSHA has decided to enforce the prior standard of 200 μg/m^3 until the Court has completed a full judicial review of the new standard.[191]

FOOD AND DRUG ADMINISTRATION: LIMITATIONS ON LEAD IN FOODS AND HOUSEWARES

LEGISLATIVE AUTHORITY

The Food, Drug and Cosmetic Act is a confusing, cumbersome, and inflexible body of legislation that has as its central objective the prevention of human exposure to poisonous or deleterious substances in foods. Recent analysis of the law—and of the FDA's actions in implementing it—point out that current food safety statutes are a patchwork of legislative policies that invite inconsistent treatment of comparable risks to human health from exposure to harmful substances in food.[192,193] This potential for inconsistency arises from the disparate treatment of different classes of food constituents that Congress has infused into the food and drug laws during the last 4 decades. Consequently, a brief legislative history of food and drug laws is essential in explaining the basis for FDA's current tolerances for lead in food, as well as the potential for future agency programs to reduce present lead levels in food.

The first federal food safety law, passed in 1906, authorized FDA to declare as adulterated any food that contained any added poisonous or added deleterious substance which made such article injurious to health. FDA, which was then an enforcement agency in the Department of Agriculture, interpreted this prohibition as applying exclusively to substances that were purposely incorporated into food or intentionally applied during processing.[194]

In 1938, Congress revised the Food and Drug Act to expand FDA's ability to control hazardous substances in foods. The amendments established three standards that are still used in controlling toxicants in food:

1. The basic authority of Section 402 of the law to declare as adulterated a food containing any "added" poisonous or deleterious substance that is injurious to health and unnecessary or avoidable in food production.[195]

2. The "ordinarily injurious" standard, which applies to constituents that fall outside the category of "added."[196]

3. The tolerance-setting procedures of Section 406, which apply to "added" constituents that are "necessary" in the production of food or "cannot be avoided by good manufacturing practice."[197]

Although these Sections clearly establish a distinction between substances that are "added" and those that are not, Congress did not define the term "added" or the concepts of "necessary" and "unavoidable."

Subsequent amendments to the 1938 act have significantly increased the complexity of the three legal standards of control. Each amendment expanded FDA's authority to regulate a subcategory of "added" food contaminants, such as pesticide residues (1954),[198] food additives (1958),[199] color additives (1960),[200] and animal drug residues (1968),[201] without replacing or, in many cases, modifying existing legal authority.[202] The specific amendments that are relevant to FDA efforts to control lead in food include the Pesticide Residues Amendment of 1954 and the Food Additives Amendment of 1958. Because tolerances for insecticidal lead compounds were established before enactment of the Pesticide Residues Amendment, only the Food Additives Amendment is discussed here.

The Food Additives Amendment authorizes FDA in effect to license the use of substances used as food additives. Under the provisions of the amendment, food processors must receive FDA approval for both types and quantities of substances intended for use as ingredients in formulated foods. To obtain approval for use, processors must provide FDA with technical information, including the conditions under which the additive can be safely used, the intended effect of the additive, and the chemical composition of the additive required to produce this effect.[203] Any food that bears or contains an additive that FDA has not approved, or that contains an additive in excess of FDA use specifications, shall be declared adulterated under Section 402(a)(2)(C) of the act.

The amendment[204] broadly defines the term "food additive" to mean any substance:

. . . the intended use of which results or may reasonably be expected to result, directly or indirectly, in its becoming a component or otherwise affecting the characteristics of any food (including any substance intended for use in producing, manufacturing, packing, processing, preparing, treating, packaging, transporting, or holding food; and including any source of radiation intended for any such use).

It is clear that this definition includes materials used in the production of containers and packages that may migrate into food. (If there is no migration of a packaging component from the package to the food, it does not become a component of the food and therefore is not a food additive.) The lead that enters canned food from solder in the can seam is a prime example of a migrating packaging material.

Two important categories of substances are, by law[205] exempted from FDA regulations on food additives. The first of these includes substances whose use in food processing and packaging is "generally recognized as safe" (GRAS) by qualified experts. This category embraces a large number of substances—sugar and salt are common examples—many of which also require contaminant limitations in order to be regarded as safe. The second category of exceptions includes food additives demonstrated to be safe under conditions of intended use through scientific procedures or use experience developed prior to 1958. Substances in this category have been effectively exempted from action by the additives amendment, and FDA has operated under the assumption that they are permanently exempt as long as they are used for the intended purposes of the prior sanction, even if new scientific evidence casts doubt on their safety.[206] Both the GRAS and prior-sanction categories of exceptions are use-specific; and both exceptions are important to FDA's approach to controlling lead in food.

The Food Additives Amendment also contains the so-called Delaney Clause (named for its author), which stipulates that FDA cannot grant use approval to any food additive found to be carcinogenic in humans or animals. The law states:[207]

. . . no additive shall be deemed to be safe if it is found to induce cancer when ingested by man or animal, or if it is found, after tests which are appropriate for the evaluation of the safety of food additives, to induce cancer in man or animal. . . .

The Delaney Clause does not allow FDA latitude in controlling trace levels of carcinogenic substances in food additives. The clause carries the presumption that no level of human exposure to a carcinogen can be considered safe.

Finally, FDA does not view its authority to regulate "added" substances in food as being entirely limited by the amendments passed since 1938.[208] For example, the agency has become increasingly concerned with environmental contaminants whose occurrence in food is unintended, undesired, and to a large extent uncontrollable—a problem that Congress has not yet addressed. Although FDA has authority to regulate such contaminants under the "injurious to health" or "ordinarily injurious" standards of Section 402, the agency has classified environmental contaminants as "added poisonous substances" whose occurrence cannot entirely be avoided, in order to use the tolerance-setting authority of Section 406.

AGENCY PROGRAMS

FDA's current program for controlling lead in foods developed in a piecemeal fashion that reflects the historic development of the Food and Drug Act. To date, the agency has implemented selective, direct controls on lead in pesticide spray residues on fruits and vegetables and on leachable lead from certain ceramic and silver-plated eating and cooking utensils. FDA also has implemented some indirect controls on lead in foods in the form of allowable lead contaminant levels in GRAS substances. Finally, although FDA has not promulgated tolerances for lead in canned foods, the agency informally has encouraged the canning industry to adopt quality-control procedures to reduce lead levels in canned foods as much as is practicable.

Tolerance for Lead in Pesticide Residues

FDA first established controls on lead in foods in the 1930s, when the agency established informal guideline tolerances for lead arsenate spray residues on fresh fruits and vegetables. Based mainly on the results of in-house research, the tolerances were initially set at 3.5 $\mu g/g$ of combined lead. In 1937, Congress directed the Public Health Service to investigate the lead arsenate tolerance, and on the recommendation of that agency,[209] FDA increased the tolerance to its present level of 7.0 $\mu g/g$.[210]

Maximum allowable lead arsenate residues apparently were changed again in the 1960s. The current tolerances are 1 $\mu g/g$ on citrus fruits and 7 $\mu g/g$ on other fruits and vegetables.[211] The current tolerances are enforced under provisions of the 1954 Pesticide Residue Amendment,[212] and authority to enforce them was transferred to the EPA in the 1970 reorganization plan that created that agency.[213]

Tolerances on Lead in Food Containers

FDA's interest in the problem of lead migration into foods from the solder in cans also dates from the 1930s. There are indications in FDA correspondence issued after 1940 that the 7.0 $\mu g/g$ pesticide tolerance became an unofficial guideline in developing controls for permissible lead levels in canned foods.[214] The question of what would be the maximum functional and safe level of lead in lead–tin solder was of extreme importance during World War II, when there was a critical shortage of tin for the war effort. In this regard, studies by the War Metallurgy Committee of the NAS/NRC determined that it was safe to change the formula for solders from a lead/tin ratio of 63/37 to one of 98/2 for use in soldering tin-plated cans for food packaging.

The procedures and scientific basis for setting these early tolerances were not published, but are contained in the files and official correspondence of the FDA. Because of the difficulty of obtaining those documents, the rationales for these controls are not examined here. Only those regulations promulgated since the enactment of the Food Additive Amendment of 1958 and for which public documentation is readily available are discussed below.

FDA promulgated principles for evaluating the safety of food additive uses in 1959.[215] The principles specify that the "safe" use of an additive—as defined in the 1958 amendments[216]—means that there is a reasonable certainty in the minds of competent scientists that a substance is not harmful under the intended conditions of use.[217] In determining a safe use, the agency considers the following:

1. The probable consumption of the substance and of any substance formed in or on food because of its use.
2. The cumulative effect of the substance in the diet, taking into ac-

count any chemically or pharmacologically related substance or substances in such diet.

3. Safety factors which, in the opinion of experts qualified by scientific training and experience to evaluate the safety of food and food ingredients, are generally recognized as appropriate.

In reaching a decision on any request to declare a specific use of a food additive safe, FDA considers the specific biological properties of the compound and the adequacy of the methods employed to demonstrate safety for the proposed use.[218] In this regard, FDA is guided by principles and procedures for establishing the safety of food additives as stated in current publications of the NAS/NRC. Procedures other than those outlined by NAS/NRC are also acceptable if FDA finds that such procedures give comparable or more reliable results.

FDA has also adopted procedures for determining the eligibility of substances for classification as GRAS.[219] General recognition of safety may be based only on the views of experts, and the basis for these views may be either: (a) scientific procedures; or (b) in the case of a substance used in food prior to January 1, 1958, through experience based on common use in food. With respect to scientific procedures, the designation of a substance as GRAS shall require the same quantity and quality of scientific evidence as is required to obtain approval of a food additive status for the ingredient. With respect to use of the substance in food prior to 1958, the status of a substance as GRAS shall ordinarily be based upon generally available data and information.

In implementing the GRAS classification procedures, FDA has distinguished between "direct" and "indirect" food substances that are generally recognized as safe. Direct food ingredients refer to substances added directly to human food[220] and indirect human food ingredients refer to substances that migrate into food from food-contact surfaces.[221] This latter category contains limitations that are applicable to controlling lead in food.

Indirect food substances that are GRAS are for the most part packaging materials. The affirmation as GRAS of an indirect food ingredient does not authorize direct addition of that ingredient to food. Affirmation only authorizes the use of these ingredients as additives because of their potential migration from food wrappers, containers, or other contact surfaces.

To date, three indirect food additives that have been affirmed as GRAS are subject to grade specifications that limit the content of lead and other heavy metals. Guar gum (technical grade), locust (carob) bean gum, and sorbose are substances affirmed as GRAS for intended uses as constitutents of food-contact surfaces. In each of these the lead content is limited to 20, 10, and 40 parts per million (ppm), respectively.

Lead in Ceramic and Hollowware Products. FDA applied the principle for evaluating food additives in developing controls for lead that migrates into food from food-contact surfaces, such as ceramic cookware and silver-plated hollowware. The agency's concern with the problem of lead migration from pottery glazes into food began in the late 1960s. On the basis of a survey of imported pottery, FDA determined that improperly glazed ceramic ware can be a source of significant quantities of lead in the diet, especially if utensils of this kind are used continuously to prepare or serve acidic foods.

FDA initially implemented an administrative guideline of 7.0 ppm of leachable lead from domestic and imported pottery in 1973. Recent amendments to that guideline have reduced the action level to 5.0 and 2.5 ppm for small and large ceramic hollowware (bowls), respectively.[222] In addition to ceramic ware, FDA has established administrative guidelines for leachable lead from enamelware, pewter, and silver-plated hollowware at the 7.0 ppm level. For silver-plated cups intended for use by infants, the action level is 0.5 ppm.

Under these guidelines, FDA analyzes samples of domestic and imported ceramic, pewter, and silver-plated hollowware. Those articles that exceed specified action levels are designated as adulterated under Section 402(1)(2)(C) of the Food, Drug and Cosmetic Act[223] because they contain a food additive, in this case lead, that is unsafe within the meaning of Section 409(a).[224]

FDA has not yet published in the *Federal Register* or any other public document a rationale for the leachable lead guidelines. The guidelines were apparently derived from a report of an expert panel convened by the World Health Organization in 1976.[225] The panel stated that the problem of lead release from ceramic foodware requires effective control measures to assure protection of health. As a secondary consideration, the panel also noted that varying standards from country to country over the release of heavy metals from glazed pottery surfaces present nontariff barriers to international trade in these comodities. The panel's main concerns were to establish limits for lead release and internationally accepted uniform pottery sampling and leachate testing procedures.

Tolerances for Lead in Foods. In the 1970s, FDA undertook efforts to reduce lead in canned food, and in particular, the agency has focused its attention on foods that are consumed in large quantities by infants, such as canned evaporated milk and juices. In 1974 FDA proposed, under the provisions of Section 406, a tolerance of 0.3 ppm lead in canned evaporated milk.[226] The proposal was based on investigations of evaporated milk processing plants that determined that the differences between the average concentration of lead in raw milk and in canned evaporated milk were higher than could be caused by the normal procedure of concentrating milk in the evaporation process. The agency concluded that a substantial portion of the lead in evaporated milk was added during or as a result of processing.

In proposing to limit lead in canned milk as an unavoidable substance requiring a tolerance (rather than as a food additive requiring an action level), FDA noted that a tolerance is appropriate when there are no changes foreseeable in the near future that might affect the appropriateness of the proposed limitation. FDA concluded that improvements in can technology that could further reduce lead levels in evaporated milk were not expected in the near future. The agency also stated that scientific evidence on the toxicity of lead was sufficiently well established and that no data were expected to be developed in the near future that would cause the Commissioner to alter the proposed limit.[227]

The proposed 0.3 ppm lead tolerance was based on calculations that daily lead intake for infants could range from 70 μg for infants from birth to 3 months, who obtain 80 to 90 percent of their total caloric intake from formula, to about 170 μg for 9-to-12-month-olds, who obtain 80 percent of their caloric intake from formula.[228] The agency noted that these intake levels are significantly lower than the 300 μg of lead per day suggested by the HEW Ad Hoc Committee on Pediatric Lead Toxicity[229] as a maximum permissible lead intake level from all sources for children between 1 and 3 years of age.

At approximately the same time as the tolerance proposal, FDA informed the evaporated milk industry of the seriousness of the problem of added lead in canned milk and encouraged the industry to develop a quality-control program. As a result of its own studies, the industry made modifications in can manufacturing procedures and introduced new techniques to reduce lead levels in evaporated milk.[230] As a result of these changes, the average lead level in evaporated milk declined from 0.52 ppm in 1972 to 0.10 ppm in 1978.[231] The tolerance proposal is still pending; it was never enacted in final form.

FDA has also pressed manufacturers of infant juices to lower lead levels in their products.[232] Largely as a result of these efforts, lead levels in canned juices have been reduced significantly since 1973. Recently, all infant juice manufacturers voluntarily switched from tin cans to glass jars, presumably bringing about further reductions of lead levels in this product.

OTHER RECENT AND PENDING DECISIONS BY FEDERAL AGENCIES ON LEAD IN THE ENVIRONMENT

The case studies presented here represent major programs undertaken by the federal government in recent years to control human exposure to lead, but several additional regulatory efforts are currently under way or recently completed. Because most of them are less directly related to significant human exposures to lead, and because the basis for actions to be taken has not yet been fully developed or made public in all cases, it was not practical to include detailed discussion on every action. However, several current and pending activities are briefly described here.

FURTHER REGULATIONS OF LEAD CONTENT OF FOODS

FDA is gathering information to support broader regulations on the lead content of foods,[233] and has published an advance notice of proposed rulemaking on this problem.[234] It is FDA's intent eventually to propose comprehensive tolerance limits for lead in all foods; however, the agency's initial top priority is to reduce lead levels in foods intended for consumption by infants and young children.[234,235] According to the advance notice, FDA will attempt to reduce the contribution of lead in canned foods by 50 percent over a 5-year period.[236]

The manner in which FDA will go about regulating lead in foods is currently subject to uncertainty. In another regulatory matter concerning the use of lead acetate in cosmetics (discussed below), FDA has raised the issue of the possible carcinogenicity of lead. The agency recognizes that although animal data show rather convincingly that lead causes cancer when ingested in large doses, data on humans are contradictory (see Chapter 2). In August 1979, FDA published in the *Federal Register* a statement of its concerns on the matter of carcinogenicity and other questions about lead in foods.[237] The agency has appealed to the scientific community and others for assistance in resolving several scientifically difficult concerns about the risk to humans posed by lead in foods. If FDA ultimately determines that lead is a carcinogen under terms of the Delaney Clause (see case study on FDA), it would have little choice but to ban all avoidable additions of the metal to foods.

EFFLUENT GUIDELINES FOR INDUSTRIAL SOURCES OF LEAD DISCHARGE INTO WATERS

Under the Clean Water Act of 1977, EPA is currently preparing to issue effluent limitations on the discharge of lead in wastewaters from 36 categories of industries. Promulgation of the regulations is scheduled to begin in mid-1979, and to continue through 1981. Under the terms of the law, guidelines are to be based on "best available technology."[238]

FINAL WATER QUALITY CRITERIA AND PRIMARY DRINKING WATER STANDARD FOR LEAD

EPA expects to publish a revised water quality criteria document for lead in late 1979. The draft document (see Appendix A for a synopsis) is being revised, following a 60-day period of public comment. In late 1979, EPA is also expected to publish its proposed final drinking water standard for lead. The agency has been studying the recommendation of the National Research Council that the standard be lowered from its present level (50 μg/l) to 25 μg/l.[239] EPA proposed that a study be done on the corrosion of lead pipe in distribution systems before the agency revised its standard, but according to the IRLG no such study has yet been initiated.[240]

REGULATIONS ON LEAD IN SOLID WASTES, SLUDGES, AND HAZARDOUS WASTES

EPA published proposed regulations for solid waste disposal in February 1978;[241] they included consideration of disposal of wastes on lands used for production of food-chain crops. In this context, limits were proposed on the cadmium content of wastes, but not the lead content. In December 1978, EPA published proposed hazardous waste management rules.[242] Lead is listed as a hazardous contaminant in the proposed rules. The rules are intended to provide for proper management of hazardous wastes to prevent human exposure to toxic contaminants, either by leaching into water supplies or by uptake from soil into food chains. Final regulations are anticipated early in 1980.

Under the Clean Water Act of 1977, EPA is obligated to develop a comprehensive strategy for the management and utilization of municipal sludges. The agency has concentrated its efforts to date on the development of proposed rules for the use and disposal of sludges; the proposals were expected to be published in the summer of 1979.[243] The proposed rules will include guidelines for the disposal of sludges on croplands, and recommendations for the use of sludges as fertilizers or soil conditioners in lawns and gardens. EPA's chief concern in regard to lead is that the lead in sludge used in home gardens might be ingested by children who play in the soil[244] (see Chapter 2).

FDA has announced its intent to develop food contaminant levels for foods grown on land fertilized with solid wastes. No date has been set for the proposed action.[245]

NEW SOURCE PERFORMANCE STANDARDS FOR LEAD EMISSIONS FROM LEAD–ACID BATTERY MANUFACTURE

Under the authority of the Clean Air Act, EPA proposed in May 1979 to require operators of new, modified, or reconstructed lead-acid battery manufacturing facilities to employ the best demonstrated systems for continuous emission reduction. The purpose of the regulation is to prevent emissions of lead that are deemed a potential hazard to public health.[246] Emission standards were geared to provide for compliance with EPA's national ambient air quality standard for lead (see earlier case study). EPA has used the NSPS rulemaking procedure before in regard to emissions from other sources of lead in the atmosphere; the new rule represents extension of the approach to a new industrial source category. EPA estimates that about 100 large battery manufacturing plants would be affected, most of them in urban areas.[247]

REGULATION OF LEAD ACETATE IN COSMETICS

Lead acetate is a cosmetic ingredient used in hair dyes and mascara. FDA is in the process of regulating the compound as a color additive; action was begun in 1978[248], but a final decision has been postponed at least until March 1980.[249] FDA extended the closing date for its action in order to allow more time to consider the question of whether lead salts are animal carcinogens. If the eventual decision by FDA is that lead compounds may be regulated under the Delaney Clause (see FDA case study), the use of lead acetate as a hair dye might still be permitted, since the Delaney Clause is discretionary when it applies to substances that are not ingested. FDA-supported research has shown that only about 0.5 μg of lead is absorbed through the scalp under normal conditions of use (one application of a hair dye containing lead acetate),[250] and the agency indicated that, except for the question of carcinogenicity, this use of lead would not be deemed a hazard.[251]

LIMITATIONS ON LEAD ON DECORATED GLASSWARE

Concerns abut exposure of children to lead in decals on decorated glassware prompted the formation of an interagency task force under the IRLG to look into the problem. The task force, consisting of representatives of FDA, EPA, and CPSC, recommended in October 1978 that the agencies support a voluntary standard limiting leachable lead to 50 μg/g on the lip and rim of such glassware, and that industry initiate a monitoring program for cadmium and lead in such products. The recommendations were published in the *Federal Register* in December 1978.[252]

ACTIONS CURRENTLY UNDER COURT REVIEW

Two of the standards adopted in 1978, described in earlier case studies in this appendix, are presently being reviewed by the courts. The Lead Industries Association and the Battery Council International petitioned for review of OSHA's standards for occupational exposures; the Court of Appeals for the District of Columbia issued a partial stay of the standard pending completion of its review. In a separate action, the Lead Industries Association challenged EPA's national primary ambient air quality standard for lead. That issue has not been resolved to date.

INTERAGENCY COORDINATION OF REGULATORY ACTIVITIES ON LEAD

About 2 years ago, the Interagency Regulatory Liaison Group was formed to improve the coordination of federal regulatory activities. IRLG has a work group on lead that collects and publishes information about regulatory activities of the various agencies,[253] and several lead-related activities have recently been undertaken as joint, interagency projects. For example, the task force on lead and cadmium on decorated glasses, mentioned above, was formed under IRLG auspices. A number of other actions have included multi-agency comments on regulations proposed by one of the agencies; for instance, EPA's proposed air quality standard was reviewed by eight agencies (CDC, PHS, CPSC, FDA, OSHA, the Department of Transportation, the Department of the Interior, and the Department of Commerce).[254] A number of agencies, including FDA, DOE, and DOT, participated in the development of EPA's regulations on hazardous waste disposal. In general, even before the creation of IRLG, there was significant communication and informal exchange of information between and among agencies whose regulatory concerns overlap; since IRLG, that coordination has improved.

Nevertheless, there are still opportunities for better coordination. Two agencies (CDC and HUD) with major programs related to lead, discussed in earlier case studies in this appendix, are not members of IRLG, because neither is a "regulatory agency" in its primary mission. Both have been able to participate in some IRLG activities informally, and have commented on actions by other agencies, but have not been formally included in study groups or task forces.

The descriptions in the case studies presented here of the diverse legislative authorities given the various agencies to regulate lead under different laws show that the mandates under which each agency operates give different weight to specific considerations, differ in standards of proof employed, and diverge in a number of other respects. Some agencies—especially EPA and FDA—are subject to several laws with internal inconsistencies, and effective coordination of actions even within the agency is sometimes difficult. Few of the laws require one agency to take into account what the other agencies have done or are doing, even though such consideration may be vital to the development of strategies to respond to problems. Most of the coordination that has been achieved has come about in spite of, rather than because of, divergent legislative mandates.

The problem of coordination of decisions on lead is addressed in Chapter 3 of this report as well.

NOTES

1. The main laws that currently provide for federal control of human exposure to lead include the Clean Air Act Amendments of 1970 and the Amendments of 1977 (42 USC 7401 et seq., 1977; PL 91-604, 84 Stat. 1676–1713; PL 95-95, 91 Stat. 685–796); the Safe Drinking Water Act of 1974 (42 USC 300 et seq.; PL 92–523, 88 Stat. 1660–1694); the Food and Drug Act (21 USC 336, 341, 342, 346, 371, 52 Stat. 1045-1046 as amended, 1049, 1055–1056 as amended by 70 Stat. 919 and 72 Stat. 948); the Lead-Based Paint Poisoning Prevention Act of 1971 and Amendments of 1973 and 1976 (42 USC 4801–4846, 1976; PL 91-695, 84 Stat. 2078–2080; PL 93-151, 87 Stat. 565–568; PL 94-317, 90 Stat. 705–706); the Occupational Safety and Health Act of 1974 (29 USC 651 et seq.; PL 91–596, 84 Stat. 1593, 1599); the Resource Conservation Recovery Act of 1976 (42 USC 6901 et seq.; PL 94-580, 90 Stat. 2795–2841); the Toxic Substances Control Act of 1976 (15 USC 2601 et seq.; PL 94-469, 90 Stat. 2003); and the Consumer Product Safety Act as amended (15 USC 2051 et seq.; PL 92-573, 86 Stat. 1207).
2. U.S. Congress, Senate (1970) Lead-Based Paint Elimination Act of 1970. Report to Accompany H.R. 19172. Committee on Labor and Public Welfare, S. Report 91-1432:2. 91st Congress, 2nd Session.
3. U.S. Congress, Senate (1970) Lead-Based Paint Poisoning. Committee on Labor and Public Welfare, 1970, hearings on S. 3216 and H.R. 19172. 91st Congress, 2nd Session.
4. U.S. Congress, Senate (1972) Lead-Based Paint Poisoning Amendments of 1972. Committee on Labor and Public Welfare, hearings on S. 3080. 92nd Congress, 2nd Session.
5. U.S. Congress, Senate (1975) Lead-Based Paint Poisoning Prevention Act of 1975. Committee on Labor and Public Welfare, hearings on S. 1664. 94th Congress, 1st Session.
6. Lead-Based Paint Poisoning Prevention Act of 1971 and Amendments of 1973 and 1976. 42 USC 4801 (c)(1).
7. *Ibid.*, 4801 (c)(2).
8. *Ibid.*, 4801 (c)(3).
9. *Ibid.*, 4811 (a)(1).
10. *Ibid.*, 4811 (a)(2).
11. U.S. Congress, Senate (1970) Hearings on S. 3216 and H.R. 19172:42 ff.
12. U.S. Congress, Senate (1972) Hearings on S. 3080:23 ff.
13. *Ibid.*, 12 ff.
14. U.S. Congress, House (1970) Lead-Based Paint Poisoning Prevention Act. Conference Report to Accompany H.R. 19172, H. Report 91-1802:5. 91st Congress, 2nd Session.

15. U.S. Congress, Senate. Lead-Based Paint Elimination, S. Report 91-1432:3.

16. *Ibid.*, 5.

17. U.S. Congress, House (1973) Lead-Based Paint Poisoning Prevention Act Amendments of 1973. Report to Accompany S. 607. Committee on Labor and Public Welfare, S. Report 93-130:4. 93rd Congress, 1st Session.

18. U.S. Public Health Service: Grants for prevention of lead-based paint poisoning. 37 Federal Register 1116 (January 25, 1972).

19. U.S. Public Health Service. Grants for prevention of lead-based paint poisoning, U.S. Department of Health, Education, and Welfare. 42 CFR 91, 37 Federal Register 9188 (May 5, 1972).

20. U.S. Public Health Service. Lead-based paint poisoning prevention. 42 CFR 91.5.

21. *Ibid.*, 91.8

22. Steinfeld, J.L. (1971) Medical aspects of childhood lead poisoning. Pediatrics 48(3):464–468.

23. Center for Disease Control, U.S. Department of Health, Education, and Welfare (1975) Increased lead absorption and lead poisoning in young children; (1978) Preventing lead poisoning in young children.

24. Steinfeld (1971) see Note 22.

25. Center for Disease Control (1975, 1978) see Note 23.

26. *Ibid.*

27. U.S. Congress, Senate. Hearings on S. 1664, 7.

28. *Ibid.*, 9.

29. *Ibid.*, 13.

30. Center for Disease Control (1975, 1978) see Note 23.

31. Center for Disease Control (1978) see Note 23.

32. The term "HUD-associated housing" refers to any structures owned or financially assisted by HUD, when such structures are being constructed, sold, purchased, leased, rehabilitated (including routine maintenance work), modernized, or improved with any form of HUD financial assistance, whether by grant, loan, advance, housing assistance payments, HUD-guaranteed loans, or HUD-insured mortgages.

33. Lead-Based Poisoning Prevention Act of 1971 and Amendments of 1973 and 1976. 42 USC 4822.

34. *Ibid.*

35. *Ibid.* 4831.

36. U.S. Department of Housing and Urban Development. Prohibition of use of lead-based paint and elimination of lead-based paint hazard. 24 CFR 35, 37 Federal Register 22732 (October 21, 1972).

37. U.S. Congress, House (1973) Lead-Based Paint Poisoning Prevention Act Amendments. Conference Report to Accompany S. 607, H. Report 93-522:7. 93rd Congress, 1st Session.

38. Lead-Based Paint Poisoning Prevention Act of 1971, 42 USC 4841 (3).

39. U.S. Department of Housing and Urban Development (1976) Lead-based paint poisoning prevention in HUD-associated housing and federally owned property to be sold for residential habitation. 24 CFR 35, 41 Federal Register 28876 (July 13, 1976).

40. U.S. Department of Housing and Urban Development (1975) Lead-based paint poisoning prevention in federally owned and federally assisted housing. 40 Federal Register 26974 (June 25, 1975).

41. In 1976, there were approximately 35,000,000 housing units in the United States that were constructed prior to 1950. (See U.S. Department of Commerce, Bureau of the Census, Annual Housing Survey, 1976, United States and Regions, Part A: General Housing Characteristics, Current Housing Reports, Series H-150-76.) Although the

number of dwelling units in HUD-assisted programs is constantly changing, the Department estimated that approximately 863,000 (or 2.5 percent) of all units constructed before 1950 were in HUD-financed assistance and insurance programs in 1976. (Irwin H. Billick, personal communication, April 9, 1979.)

42. U.S. Department of Housing and Urban Development. 41 Federal Register 28876 (July 13, 1976).
43. U.S. Department of Housing and Urban Development. 40 Federal Register 26974 (June 25, 1975).
44. U.S. Department of Housing and Urban Development. 41 Federal Register 28876 (July 13, 1976).
45. *Ibid.*, page 28877.
46. U.S. Department of Housing and Urban Development. Lead-based paint poisoning prevention in certain residential structures. 24 CFR 35, 42 Federal Register 5042 (January 27, 1977).
47. U.S. Department of Health, Education, and Welfare. Lead-based paint poisoning prevention in federal and federally assisted construction. 42 CFR 90, 37 Federal Register 4915 (March 7, 1972).
48. Billick, I. and E. Gray (1978) Lead Based Paint Poisoning Research, Review and Evaluation 1971–1977. Washington, D.C.: U.S. Department of Housing and Urban Development.
49. U.S. Department of Housing and Urban Development. 40 Federal Register 26974 (June 25, 1975) and 41 Federal Register 28876 (July 13, 1976).
50. Consumer Product Safety Act, 15 USC 2057.
51. Consumer Product Safety Commission. Regulation of products subject to other acts under the Consumer Products Safety Act, 16 CFR 1145; Lead-containing paint and certain consumer products bearing lead-containing paint, 16 CFR 1303; Hazardous substances and articles, administration and enforcement regulations. 16 CFR 1500, 42 Federal Register 44192–44202 (September 1, 1977).
52. Lead-Based Paint Poisoning Prevention Act of 1971. 42 USC 4831 (c).
53. Consumer Product Safety Commission. Lead-based paint and certain consumer products bearing lead-based paint. 41 Federal Register 33638 (August 10, 1976).
54. 42 USC 4841.
55. Consumer Product Safety Commission (1974) A Report to Congress in Compliance with the Lead-Based Paint Poisoning Prevention Act, as Amended, December 23, 1974.
56. Purdy, R. et al. (1974) Toxicological Investigation of Chronic Lead Paint Ingestion in the Juvenile Baboon, Final Report. Southwest Foundation for Research and Education, December.
57. Kniep, T. et al. (1974) Lead Toxicity Studies in Infant Baboon: A Toxicological Model for Childhood Lead Poisoning, Draft of Final Report. New York: Institute of Environmental Medicine, New York University.
58. Consumer Product Safety Commission. (1974) A report to Congress.
59. National Research Council (1976) Recommendations for the Prevention of Lead Poisoning in Children. Committee on Toxicology, Assembly of Life Sciences. Washington, D.C.: National Academy of Sciences.
60. Consumer Product Safety Commission. Determination of safe level of lead in paint. 42 Federal Register. 9404 (February 16, 1977).
61. National Research Council (1976), 9.
62. *Ibid.*, 10.
63. Consumer Product Safety Commission. 42 Federal Register 9406 (February 16, 1977).
64. *Ibid.*, 9404.
65. Consumer Product Safety Commission. 42 Federal Register 44193 (September 1, 1977).

66. U.S. Food and Drug Administration. Hazardous substances. Definitions and procedural and interpretative regulations, classification of certain lead-containing paints and other similar surface-coating materials as banned hazardous substances. 21 CFR 191.9, 37 Federal Register 5229-5231 (March 11, 1972).

67. Consumer Product Safety Commission. Federal Hazardous Substances Act Regulations, Revision and Transfer. 16 CFR 1500 and 1505, 38 Federal Register 27012 et seq. (September 27, 1973).

68. Consumer Product Safety Commission. 41 Federal Register 33638 (August 10, 1976).

69. Consumer Product Safety Act. 15 USC 2079 (d).

70. Consumer Product Safety Commission. 42 Federal Register 44193 (September 1, 1977).

71. Consumer Product Safety Act. 15 USC 2058.

72. Consumer Product Safety Commission. 42 Federal Register 44198-44199 (September 1, 1977).

73. *Ibid.*, 44200.

74. National Research Council (1976) see Note 59.

75. Steinfeld, J.L. (1971) Medical aspects of childhood lead poisoning. Pediatrics 48(3):464-468.

76. National Bureau of Standards (1972) Estimates of the Nature and Extent of Lead Poisoning in the United States. National Bureau of Standards Technical Note 746. Washington, D.C.: U.S. Department of Commerce.

77. Consumer Product Safety Commission. 42 Federal Register 44197 (September 1, 1977).

78. *Ibid.*, 44199.

79. *Ibid.*, 44201.

80. *Ibid.*

81. Clean Air Act Amendments of 1970 and 1977. 42 USC 7545 (c)(1).

82. U.S. Environmental Protection Agency. Regulation of fuels and fuel additives. 40 CFR 80, 38 Federal Register 1254-1256 (January 10, 1973).

83. U.S. Environmental Protection Agency. Regulation of fuels and fuel additives. 40 CFR 80, 38 Federal Register 33734-33741 (December 6, 1973).

84. U.S. Environmental Protection Agency. 37 Federal Register 3882-3884 (February 23, 1972).

85. U.S. Environmental Protection Agency. Regulation of fuels and fuel additives. 40 CFR 80, 38 Federal Register 1254 (January 10, 1973).

86. *Ibid.*

87. U.S. Environmental Protection Agency. 38 Federal Register 33740 (December 6, 1973).

88. John R. Quarles, Jr. Press conference on reducing lead in gasoline. Environmental News, November 28, 1973.

89. U.S. Environmental Protection Agency. 38 Federal Register 33737 (December 6, 1973).

90. U.S. Environmental Protection Agency. EPA's position on the health implications of airborne lead. Federal Register (November 28, 1973).

91. U.S. Environmental Protection Agency. Regulation of fuels and fuel additives. 40 CFR 80.20.

92. U.S. Environmental Protection Agency. Regulation of fuels and fuel additives. 40 CFR 80, 41 Federal Register 42675 (September 28, 1976).

93. U.S. Environmental Protection Agency. Regulation of fuels and fuel additives: Lead phase-down regulations. 44 Federal Register 33116 (June 8, 1979).

94. U.S. Environmental Protection Agency. 38 Federal Register 33740 (December 6, 1973).

95. *Ibid.*, 33734.

96. Clean Air Act Amendments of 1970 and 1977. 42 USC 7408 (a)(1).

97. *Ibid.*, 7408 (a)(2).

98. *Ibid.*, 7408 (b)(1).

99. *Ibid.*, 7409 (b)(1).

100. *Ibid.*, 7409 (a)(1).

101. *Natural Resources Defense Council, Inc. et al.* v. *Russell Train, Administrator* EPA (1976) 6 ELR 20366.

102. U.S. Congress, House (1977) Clean Air Act Amendments of 1977, Report to Accompany H.R. 6161, H. Report. 95-294, 49. 95th Congress, 1st Session.

103. U.S. Environmental Protection Agency (1977) Air Quality Criteria for Lead. Office of Research and Development. EPA-600/8-77-017. Washington, D.C.: U.S. Environmental Protection Agency.

104. U.S. Environmental Protection Agency. National primary and secondary ambient air quality standards for lead. 43 Federal Register 46247 (October 5, 1978).

105. U.S. Office of the President. Executive Order 11821. Inflation Impact Statements. 39 Federal Register 41502 (November 29, 1974); Executive Order 11949, Economic Impact Statements. 42 Federal Register 1017 (December 31, 1976).

106. U.S. Environmental Protection Agency (1977) Economic Impact Assessment for the National Ambient Air Quality Standard for Lead. Office of Air Quality Planning and Standards. Research Triangle Park, N.C.: U.S. Environmental Protection Agency.

107. U.S. Environmental Protection Agency. Lead, proposed national ambient air quality standard. 42 Federal Register 63077 (December 14, 1977).

108. *Ibid.*, 63077-63078.

109. U.S. Environmental Protection Agency. 43 Federal Register 46252 (October 5, 1978).

110. U.S. Environmental Protection Agency. Air Quality Criteria for Lead, 10-6.

111. *Ibid.*, 11-4.

112. *Ibid.*, 11-32.

113. *Ibid.*, 11-36.

114. U.S. Environmental Protection Agency. 43 Federal Register 46253 (October 5, 1978).

115. U.S. Environmental Protection Agency. Air Quality Criteria for Lead, 1-13.

116. U.S. Environmental Protection Agency. 43 Federal Register 46249 (October 5, 1978).

117. *Ibid.*, 46254.

118. *Ibid.*, 46253.

119. *Ibid.*

120. U.S. Environmental Protection Agency. Air Quality Criteria for Lead, Chapter 12.

121. U.S. Environmental Protection Agency. 43 Federal Register 46252 (October 5, 1978).

122. *Ibid.*, 46255.

123. *Ibid.*, 46253.

124. Azar, A., R.D. Snee, and K. Habibi (1975) An epidemiologic approach to community air lead exposure using personal air samplers. Pages 254–288, Environmental Quality and Safety. Supplement II:Lead.

125. U.S. Environmental Protection Agency. 43 Federal Register 46254 (October 5, 1978).

126. *Ibid.*

127. *Ibid.*, 46253.

128. U.S. Environmental Protection Agency. Air Quality Criteria for Lead, Chapter 12.

129. U.S. Environmental Protection Agency (1978) 43 Federal Register 46253.

130. *Ibid.*, 46254.

131. *Ibid.*

132. Safe Drinking Water Act (1974) 42 USC 300 g-1 (a).

133. *Ibid.*, 300 g-1 (e).

134. *Ibid.*, 300 g-1 (b).

135. *Ibid.*, 300 f (1).

136. *Ibid.*, 300 g-1 (b) (3).
137. U.S. Environmental Protection Agency. National Interim Primary Drinking Water Regulations. 40 CFR 141, 40 Federal Register 59566 et seq. (December 24, 1975).
138. U.S. Environmental Protection Agency (1976) Appendix A: Background used in developing the National Interim Primary Drinking Water Regulations, Pages 69–75, National Interim Primary Drinking Water Regulations. Office of Water Supply. EPA-570/9-76-003. Washington, D.C.: U.S. Environmental Protection Agency.
139. *Ibid.*, 71.
140. *Ibid.*, 72.
141. U.S. Environmental Protection Agency. Primary drinking water proposed interim standards. 40 Federal Register 11991 (March 14, 1975).
142. U.S. Environmental Protection Agency. Drinking Water Regulations, 70–71.
143. Medical aspects of childhood lead poisoning (1971) HSMSHA Health Reports 86:140.
144. National Research Council (1972) Lead: Airborne Lead in Perspective. Committee on Biologic Effects of Atmospheric Pollutants, Division of Medical Sciences. Washington, D.C.: National Academy of Sciences.
145. U.S. Environmental Protection Agency. Drinking Water Regulations, 71.
146. *Ibid.*
147. U.S. Environmental Protection Agency (1975) 40 Federal Register 59575.
148. U.S. Environmental Protection Agency. Drinking Water Regulations, 72.
149. National Research Council (1977) Drinking Water and Health. Part I, Chapters 1–5. A Report of the Safe Drinking Water Committee. Advisory Center on Toxicology. Assembly of Life Sciences. Washington, D.C.: National Academy of Sciences.
150. U.S. Environmental Protection Agency. Drinking water and health: Recommendations of the National Academy of Sciences. 42 Federal Register 35764 et seq. (July 11, 1977).
151. *Ibid.*, 35771.
152. *Ibid.*, 35764.
153. U.S. Environmental Protection Agency. National secondary drinking water regulations. 42 Federal Register 17143 et seq. (March 31, 1977).
154. U.S. Environmental Protection Agency. Water quality criteria. 44 Federal Register 15956 (March 15, 1979).
155. Clean Water Act, 33 USC 1314 (a).
156. U.S. Environmental Protection Agency (1979) Lead: Ambient Water Quality Criteria. Washington, D.C.: U.S. Environmental Protection Agency.
157. U.S. Environmental Protection Agency (1977) Air Quality Criteria for Lead. Office of Research and Development. EPA-600/8-77-017. Washington, D.C.: U.S. Environmental Protection Agency.
158. World Health Organization (1977) Environmental Health Criteria 3. Lead. Geneva: World Health Organization.
159. U.S. Environmental Protection Agency. Ambient Water Quality Criteria, C-75 to C-76.
160. *Ibid.*, C-78.
161. Occupational Safety and Health Act of 1970. 29 USC 651 et seq.
162. Occupational Safety and Health Administration. Occupational safety and health standards. 29 CFR 1910, 43 Federal Register 52952 (November 14, 1978).
163. 29 USC 651(b).
164. 29 USC 652(8).
165. 29 USC 655(b)(5).
166. 29 USC 655(a).

167. U.S. Congress, Senate (1970) Occupational Safety and Health Act of 1970: Report to Accompany S. 2193, Committee on Labor and Public Welfare, S. Report 91-1432. 91st Congress, 2nd Session.
168. Occupational Safety and Health Administration. Occupational exposure to lead. 40 Federal Register 45934 (October 3, 1975).
169. National Institute for Occupational Safety and Health (1978) Criteria for a Recommended Standard Occupational Exposure to Inorganic Lead, Revised Criteria—1978. HEW (NIOSH) Publication No. 78-158. Washington, D.C.: U.S. Department of Health, Education, and Welfare.
170. 43 Federal Register 52953 (November 14, 1978).
171. 40 Federal Register 45934 (October 3, 1975).
172. *Ibid.*, 45937.
173. U.S. Congress, House (1970) Occupational Safety and Health Act of 1970: Report to Accompany H.R. 16785. Committee on Education and Labor. 91st Congress, 2nd Session, H. Report 91-1291, 18.
174. *Society of the Plastics Industry Inc.* v. *Occupational Safety and Health Administration* 509 F. 2d 1301,1308 (2nd Cir. 1975).
175. *Industrial Union Department, AFL–CIO* v. *Hodgson* 499 F. 2d 467, 474 (D.C. Cir. 1974).
176. 43 Federal Register 52954 (November 14, 1978).
177. *Ibid.*
178. *Ibid.*, 52955.
179. *Ibid.*, 52957.
180. *Ibid.*, 52958.
181. *Ibid.*, 52959.
182. *Ibid.*, 52961.
183. *Ibid.*
184. *Ibid.*, 52971.
185. *Ibid.*, 52972.
186. *Ibid.*
187. *Ibid.*, 52973.
188. *Ibid.*
189. *Ibid.*, 52978.
190. *United Steelworkers of America, AFL–CIO–CLC* v. *Marshall* No. 79-1048 (D.C. Cir., March 1, 1979).
191. Occupational Safety and Health Administration. Occupational safety and health standards. 29 CFR 1910, 44 Federal Register 14554 (March 13, 1979).
192. Merrill, R.A. (1979) Regulating Carcinogens in Food: A Legislator's Guide to the Food Safety Provisions of the Federal Food, Drug, and Cosmetic Act. In Appendix BB, Food Safety Policy: Scientific and Societal Considerations. Part 2 of a Two-Part Study by the Committee for a Study on Saccharin and Food Safety Policy, March 1, 1979, National Academy of Sciences.
193. Merrill, R.A. (1979) Regulating carcinogens in food: A legislator's guide to the food safety provisions of the Federal Food, Drug, and Cosmetic Act. Michigan Law Review: (In press).
194. *Ibid.*
195. The Food and Drug Act, 21 USC 342 (a)(1).
196. *Ibid.*
197. *Ibid.*, 21 USC 346.

198. Pesticide Residue Amendments of 1954. PL 518, 83rd Congress, 2nd Session, now codified at 21 USC 346a.

199. Food Additives Amendment of 1958. PL 85-929, 85th Congress, 2nd Session, now codified at 21 USC 348.

200. Color Additive Amendments of 1960. PL 86-618, 86th Congress, 2nd Session, now codified at 21 USC 376.

201. Animal Drug Amendments of 1968. PL 90-399, 90th Congress, 2nd Session, now codified at 21 USC 306b.

202. Merrill, R.A. (1979) see Note 193.

203. 21 USC 348 (b).

204. 21 USC 321 (s).

205. *Ibid.*

206. Merrill, R.A. (1979) see Note 193.

207. 21 USC 348 (c)(3)(A).

208. Merrill, R.A. (1979) see Note 193.

209. U.S. Public Health Service (1941) A Study of the Effect of Lead Arsenate Exposure on Orchardists and Consumers of Sprayed Fruit. Bulletin No. 267. Washington, D.C.: U.S. Public Health Service.

210. McAuliffe, J. (1978) Statement regarding FDA's programs for controlling lead in food, made to the Committee on Lead in the Human Environment, National Academy of Sciences, Washington, D.C., October 1978.

211. U.S. Environmental Protection Agency. Tolerances and exemptions from tolerances for pesticide chemicals in or on raw agricultural commodities. 40 CFR 180.194.

212. 21 USC 346(a).

213. U.S. Environmental Protection Agency. 36 Federal Register 22540 (November 25, 1971).

214. McAuliffe (1978) see Note 210.

215. U.S. Department of Health, Education, and Welfare. Food and Drug Administration. Food and drugs, food additives. 21 CFR 121, 24 Federal Register 2434 (March 28, 1959).

216. 21 USC 321(s).

217. U.S. Department of Health, Education, and Welfare. Food and Drug Administration. Food and drugs, food additives. 21 CFR 170.3(i).

218. *Ibid.*, 170.20.

219. *Ibid.*, 170.30.

220. U.S. Department of Health, Education, and Welfare. Food and Drug Administration. Food and drugs, direct food substances affirmed as generally recognized as safe. 21 CFR 184.

221. U.S. Department of Health, Education, and Welfare. Food and Drug Administration. *Ibid.* Indirect food substances affirmed as generally recognized as safe. 21 CFR 186.

222. U.S. Food and Drug Administration (1979) Guideline 7417.03, Administrative Guidelines Manual, April 23.

223. 21 USC 342 (a)(2)(C).

224. 21 USC 348 (a).

225. World Health Organization (1976) Ceramic Foodware Safety, Sampling, Analysis and Limits for Lead and Cadmium Release. Report of a WHO Meeting, Geneva, June 8–10, 1976. Geneva: World Health Organization.

226. U.S. Department of Health, Education, and Welfare. Food and Drug Administration. Lead in evaporated milk and evaporated skim milk. 39 Federal Register 42740–42743 (December 6, 1974).

227. *Ibid.*, 42742.

228. *Ibid.*

229. King, B.G. (1971) Maximum daily intake of lead without excessive body lead burden in children. American Journal of Diseases of Children 122:337-340.

230. U.S. Department of Health, Education, and Welfare. Food and Drug Administration. 39 Federal Register 42740 (December 6, 1974).

231. Merrill, R.A. (1979) see Note 193.

232. *Ibid.*

233. Interagency Regulatory Liaison Group (1979) Regulatory Reporter 1(1):43.

234. U.S. Department of Health, Education, and Welfare. Food and Drug Administration. Lead in food; advance notice of proposed rulemaking; Request for data. 44 Federal Register 51233–51242 (August 31, 1979).

235. McAuliffe (1978) see Note 210.

236. *Ibid.*

237. U.S. FDA (as in Note 234). 44 Federal Register 51234–51236 (August 31, 1979).

238. IRLG (1979) Regulatory Reporter 1(1):43–44.

239. National Research Council (1977) Drinking Water and Health. Safe Drinking Water Committee, Advisory Center on Toxicology, Assembly of Life Sciences. Washington, D.C.: National Academy of Sciences.

240. Interagency Regulatory Liaison Group (1979) Regulatory Reporter 1(1):44.

241. U.S. Environmental Protection Agency. Proposed regulations for disposal of hazardous wastes on food chain lands. 43 Federal Register 4942 (February 6, 1978).

242. U.S. Environmental Protection Agency. Proposed rules for the management of hazardous wastes. 43 Federal Register 58946 (December 18, 1978).

243. Interagency Regulatory Liaison Group (1979) Regulatory Reporter 1(1):71.

244. James Brockmaier, Office of Solid Wastes, U.S. Environmental Protection Agency, personal communication, April 1979.

245. Interagency Regulatory Liaison Group (1979) Regulatory Reporter 1(1):72.

246. U.S. Environmental Protection Agency (1979) Lead-Acid Battery Manufacture. New Source Performance Standards. Background Information for Proposed Standards. Office of Air Quality Programs and Standards, Office of Air, Noise, and Radiation. Research Triangle Park, N.C.: U.S. Environmental Protection Agency.

247. *Ibid.*

248. U.S. Department of Health, Education, and Welfare. Food and Drug Administration. Advance notice of proposed rulemaking; lead acetate as a color additive in hair dyes. 43 Federal Register 8790 (March 3, 1978).

249. U.S. Department of Health, Education, and Welfare. Food and Drug Administration. Lead acetate: Postponement of closing date, advance notice of proposed rulemaking. 44 Federal Register 12205–12208 (March 6, 1979).

250. *Ibid.*, 12206.

251. *Ibid.*, 12206–12207.

252. Interagency Regulatory Liaison Group (EPA, FDA, and CPSC). Lead and Cadmium on Decorated Glassware. 43 Federal Register 58633 (December 15, 1978).

253. Interagency Regulatory Liaison Group (1979) Regulatory Reporter 1(1):43–46.

254. U.S. Environmental Protection Agency (1978) National Ambient Air Quality Standard for Lead. Office of Air, Noise, and Radiation and Office of Air Quality Planning and Standards. Research Triangle Park, N.C.: U.S. Environmental Protection Agency.

D Common Problems that Affect the Accuracy of Chemical Analyses for Lead

INTRODUCTION

Accurate measurements of lead in environmental and clinical samples are an important component of evaluations of environmental problems and of gauging the state of well-being of individuals. Unfortunately, investigative conclusions and actions based on them have not always considered the possible inaccuracies of the analytical procedures used. A growing awareness of the questionable quality of analytical results from some, and perhaps many, analytical laboratories has enhanced the interest in and concern for the reliability of the data.

The actual magnitude of the inaccuracy problem is difficult to grasp and impossible to estimate. The proliferation of analytical laboratories engaged in environmental and health studies, the development of more sophisticated analytical instrumentation, the tendency to hire scientists with inadequate training as analysts, the failure of many laboratories to incorporate quality assurance procedures into their analytical programs, and the paucity of reliable standard reference materials are all factors that contribute to the problem. One need only examine the results of interlaboratory or collaborative test programs to develop a sobering realization of the inadequacies common to the use of analytical methods.

Such problems prompted a recent critical evaluation of methods of monitoring for lead in a variety of materials (Skogerboe et al. 1977). Another publication (Pierce et al. 1976) specifically reviewed and critiqued the determination of lead in blood. Both have emphasized those analytical methods and practices most widely used. Although numerous other publications deserve recognition, these two are reasonably comprehensive overviews and provide references to a majority of recently published work on lead analysis. This appendix will focus on particular problem areas with emphasis on those referred to in various sections of the report.

NATURE OF ANALYTICAL PROBLEMS

Sample collection, sample storage and preparation, analysis, and interpretation of results are distinct but inseparable phases of any analysis. A dozen or more variables that can affect the analysis and the decisions based thereon are distributed over these phases and must be carefully considered. While there are exceptions, the importance of careful attention to controlling the analytical variables is generally diminished when the lead concentrations to be determined are relatively high, e.g., greater than approximately 100 to 1,000 parts per million (ppm). The major problems occur when the lead concentrations are low; in general the extents of the problems increase sharply with decreasing concentration. Essentially three factors contribute to this enhancement: (1) storage and preparation of low-concentration samples become more difficult; (2) contamination control requirements become more stringent; and (3) the analyses are based on measurement of an analytical signal that approaches the inherent noise or background level of the analytical technique as the concentration becomes lower.

CONTAMINATION OF SAMPLES

The possibility of contamination of the sample is a factor too often overlooked by analysts. Laboratory air, furnishings, apparatus, containers, reagents, and the analyst himself all become increasingly important sources of contamination as the analytical concentrations of interest decrease. The extent of this problem has been discussed in depth elsewhere (LaFleur 1976). It can be illustrated by general consideration of procedures often used for analysis of foods.

Methods for the determination of lead in foods (e.g., fish tissue) usually rely on the use of a 1 to 5 g sample, which is wet-oxidized in one or more concentrated acids in preparation for analysis. Acid volumes ranging from 10 to 50 ml are required to complete the wet-oxidation process. To be classified as Analytical Reagent Grade acids by American Chemical Society standards, most mineral acids must have lead contamination levels less than 50 μg/l (50 ng/ml). Although the concentration of lead present is likely less than this, it should be emphasized that higher-purity acids (e.g. ULTREX or TransistAR grades) typically have lead levels approximating 1 ng/ml and that concentrations around 20 ng/ml are fairly typical of the AR grade. Thus, the acid blanks used in analysis may contain from approximately 100 to 1,000 ng of lead when AR acids are used.

When these estimates are converted to the blank equivalent for the 1 to 5 g food sample, values lying in the 0.02 to 1 μg/g (ppm) range are obtained; these depend on the size of the sample and the volume of acid used. Clearly, it is relatively foolhardy to attempt to analyze a sample having a lead concentration that is much lower than that of the acid blank, yet this has often been done. For instance, in one food survey, the lead levels of blanks were typically in the 0.2 to 0.5 ppm range, even though many of the samples analyzed had concentrations far less than 0.1 ppm and many others had concentrations in the blank range.

Analyses carried out under such conditions are tenuous at best. The practice often leads to the erroneous reporting of numerous "zero" concentrations which are actually nonzero. When such values are used in computing mean values, the latter are underestimates. At the other extreme are cases in which the lead content of blanks was not adequately determined, and as a result inordinately high concentrations were reported.

The problem of contamination of reagent blanks is reduced by the use of high-purity acids (e.g., ULTREX Grade), but even then it can be a serious limitation. For example, a procedure used by FDA called for the digestion of 5 g of fish tissue in 25 ml of nitric acid plus 25 ml of sulfuric acid. High-purity acids could contribute about 50 ng of lead to the blank; this is equivalent ot 0.01 ppm in the tissue. As Patterson and associates have suggested, the actual concentrations in fresh fish may be much lower than 0.01 ppm (Settle and Patterson 1979), and such a blank serves as a distinct analytical limitation.

Other reagents often used in lead analyses also can serve as sources of lead contamination. These include masking agents such as ammonium citrate and potassium cyanide, extraction agents such as dithizone, organic solvents such as chloroform and methyl isobutyl ketone, fluxing or ashing agents such as nitrates or carbonates, and distilled water. Virtually all chemical reagents are sources of lead blanks. While some are more seriously contaminated than others, all should be used in highly pure form to minimize the blank problem.

Lead has become a ubiquitous element primarily because it is used in gasoline burned by the ubiquitous automobile. Lead in air must be recognized as a potentially serious source of contamination for all analyses.

Ambient air concentrations in the 1 to 5 $\mu g/m^3$ range are not unusual; similar concentrations in the air of urban laboratories have been reported. Dustfall measurements in some analytical labs have indicated fallout levels approximating 1 to 10 $\mu g/m^2/day$. Although many lab buildings have filtered air and air conditioning, such systems are not always effective in removing particles in the size range characteristic of those that contain lead. One report has shown that the air particle count indoors can be greater than that outdoors (Thomson 1972). While contamination by lead from the air is less serious for those labs located in nonurban areas, all laboratories involved in lead analyses at low concentrations should be encouraged (if not required) to use clean-room, clean-hood, or enclosed-sample processing facilities to reduce contamination.

The containers used for sample collection, storage, and preparation are often sources of contamination. The use of soft (flint) glassware and certain plastics should be avoided because of their propensity for contributing lead to the sample. Pyrex glassware contributes less lead, and the use of Teflon or quartz ware sharply reduces the problem, but even these must be judiciously cleaned with pure acids and stored sealed prior to use. All containers and utensils used for the determination of trace concentrations of lead should be segregated from general-purpose equipment. Mechanical grinding equipment such as impact and rotary mills or high-speed blenders will contaminate the sample to some degree with the materials of construction. Too often, these materials contain lead. Mills of the Wiley type, for example, often have their sizing screens fixed in place by a lead solder, which can cause extensive contamination.

The evolutionary development of more sensitive methods of analysis has enhanced awareness of contamination problems and has led many lab- oratories to seek to alleviate the blank contribution and/or to be more judicious in measuring the actual blank level. While such efforts are to be strongly encouraged, they often tend to be handicapped by erroneous concepts that have proliferated in the literature. It is often stated that it is the variability or uncertainty in the blank correction, and not the absolute value of the blank, that affects the accuracy of the analysis (Murphy 1976, Grant 1969). Unfortunately, this statement is often interpreted to mean that only the variation in the blank and not its value limits the ability to differentiate between the sample and the blank concentrations. This interpretation deserves only one comment: NONSENSE!

It is true that the variability of the blank limits the ability to discriminate between the blank concentration and the sample plus blank concentration. It is not true, however, that the blank level is unimportant. To illustrate, consider two cases: (1) the blank level is equivalent to 0.01 ppm and the variation of this blank (the standard deviation) is 0.005

ppm, i.e., ±50 percent; and (2) the blank level is equivalent to 1 ppm with a 10-fold reduction in the relative variation, i.e., ±5 percent or ±0.05 ppm.

For analysis of samples under each of the above conditions, the pertinent question is the minimum sample concentration that can be reliably estimated. Although different criteria could be applied in making this decision, depending on the confidence one wishes to assign to the results, the decision in any case must be based on the objective application of statistics, i.e., that sample concentrations should exceed blank concentration by k times the variation in the blank concentration. If k is set at 5 to ensure a reasonably high level of confidence in the decision, the sample concentration in the present example would have to exceed the blank concentration by 5×0.005 or 0.025 ppm to be considered significant in Case 1, and by 0.25 ppm in Case 2. Thus, the higher blank level clearly limits the ability to analyze for lower sample concentrations even though the relative variation in the higher blank level is 10 times less than that for the lower blank level. This general principle applies regardless of the value of k selected.

The above example also illustrates the potential effect of blank variability on analytical accuracy. If it is assumed that the sample concentration for Case 1 above was at the minimum discrimination level of 0.025 ppm, the mean sample-plus-blank concentration measured would be $0.025 + 0.01 = 0.035$ ppm. The measured sample concentration, which is obtained by subtraction of the blank concentration from the observed value, is subject to the uncertainties of both the blank and the sample-plus-blank measurements. If both measurements were based on the same number of replicates and if variations characteristic of both measurement sets were equivalent, the standard deviation of the sample concentration would be the added variances, i.e.,

$$s_s = ((0.005)^2 + (0.005)^2)^{1/2} = 0.007 \text{ ppm.}$$

The estimated relative standard deviation for the blank-corrected sample concentration would therefore be ±28 percent. The same assumptions and approach also yield a relative standard deviation estimate of ±28 percent for the higher blank concentration in Case 2. It must be recognized that the precision (reproducibility) of measurements limits the accuracy of the analysis in the absence of systematic errors, and that the limitations imposed by precision on the accuracies of analyses should be considered in relative, rather than absolute, terms. The present examples demonstrate that equivalent accuracy estimates may be obtained under quite divergent conditions of precision and blank concentrations.

The examples emphasize the importance of contamination control to permit reliable analyses at low concentration levels, and point out a common misconception that justifiably calls into question the integrity of analytical results from some laboratories.

PROBLEMS OF MEASUREMENT ACCURACY

Given the reduction of the blank problem through the use of judicious analytical procedures, the accurate measurement of lead can be carried out by any of several techniques. It is not the purpose of this report to recommend one over the other. Experience suggests, however, that some comment regarding the potential deficiencies of certain popular techniques is advisable.

Anodic-stripping voltammetry and differential-pulse polarography can be sensitive and reliable lead measurement techniques. Problems arise from: the use of impure electrolyte media for the analyses, so that the lead blank becomes limiting; the use of the method of standard additions for calibration purposes; and the all-too-common failure to recognize that these techniques measure only electroactive (ionic) lead. The latter problem can be overcome only by treating the sample to ensure that all lead present is converted to the electroactive form. Calibration by the method of standard additions, to be valid, requires linearity of response. Yet, some analysts rely on a two-point measurement even though they know intuitively that this is insufficient proof of linearity.

Atomic absorption analysis using furnace vaporization is also widely used. Numerous lead analyses by this technique during the early 1970s were subject to positive errors due to interferences caused by molecular absorption and/or light scattering. For example, one clinical laboratory measured blood lead levels for 1,000 patients and obtained a mean value of 42 $\mu g/100$ ml. When the analyses were repeated using a dual-beam system designed to correct for the scattering and absorption interferences, the mean value was reduced to 22 $\mu g/100$ ml. Analyses from labs that fail to use this means of interference correction should be labelled suspect. However, the correction units are typically applicable only within certain ranges. If the interference signal accounts for a reading that is equal to or greater than a full-scale absorbance reading (approximately 1.0 absorbance units), the correction accuracy is diminished and the analysis may be highly inaccurate. Too many laboratories have been unaware of this problem.

Although other problems with other lead analysis methods could be discussed, the above examples are representative of errors often associated with the most commonly used measurement techniques. They illustrate a general inadequacy in analytical practice. The spreads in the results of interlaboratory comparison studies emphasize the potential seriousness of such deficient practices.

OPPORTUNITIES FOR IMPROVEMENTS

Dramatic improvements in the quality of lead analyses are unlikely to come from any single source. A good quality-control program would surely make an important contribution. Such a program should rely on replicate analyses, recovery of known additions, analysis of known materials, and continued participation in collaborative test programs. The program must be organized so that an appreciable portion of the control checks are performed on an incognito basis to avoid biasing the analysts. Finally, adequate records must be kept to ensure the rejection of suspect results, the detection of systematic errors, and the continual evaluation of lab performance and changes therein.

It should also be emphasized that there are analytical methods that are less susceptible to the types of problems discussed above. These are essentially limited to the isotope measurement methods, e.g., activation analysis and stable-isotope mass spectrometry. Properly used, such methods can produce results that approach the absolute in terms of analytical accuracy. In the case of lead, the unique isotopic compositions associated with mineral deposits of different geologic ages often provide a highly specific method of differentiating between the sources of lead in the environment. Such isotope tracing measurements generally must rely on high-precision isotope mass spectrometry. Future research efforts might give isotope tracing measurements prominent consideration. A few carefully planned, highly specific, and accurate measurements often prove more valuable than hundreds of less specific and accurate measurements.

It is certain that the ability to measure lead has improved appreciably over the past decade or two. It is equally certain that considerable room for improvement still exists. This problem and how to solve it have been under discussion for some time. Some of the means of reducing the uncertainties in analysis have been mentioned above. The blank problem must be addressed, sources of error associated with commonly used techniques must be recognized, quality-assurance programs must become common requirements, and demands for continued demonstration of laboratory competence must receive serious consideration. The widespread use of such practices would have prevented many of the negative evaluations of lead analytical data that appear in this and other reports.

REFERENCES

Grant, C.L. (1969) Pages 1–9, Purification of Inorganic and Organic Materials, edited by M. Zief. New York: Marcel Dekker.

LaFleur, P., ed. (1976) Accuracy in Trace Analysis: Sampling, Sample Handling, and Analysis. National Bureau of Standards, Special Publication No. 422. Washington, D.C.: U.S. Department of Commerce.

Murphy, T.J. (1976) The role of the analytical blank in accurate trace analysis. Pages 509–539, Accuracy in Trace Analysis, Volume 1, edited by P. LaFleur. National Bureau of Standards. Special Publication No. 422. Washington, D.C.: U.S. Department of Commerce.

Pierce, J.O., S.R. Koirtyohann, T.E. Clevenger, and F.E. Lichte (1976) The Determination of Lead in Blood. New York: International Lead Zinc Research Organization, Inc.

Settle, D.M. and C.C. Patterson (1979) Lead in albacore: Guide to lead pollution in Americans. Science: (In press).

Skogerboe, R.K., A.M. Hartley, R.S. Vogel, and S.R. Koirtyohann (1977) Monitoring for lead in the environment. Pages 33–70, Lead in the Environment, edited by W.R. Boggess and B.G. Wixson. National Science Foundation, Report No. NSF/RA-770214. Washington, D.C.: U.S. Government Printing Office.

Thomson, Q.R. (1972) Indoor versus outdoor air pollution. Contamination Control Biomedical Environments 11:22–28.

Individuals
Who Provided Information
for the Study

NOTE: The Committee on Lead in the Human Environment held the Workshop on Lead in the Human Environment on September 11–12, 1978, in order to solicit and consider the diverse knowledge and opinions of a broad range of individuals with expertise on lead issues. The participants in the workshop provided information upon which the Committee may later have based some of its conclusions, but this report and the judgments it contains are the sole responsibility of the Committee on Lead in the Human Environment. Attendance at the workshop should not be taken as evidence that an individual endorses the findings or recommendations of this report. Not all of those who attended participated actively in discussions, and while the Committee was exposed to many views, it did not necessarily agree with all that was said.

Individuals marked with a single asterisk provided written comments or publications. Daggers indicate members of the Committee on Lead in the Human Environment.

MODERATOR

†BEN B. EWING, Institute for Environmental Studies, University of Illinois, Urbana

KEYNOTE SPEAKER

†EMIL A. PFITZER, Division of Toxicology, Hoffmann-LaRoche, Inc., Nutley, N.J.

PANEL ON CRITICAL ENVIRONMENTAL PATHWAYS AND EXPOSURES

†NORD L. GALE (*Moderator*), Department of Life Sciences, University of Missouri, Rolla
*T.J. CHOW, Scripps Institute of Oceanography, La Jolla, Calif.

PAUL CORNELIUSSEN, Bureau of Foods, U.S. FDA, Washington, D.C.

MYRON L. CORRIN, Department of Atmospheric Science, Colorado State University, Fort Collins

*TED J. KNEIP, New York University Medical Center

WILLIAM MARCUS, Office of Drinking Water, U.S. EPA, Washington, D.C.

*GEORGE W. WETHERILL, Department of Terrestrial Magnetism, Carnegie Institute of Washington, Washington, D.C.

PANEL ON LEAD AND HUMAN HEALTH

†LLOYD B. TEPPER (*Moderator*), Air Products and Chemicals Inc., Allentown, Pa.

*J. JULIAN CHISOLM, JR., Department of Pediatrics, Johns Hopkins University School of Medicine, Baltimore, Md.

ANITA S. CURRAN, Department of Health, Westchester County, N.Y.

*ROBERT A. GOYER, Department of Pathology, University of Western Ontario, London

*HERBERT L. NEEDLEMAN, Children's Hospital Center, Boston, Mass.

PANEL ON CONTROL STRATEGIES

†CLIFF I. DAVIDSON (*Moderator*), Department of Civil Engineering, Carnegie-Mellon University, Pittsburgh, Pa.

*KENNETH BRIDBORD, Office of Extramural Coordination and Special Projects, NIOSH, Washington, D.C.

*LAWRENCE CHADZYNSKI, Lead Poisoning Control Program, Department of Health, Detroit, Mich.

J. CHARLES JENNETT, Department of Civil Engineering, Syracuse University, Syracuse, N.Y.

*PHILIP LANDRIGAN, Center for Disease Control, U.S. HEW, Atlanta, Ga.

*FRANCES K. MILLICAN, pediatric psychiatrist, Bethesda, Md.

*GEORGE PROVENZANO, Institute for Environmental Studies, University of Illinois, Urbana

PANEL ON OTHER ISSUES AND PERSPECTIVES

†BEN B. EWING (*Moderator*), Institute for Environmental Studies, University of Illinois, Urbana

JOHN ELLIOTT, Office of Toxic Substances, U.S. EPA, Washington, D.C.

*EMMETT S. JACOBS, Additives and Environmental Studies Division, E.I. du Pont de Nemours & Co., Wilmington, Del.

*DAVID SCHOENBROD, Natural Resources Defense Council, New York

OTHER MEMBERS OF THE COMMITTEE ON LEAD IN THE HUMAN ENVIRONMENT WHO ATTENDED THE WORKSHOP

†JOHN M. HUNTER, Departments of Geography and Community Medicine, Michigan State University, East Lansing

†A. HAROLD LUBIN, Childrens Hospital, Columbus, Ohio

†KATHRYN R. MAHAFFEY, Bureau of Foods, U.S. FDA, Cincinnati, Ohio

†JEROME O. NRIAGU, Canada Center for Inland Waters, Burlington, Ontario

†CLAIR C. PATTERSON, Division of Geological and Planetary Sciences, California Institute of Technology, Pasadena

†RODNEY K. SKOGERBOE, Department of Chemistry, Colorado State University, Fort Collins

OTHERS WHO ATTENDED THE WORKSHOP

W.H. ALLAWAY, Department of Agronomy, Cornell University, Ithaca, N.Y.

*CAROL ANGLE, College of Medicine, University of Nebraska, Omaha

G.N. BIDDLE, Bureau of Foods, U.S. FDA, Washington, D.C.

IRWIN H. BILLICK, Office of Policy Development and Research, U.S. HUD, Washington, D.C.

ALVIN BLOCK, Environmental Sciences Associates, Bedford, Mass.

RITA BOGOROCH, Bureau of Chemical Hazards, National Health and Welfare Canada, Ottawa

SHERRY BOLTZ, National Paint and Coatings Association, Washington, D.C.

KENNETH BOYER, Bureau of Foods, U.S. FDA, Washington, D.C.

WILLIAM BRADLEY, The Proprietary Association, Washington, D.C.

*RICHARD J. BULL, Health Effects Research Lab, U.S. EPA, Cincinnati, Ohio

*RICHARD A. BURGESS, JR., Graduate School of Public Health, University of Pittsburgh, Pittsburgh, Pa.

ELLEN BURSTYN, Cosmetic, Toiletry and Fragrance Association, Inc., Washington, D.C.

STEPHEN G. CAPAR, Bureau of Foods, U.S. FDA, Washington, D.C.

C.W. CARLSON, SEA-AG Research, USDA, Washington, D.C.

SANDRA CARPENTER, Lead Poisoning Division, Government of the District of Columbia, Washington, D.C.

PETER CHICHILO, Bureau of Foods, U.S. FDA, Washington, D.C.

STANTON COERR, Office of Air Quality Planning and Standards, U.S. EPA, Research Triangle Park, N.C.

*GEORGE J. COHEN, Children's Hospital, Washington, D.C.

CHARLES COLBERT, Greene Memorial Hospital, Yellow Springs, Ohio.

*JEROME F. COLE, International Lead Zinc Research Organization, Inc., New York

MARGARET COLLINS, Department of Zoology, Howard University, Washington, D.C.

JOSEPH CRISLER, Department of Human Resources, Washington, D.C.

*ELBERT L. DAGE, Office of Toxic Substances, U.S. EPA, Washington, D.C.

LESLIE DUNN, U.S. EPA, Las Vegas, Nev.

*HARRY W. EDWARDS, Department of Mechanical Engineering, Colorado State University, Fort Collins

EDGAR ELKINS, National Food Processors Association, Washington, D.C.

RONALD M. ENG, League of Women Voters of D.C., Washington, D.C.

N.F. ESTRIN, Cosmetic, Toiletry and Fragrance Association, Inc., Washington, D.C.

WILLIAM F. FINN, Department of Medicine, University of North Carolina, Chapel Hill

*ALF FISCHBEIN, Environmental Sciences Laboratory, Mt. Sinai School of Medicine, New York

TOM FOX, Institute for Local Self-Reliance, Washington, D.C.

CARL L. GIANETTA, Bureau of Foods, U.S. FDA, Washington, D.C.

*ABRAHAM GOLDBERG, Department of Materia Medica, University of Glasgow, Scotland

ALAN M. GOLDBERG, Department of Environmental Health Sciences, Johns Hopkins University, Baltimore, Md.

V. EUGENE GRAY, Office of Policy Development and Research, U.S. HUD, Washington, D.C.

*PAUL B. HAMMOND, Department of Environmental Health, University of Cincinnati Medical Center, Cincinnati, Ohio

ROBERT HARRISS, NASA Langley Research Center, Hampton, Va.

DELBERT D. HEMPHILL, Environmental Trace Substances Research Center, University of Missouri, Columbia

ROBERT J.M. HORTON, Health Effects Research Laboratory, U.S. EPA, Research Triangle Park, N.C.

*VERNON N. HOUK, Center for Disease Control, U.S. HEW, Atlanta, Ga.

ROBERT E. HRUSKA, Behavioral Neuropharmacology Unit, National Institute of Neurological and Communicative Disorders and Stroke, Bethesda, Md.

PATRICK J. HURD, National Paint and Coatings Association, Washington, D.C.

TESSA HUXLEY, Institute for Local Self-Reliance, Washington, D.C.

CONSTANCE JACKSON, Scientists Institute for Public Information, New York

RUDOLPH E. JACKSON, Department of Pediatrics and Child Health, Howard University Hospital, Washington, D.C.

HELEN JOHANSEN, Epidemiology Branch, National Health and Welfare Canada, Ottawa

REBECCA JOHNSON, Office of Regulatory Functions, Lead Paint Poisoning Prevention, U.S. HUD, Washington, D.C.

KENNETH D. KEISER, Environmental Health Letter, Washington, D.C.

ROBERT G. KELLAM, Office of Air Quality Planning and Standards, U.S. EPA, Research Triangle Park, N.C.

DAVID E. KOEPPE, Department of Agronomy, University of Illinois, Urbana

S. ROY KOIRTYOHANN, Department of Chemistry, University of Missouri, Columbia

*PETER LASSOVSZKY, Office of Drinking Water, U.S. EPA, Washington, D.C.

YUEN SAN LEE, Interdisciplinary Science Department, University of the District of Columbia, Washington, D.C.

MILTON A. LESSLER, Department of Physiology, Ohio State University, Columbus

*ORVILLE LEVANDER, Nutrition Institute, USDA, Beltsville, Md.

*RUTH LILIS, Environmental Sciences Laboratory, Mt. Sinai School of Medicine, New York

*JANE S. LIN-FU, Bureau of Community Health Services, Health Services Administration, Rockville, Md.

FRANK C. LU, Department of Pharmacology, University of Miami, Florida

*DONALD R. LYNAM, International Lead Zinc Research Organization, Inc., New York

EDWARD B. McCABE, Department of Pediatrics, University of Wisconsin, Madison

HARRY MAHAR, MITRE Corporation, McLean, Va.

*J. WISTER MEIGS, Connecticut Cancer Epidemiology Program, New Haven

DAVID J. MILLER, Washington, D.C.

WINSTON MILLER, City Health Department, Baltimore, Md.

K.D. MILLS, Associated Octel Industries, Ann Arbor, Mich.

SAM MOLINAS, Consumer Product Safety Commission, Washington, D.C.

K.W. NESLON, ASARCO, Inc., New York

MELVIN L. OTT, The Bunker Hill, Kellogg, Idaho

RONALD K. PANKE, Doctor's Clinic, Kellogg, Idaho

*SERGIO PIOMELLI, Department of Hematology, New York University Medical Center, New York

RITA D. PITTILLO, Naval Research Laboratory, Washington, D.C.

*JAMES R. PREER, Interdisciplinary Science Department, University of the District of Columbia, Washington, D.C.

*HARRY ROELS, Institute of Hygiene and Epidemiology, University of Louvain, Brussels, Belgium

JOHN F. ROSEN, Department of Pediatrics, Montefiore Hospital, Bronx, N.Y.

WALTER G. ROSEN, Office of Toxic Substances, U.S. EPA, Washington, D.C.

*JAMES W. SAYRE, Department of Pediatrics, School of Medicine, University of Rochester, N.Y.

*NICHOLAS SCHMITT, Environmental Health Consultant, Victoria, B.C., Canada

GEORGE SCHREIBER, Health Protection Branch, National Health and Welfare Canada, Ottawa

H.S. SEKHON, Interdisciplinary Science Department, University of the District of Columbia, Washington, D.C.

EUGENE P. SESKIN, Resources for the Future, Washington, D.C.

MAURICE A. SHAPIRO, Graduate School of Public Health, University of Pittsburgh, Pittsburgh, Pa.

DOUGLAS SHIER, National Bureau of Standards, U.S. Department of Commerce, Washington, D.C.

*ELLEN SILBERGELD, Behavioral Neuropharmacology Unit, National Institute of Neurological and Communicative Disorders and Stroke, Bethesda, Md.

*THOMAS M. SPITTLER, U.S. EPA, Lexington, Mass.

BERNARD R. STEPHENS, Department of Human Resources, Washington, D.C.

MARK K. TAYLOR, COMBE, Inc., White Plains, N.Y.

*GARY TER HAAR, Toxicology and Industrial Hygiene Department, Ethyl Corporation, Baton Rouge, La.

RONALD THOMAS, Lead Poisoning Prevention Branch, Department of Human Resources, Washington, D.C.

D. TURNER, Associated Octel Co., Ellesmere Port, England

*JOSE A. VALCIUKAS, Environmental Sciences Laboratory, Mt. Sinai School of Medicine, New York

PATRICIA W. VAN BUREN, Environmental Health Administration, Government of the District of Columbia, Washington, D.C.

*WILLIAM D. WATSON, JR., Resources for the Future, Washington, D.C.

GLEN WEGNER, Boise Cascade Corporation, Boise, Idaho

*JEROME J. WESOLOWSKI, California Department of Health, Berkeley

PHYLLIS WETHERILL, Washington, D.C.

BOBBY G. WIXSON, Environmental Research Center, University of Missouri, Rolla

MURIEL WOLF, Childrens Hospital National Medical Center, Washington, D.C.

*PAUL T.S. WONG, Canada Center for Inland Waters, Burlington, Ontario

*JOHN M. WOOD, Freshwater Biological Institute, University of Minnesota, Navarre

OTHER INDIVIDUALS WHO FURNISHED INFORMATION ON LEAD IN THE ENVIRONMENT

DALE E. BAKER, Department of Agronomy, Pennsylvania State University, University Park

DONALD BARLTROP, Department of Child Health, Westminster Medical School, University of London, England

KAREN BLACKBURN, Office of Health and Ecological Effects, U.S. EPA, Cincinnati, Ohio

JOSEF EISINGER, Bell Laboratories, Murray Hill, N.J.

W.F. FORBES, Faculty of Mathematics, University of Waterloo, Ontario, Canada

LEONARD J. GOLDWATER, Consultant, Chapel Hill, N.C.

PHILIPPE GRANDJEAN, Environmental Sciences Laboratory, Mt. Sinai School of Medicine, New York

SVEN HERNBERG, Institute of Occupational Health, Helsinki, Finland

HOWARD C. HOPPS, Department of Pathology, Medical Center, University of Missouri, Columbia

T.C. HUTCHINSON, Department of Botany, University of Toronto, Ontario, Canada

JOHN F. JAWORSKI, Environmental Secretariat, National Research Council of Canada, Ottawa

JOHN KEITH, U.S. Geological Survey, Reston, Va.

STEVEN E. LINDBERG, Environmental Sciences Division, Oak Ridge National Laboratory, Oak Ridge, Tenn.

J. LARRY LUDKE, Columbia National Fishery Research Laboratory, U.S. Fish and Wildlife Service, Columbia, Mo.

FRANK McMANUS, McManus and Associates, Washington, D.C.

RONALD P. MILBERG, Soil Nitrogen and Environmental Chemistry Laboratory, USDA, Beltsville, Md.

MICHAEL R. MOORE, Department of Materia Medica, University of Glasgow, Scotland

A.L. PAGE, Department of Soil and Environmental Sciences, University of California, Riverside

JAMES W. PATTERSON, Pritzker Department of Environmental Engineering, Illinois Institute of Technology, Chicago

LLOYD E. SMYTHE, Department of Analytical Chemistry, University of New South Wales, Sydney, Australia

MARVIN STEPHENSON, National Science Foundation, Washington, D.C.

LUCILLE F. STICKEL, Patuxent Wildlife Research Center, U.S. Fish and Wildlife Service, Laurel, Md.

CLIFFORD D. STREHLOW, Department of Pediatrics, St. Mary's Hospital Medical School, London, England

ALAN W. TAYLOR, Soil Nitrogen and Environmental Chemistry Laboratory, USDA, Beltsville, Md.

RALPH R. TURNER, Environmental Sciences Division, Oak Ridge National Laboratory, Oak Ridge, Tenn.

JOHN W. WINCHESTER, Department of Oceanography, Florida State University, Tallahassee

R.L. ZIELHUIS, Coronel Laboratory of Industrial Hygiene, University of Amsterdam, The Netherlands

INDIVIDUALS WHO PROVIDED INFORMATION ON FEDERAL RESEARCH PROGRAMS RELATED TO LEAD IN THE ENVIRONMENT

CONGRESSIONAL RESEARCH SERVICE

JAMES M. McCULLOUGH, Science Policy Research Division, Library of Congress, Washington, D.C.

CONSUMER PRODUCT SAFETY COMMISSION

SAM MOLINAS, Assistant to the Deputy Associate Executive Director for Health Sciences, CPSC, Washington, D.C.

DEPARTMENT OF AGRICULTURE

RUFUS CHANEY, Waste Management Program, Agricultural Environmental Quality Institute, Agricultural Research Service, Beltsville, Md.

ORVILLE LEVANDER, Nutrition Institute, Agricultural Research Service, Beltsville, Md.

ALAN W. TAYLOR, Chief, Soil Nitrogen and Environmental Chemistry Laboratory, Agricultural Environmental Quality Institute, Beltsville, Md.

DEPARTMENT OF COMMERCE

National Bureau of Standards

PHILIP LaFLEUR, Director, Center for Analytical Chemistry, Gaithersburg, Md.
THOMAS MURPHY, Atomic Absorption Division, Center for Analytical Chemistry, Gaithersburg, Md.
DOUGLAS R. SHIER, Center for Applied Mathematics, Washington, D.C.

National Oceanic and Atmospheric Administration

BETTY M. HACKLEY, Seafood Quality and Inspection Division, National Marine Fisheries Service, Washington, D.C.
RICHARD LEHMANN, Office of Congressional Affairs, Washington, D.C.

DEPARTMENT OF ENERGY

DAVID BALLENTINE, Office of Energy Research, Germantown, Md.
W. FRANKLIN HARRIS, Terrestrial Ecology Section, Environmental Sciences Division, Oak Ridge National Laboratory, Oak Ridge, Tenn.
ROBERT A. LEWIS, Office of Health and Environmental Research, Germantown, Md.
ROBERT I. VAN HOOK, Environmental Sciences Division, Oak Ridge National Laboratory, Oak Ridge, Tenn.
HERBERT VOLCHOK, Environmental Measurement Laboratory, New York, N.Y.

DEPARTMENT OF HEALTH, EDUCATION, AND WELFARE

Center for Disease Control

VERNON N. HOUK, Director, Environmental Health Services Division, Bureau of State Services, Atlanta, Ga.
PHILIP J. LANDRIGAN, Bureau of Epidemiology, Atlanta, Ga.

National Institute for Occupational Safety and Health

KENNETH BRIDBORD, Director, Office of Extramural Coordination and Special Projects, Washington, D.C.
JACQUELINE MESSITE, Regional Consultant for Occupational Medicine, Region 2, U.S. Public Health Service, New York.

Food and Drug Administration

KENNETH W. BOYER, Division of Chemical Technology, Bureau of Foods, Washington, D.C.
PETER CHICHILO, Division of Food and Color Additives, Bureau of Foods, Washington, D.C.
PAUL CORNELIUSSEN, Division of Chemistry and Physics, Bureau of Foods, Washington, D.C.
JOHN McAULIFFE, Chief, Petitions Control Branch, Division of Food and Color Additives, Bureau of Foods, Washington, D.C.
SAMUEL SHIBKO, Division of Toxicology, Bureau of Foods, Washington, D.C.
SIDNEY WILLIAMS, Acting Director, Division of Chemical Technology, Bureau of Foods, Washington, D.C.

National Institutes of Health

MARTIN BLUMSAK, Office of the Director, Division of Research Resources, Bethesda, Md.

ALAN R. HOUGH, Program Analyst, Office of Extramural Programs, National Institute of Environmental Health Sciences, Research Triangle Park, N.C.

CHRISTOPHER SCHONWALDER, Office of Extramural Programs, National Institute of Environmental Health Sciences, Research Triangle Park, N.C.

RAYMOND E. SHAPIRO, Assistant Director for Toxicology Coordination, National Institute of Environmental Health Sciences, Research Triangle Park, N.C.

ELLEN K. SILBERGELD, Behavioral Neuropharmacology Unit, National Institute of Neurological and Communicative Disorders and Stroke, Bethesda, Md.

DEPARTMENT OF HOUSING AND URBAN DEVELOPMENT

IRWIN H. BILLICK, Program Manager, Lead-Based Paint Poisoning Prevention Research, Office of Policy Development and Research, Washington, D.C.

V. EUGENE GRAY, Lead-Based Paint Poisoning Prevention Research Program, Office of Policy Development and Research, Washington, D.C.

DEPARTMENT OF THE INTERIOR

Bureau of Mines

ROGER MARKLE, Director, Washington, D.C.

EDWIN MAUST, Chief, Office of Energy and Minerals Technology Coordination, Washington, D.C.

Fish and Wildlife Service

RICHARD SCHOETTGER, Director, Columbia National Fishery Research Laboratory, Columbia, Mo.

LUCILLE F. STICKEL, Director, Patuxent Wildlife Research Center, Laurel, Md.

Geological Survey

JOHN BREDEHOEFT, Deputy Assistant Chief Hydrologist for Research, Water Resources Division, Reston, Va.

JOHN KEITH, Deputy Chief for Geochemistry, Office of Geochemistry and Geophysics, Reston, Va.

ENVIRONMENTAL PROTECTION AGENCY

GEORGE A. ARMSTRONG, Office of Health and Ecological Effects, Office of Research and Development, Washington, D.C.

JOSEPH BEHAR, Monitoring and Technical Support Laboratory, Office of Research and Development, Las Vegas, Nev.

RICHARD J. BULL, Health Effects Research Laboratory, Office of Research and Development, Cincinnati, Ohio.

JOSEPHINE COOPER, Health Effects Research Laboratory, Office of Research and Development, Research Triangle Park, N.C.

JOHN H. ELLIOTT, Office of Program Integration and Information, Office of Toxic Substances, Washington, D.C.

STEPHEN J. GAGE, Assistant Administrator for Research and Development, Washington, D.C.

DANIEL G. GREATHOUSE, Health Effects Research Laboratory, Office of Research and Development, Cincinnati, Ohio.

JERRY STARA, Office of Environmental Criteria and Assessment (Water), Office of Research and Development, Cincinnati, Ohio.

NATIONAL SCIENCE FOUNDATION

RICHARD CARRIGAN, Program on Environmental Trace Substances, Washington, D.C.

MARVIN STEPHENSON, Division of Problem-Focused Research Applications, Washington, D.C.

CHARLES THIEL, Program on Chemical Threats to Man and the Environment (On leave to Federal Emergency Management Agency 1978–79), Washington, D.C.